cosmetics unmasked

Your family guide to safe cosmetics and
allergy-free toiletries

DR STEPHEN ANTCZAK & GINA ANTCZAK

Thorsons

Thorsons
An Imprint of HarperCollins*Publishers*
77–85 Fulham Palace Road
Hammersmith, London W6 8JB

The Thorsons website address is:
www.thorsons.com

First published 2001

10 9 8 7 6 5 4 3

A catalogue record of this book is
available from the British Library

ISBN 0 00 710568 1

Printed and bound in Great Britain by
Martins the Printers Limited, Berwick upon Tweed

To Margaret Hollins who started the ball rolling and who taught us that since we must die of something, it might as well be good food and drink.

contents

list of sample labels and cosmetic ingredients

preface

When a close friend presented me with a bottle of cleansing lotion and a tub of moisturizing cream, and asked me which ingredient was making her face blotchy and sore, I was left guessing. There were several ingredients in common and some of the simpler chemicals were quickly eliminated as suspects, but it was not reassuring for her when I admitted I had no idea what some of the other ingredients were – not reassuring, because I am a Chemist. The labels appeared to be written in some form of code using non-standard chemical terms that I could not understand. After a little detective work to crack the code, we decided she should avoid Oxybenzone (Benzophenone-3) for a while. It seemed to do the trick, but Oxybenzone is an ultra-violet (UV) light absorber used in sunscreens. Why would the manufacturer put it in cleansing lotion?

I decided to make it my business to find out more about these mysterious cosmetic ingredients. I wanted to know why there were six different preservatives in my shower gel and whether the sodium nitrite in the mouthwash was good for my teeth, or if it was there to stop the manufacturer's machinery from rusting. I was intrigued by an expensive "hypoallergenic" conditioner that seemed to have, more or less, the same ingredients as a cheap supermarket brand. Did the word "natural" splashed across the front of a bottle mean anything when the plant extract was way down the list of ingredients, hidden in a sea of synthetic chemicals? And why was sodium lauryl sulfate (SLS) the most common surfactant (cleaning chemical) used in shampoos, shower gels, foaming bath oils, and everything else that cleans, when the bottle on my laboratory shelf carries the following list of warnings:

- Avoid inhaling the dust
- Wear suitable protective clothing
- Irritating to eyes, skin, and the respiratory system
- Harmful by inhalation or if swallowed
- May cause sensitization by inhalation
- May cause serious damage to eyes
- In the event of eye contact rinse with plenty of water and seek medical advice?

Did I really want this stuff in my toothpaste?

In this age of suspicion over genetically engineered foods, it is ironic that we are not only unconcerned about the chemicals we plaster over our bodies, but have in fact embraced them with open arms in the vain hope they will relax us, make us more beautiful, or stop us from aging. People shudder at the idea of the cosmetics used in the last century, which contained arsenic and lead compounds, but they don't blink an eyelid at coloring their hair with similar lead compounds, or soaking in a bath of chemicals that cause contact dermatitis. The reason for this is largely due to a lack of information. It is our aim to put this right.

We will not be saying how bad cosmetics are. Indeed, *most* cosmetics pose no problems for *most* people. But there is a growing need for information about the things that may, and often do, cause us harm, and it is important to see through the potentially harmful misinformation fed to us daily by the advertisers who want us to buy these products. Equally, it is important to see through the literature written by the bandwagon of do-gooders who are anti everything to do with artificial ingredients in cosmetics. A number of other books we found on this subject tended to focus solely on what their authors considered to be extreme hazardous effects of cosmetics, drawing unscientific conclusions from certain studies and reports, which are out of all proportion to the true nature of the hazards. They produce sensational, scaremongering stories that may be worthy of a good read in a woman's weekly but have no place in serious scientific reporting.

It is the intention of this book to help the consumer crack the cosmetic code, to understand the laws and science behind the labels, and to allow them to make an informed choice. The book provides sufficient scientific background information to help in the understanding of what the ingredients used in cosmetics are, why they are used, and how they work. It reports the facts about cosmetic ingredients without unduly corrupting them by sensationalism or misinterpretation. Above all, it provides balanced, scientific advice to help you – the consumer – to make up your own mind in choosing the product that is best for you.

Note: To the best of our knowledge, the information contained within this book is correct at the time of writing.

Stephen Antczak

October 2000

1 introduction

In the factory we make cosmetics. In the store we sell hope.

Charles Revson

There are over 7,000 ingredients available to manufacturers for use in cosmetics and toiletries (including nearly 1,000 aromatic and perfume chemicals), of which more than a thousand are known to have harmful effects, and many of these are subject to some level of legal restriction. Another 900 ingredients may have been manufactured in such a way as to be potentially contaminated with cancer-causing chemicals. Recent tests carried out by the US Food and Drug Administration (FDA) have found that a large number of these contaminants have indeed found their way into finished products in substantial quantities. This means that more than one out of every four of the ingredients listed on the label of a bottle of shampoo, for instance, or a jar of face cream, is either on the restricted list, or may be harmful in some way. That does *not* mean that the product is harmful, but simply that there are potential dangers that the user should be aware of.

NAME STANDARDIZATION

In order to address this issue, the authorities responsible for the regulation of cosmetics and toiletries – the European Union (EU) Commission in Europe and the FDA in the USA – have introduced standards for the listing of ingredient names on product labels. Standardization has made it easier to import and export cosmetics and toiletries through the use of internationally agreed ingredient names. The EU

Commission and the FDA have clearly stated why ingredients should be listed on all products, using standard names: if ingredients are clearly listed, consumers who have an allergy or sensitivity to particular ingredients can easily identify, and so avoid, the cosmetics that contain them. To some extent, this is an acknowledgment by the regulating authorities that some cosmetic ingredients are irritants or have harmful effects.

MEANINGLESS LABELS

This standardization of ingredient names sounds all very helpful to those consumers with sensitive skin and allergies, until you actually pick up a bottle of shampoo or skin cream and try to read the label. The chemical names of many of the ingredients are completely meaningless to most people, including chemists. The formal name of a chemical can run into several lines and read like a sentence – with commas, hyphens, brackets, and numbers scattered between the unpronounceable, long words. To a chemist, the name is a precise description of the ingredient's chemical structure and yields a great deal of information about a substance. The problem is that cosmetic and toiletry manufacturers do not use formal chemical names. If they did, the list of ingredients would not fit on the label. Either shortened versions or trivial names are used, but these carry no useful information unless you are in the know, which most consumers are not.

If you become sensitized to a product, there is quite a problem of tracking down the offending chemical. Most cosmetics and toiletries contain at least a dozen ingredients. One brand of sunscreen on sale in the UK lists 46 chemicals and invites the customer to see the in-store list for further ingredients. How do you know which of these ingredients is either making you itch or your face feel as though it's been burnt?

MEANINGLESS ADVERTISING

Before using a cosmetic or toiletry product, you may want to know three things:

- What are the ingredients?
- Why are they used?

If you cannot glean this information from the labels, then you are at the mercy of the advertisers to inform you about the products. But the information on cosmetic ingredients is usually vague, often incomplete, and uninformative. Cosmetic manufacturers frequently disguise the true nature of ingredients by describing their properties with meaningless phrases, such as "reveals fresher, younger-looking skin." What this actually means is that keratolytic chemicals dissolve the protective, outer layer of skin cells. This exposes the more sensitive, deeper layers of your skin, and thus increases the risk of damage by ultraviolet radiation and the absorption of chemical ingredients that were never meant to penetrate your skin.

IS IT SAFE?

There is a widely held belief that products such as cosmetics would not be readily available to the consumer unless they were safe. The manufacturers and advertisers of the products reinforce this belief by demonstrating their "nourishing," "revitalizing," or "natural" properties. But just how safe are these products? And can they really help maintain an unblemished, youthful complexion, as the advertisers would have us believe?

In 1994 the American FDA carried out a survey into allergies caused by cosmetics and toiletries. Nearly one in four of the people questioned claimed to have suffered an allergic reaction as a result of using a cosmetic or toiletry, including make-up, foundations, and moisturizers.

On October 20, 1997, representatives of the hairdressing profession told the EU Commission that hairdressers' health was being impaired because of the large amounts of cosmetic products they were exposed to. They asked the Commission whether it had looked into this problem or if it intended to do so. The Commission responded by pointing out that, under EU law, it is the manufacturer's responsibility to ensure that a cosmetic product sold within the EU must not cause harm to human health when applied under normal or reasonably foreseeable conditions of use. But are the manufacturers' safety tests adequate? Do the new non-animal tests give reliable results, and is a product really safe to use if large or long-term exposure to the chemicals damages the health of professionals who work with them?

IS IT DANGEROUS?

This all paints a fairly bleak picture, but it is not the intention of this book to make the bathroom cabinet look like a minefield. In fact, the authors discovered much that was, in many ways, reassuring. Most cosmetics and toiletries are perfectly safe if used correctly, and relatively few people will ever suffer any real problems with them. If a particular product disagrees with you there are plenty more to choose from, and most of us can find something we like. Statistically you are more likely to scratch your eye with your mascara wand than suffer any serious effects from the chemicals in your make-up. While there are many substances which may have harmful effects, most of the ingredients used in cosmetics and toiletries are perfectly safe and have no known adverse effects.

It must be said, however, that allergies, like people, are not consistent and it is quite possible for any individual to have a sudden and unexpected adverse reaction to the most harmless ingredient imaginable.

THE AIM OF THIS BOOK

As stated above, there are three things you should know before using a cosmetic or toiletry product: what are the ingredients, why are they used, and do they have any known adverse or harmful effects? If you are a vegetarian, you may also wish to know whether a particular cosmetic contains animal products, e.g., if a conditioner contains keratin amino acids that are made from animal skin, hooves, and horns. If you are a parent, you will want to know what ingredients must not be used on infants.

The aim of this book is to help you answer all these questions in a straight-forward manner. The *A to Z of Cosmetic Terms* provides details of the nature of cosmetic ingredients, the reasons for their use and background information. The *Index of Cosmetic Ingredients* lists all the questionable ingredients, as well as some of the more common ingredients that are known to be safe. If you cannot find an ingredient in the index, it is because it has no known adverse effects. The purpose is to make you, the consumer, more informed about the products you use everyday so that you are not confused or misled by the marketing jargon in order for you to make more informed choices when buying cosmetics and toiletries.

2 marketing: myths and magic

"Anything which says it can magically take away your wrinkles is a
scandalous lie."
 "Moisturizers do work, but the rest is complete pap."

Anita Roddick, Founder and Co-Chairman of The Body Shop

Since the time that someone had something to sell, barter or trade, the art of
marketing has been practiced in one form or another. Over the years, the practice
may have become more subtle, the methods more ingenious, the marketing more
persuasive, but some vital ingredients have never changed. When it comes to the
advertising of cosmetics, the roles of vanity, misinformation, and deception play a
far greater part than providing information about the product.

You may have wondered why the models in the advertisements for anti-aging,
anti-wrinkle face creams are always young and beautiful. The message is that you
too could become or stay young and beautiful if you use these products and, of
course, it's much easier to demonstrate such a product using a model who does not
have wrinkles!

The truth of the matter is that:

- when used correctly, make-up can enhance your features or help to hide unwanted
  blemishes, wrinkles or shadows, but the effect only lasts while the make-up is applied and
  can cause an unwarranted psychological dependency on it
- suitable conditioners may be effective in many ways but they cannot magically repair
  damaged hair or make it more healthy by adding proteins, vitamins, amino acids or
  whatever else the manufacturer might throw in

face creams may help to hide the fine lines on your face or may help your skin temporarily to look and feel smoother and softer, but they cannot magically remove or reduce fine lines and wrinkles, nor can they reverse or prevent the effects of aging.

PRODUCT DEVELOPMENT

In order to stay ahead in the game, all businesses must continually focus on strategies for "growing" their business, increasing their profitability, improving their shareholder value, and keeping ahead of the competition. This means they must continually develop existing products and bring new products to the market. One way to do this is through marketing. If a shampoo was simply advertised as a product that would clean your hair, which is what in effect the basic product is all about, there would be nothing to differentiate it from any other shampoo on the shelf or to make it appear better than the other shampoos. The marketing people must continually come up with ways to do just this, and they will use a number of devices including the use of appealing design and packaging, amazing claims about what the product can do, and adding "special" ingredients not in the other shampoos. They also differentiate products by the use of pricing (see *It Must be Good – It's Expensive*, p.8).

The average market life of a new product is about two to three years, after which point the sales tend to decline sharply. To maintain or increase revenue, the product must either be periodically "improved" or replaced by a "new" one. Don't be fooled. If a manufacturer brings out a "new and improved" product, this is not because the scientists working behind the scenes in technologically advanced laboratories have made any major discoveries. It is simply a tactic to boost sales. The scientists employed by cosmetic companies are there mainly to make sure the marketing ideas work in practice, to find cheaper, more cost-effective ways of producing the product, and to ensure it conforms to the safety regulations.

Old products can be turned into new ones by changing the packaging, changing the labels, changing the image to appeal to a different age group, or by adding one or two different ingredients such as a different perfume, a different color, a plant or food extract, vitamin compounds or amino acids. Many years ago, egg and beer shampoos were all the rage. Now it's fruit, herbal extracts, vitamins, proteins, amino acids and the latest (at the time of writing) is wine and probiotics. There may be something to wine as it contains tannins and other astringents, and fruit acids such as lactic and malic acid – these being alpha-hydoxy acids (AHAs), which are mild skin peels. (See *A–Z of Cosmetic Terms – Alpha-Hydroxy Acid*.) Probiotics, on the other hand, are designed to encourage certain types of bacterial growth, which sounds contrary to the laws on cosmetics designed to protect the consumer. Sometimes, just changing the name can turn a product into a new one. For example, one manufacturer sells bath grains and foot soak grains, and for both products the ingredients, packaging, and instructions are identical!

NEW MARKETS

Another way for cosmetic manufacturers to expand their businesses is to find new markets for existing products. Deodorant sprays for example, can be turned into "intimate feminine care" products or foot-care products by changing the label. Suggesting that we need such products is a myth designed to play upon our fears. While make-up can enhance one's appearance or cover up blemishes, we do not all look ugly without make-up and can survive quite happily without it. Not using cosmetic products does not mean that we are not taking any care about our appearance, and yet the cosmetics industry would have us believe so. We do not become unhealthy if we do not use cosmetic products. Apart from carrying out the basics to keep and smell clean (washing, brushing teeth, and perhaps using a deodorant), we do not need to apply an assortment of cosmetics and toiletries to be healthy and feel human. People, however, have used make-up of one sort or another throughout history, and cosmetics' advertising has turned this into a need.

Perfumes were first used to hide unpleasant body odors in the days when deodorants did not exist and washing was not the norm. Once this reason diminished, perfume houses had to come up with other ways to convince people to buy their wares. Perfume became something you used to indicate status, and the famous brands were marketed on the basis of their exclusivity and high price – only the well off could afford to buy them. It was something you could use to make others admire you. It became an aphrodisiac and a way to impress the opposite sex. And how easy it was to convince everyone of this.

Sadly, this marketing ploy has now been extended to third world, developing countries. At least one major cosmetics company has successfully sent out representatives to outlying settlements to sell their products to people who have barely enough means to house, clothe, and feed themselves or their families.

It Must be Good – It's Expensive

Do not be lulled into thinking that an expensive product must be better than a cheaper one and pay more than you have to. While this might be true of a number of products and services, it is generally not the case with the cosmetics and toiletries we can buy in the high street. There are a number of reasons why one product might be more expensive than another, and it often has nothing to do with the quality or the capabilities of the product.

You will often have to pay more for a brand name than for an equivalent store brand, but if you check the ingredients of a store brand of shampoo against a famous brand-name product, there will be a remarkable degree of similarity. Sometimes they are even made in the same factory. The supermarket or drugstore brands are cheaper because they have fewer overheads. They do not have to pay for the expensive advertising to sell you an image. They can make huge economies in the manufacturing of vast amounts of the products and they also have enormous buying power, which reduces their costs.

Pricing may itself be used as a marketing tool, i.e. as a ploy to make you think that one brand is better than another one, or that one product is better than another made by the same company. For example, a company may sell one product at the usual price (e.g. a standard face cream) but promote a "deluxe" version of the product (e.g. a special anti-wrinkle cream) by selling it at a higher price. An exceedingly expensive, exceedingly small glass jar of anti-wrinkle cream containing a so-called special ingredient (which may not be special at all), is likely to be far more convincing than a cheap, bulky plastic tub containing exactly the same ingredients. And it will increase the company's profits.

ADVERTISING CLAIMS

As long as they can get away with it, the manufacturers will make claims about their products and use such language as to lead you to believe they can perform some pretty miraculous feats. They often resort to the "appliance of science" to sell their products, using documentary-style techniques showing graphic images of proteins or vitamins or some chemical entering into a hair shaft or the skin. They may put a graph on the back of a shampoo bottle, use language that suggests their product was developed in the most technologically advanced laboratory, or display seemingly amazing results of laboratory tests.

Some claims are not so much wrong as misleading, such as the following example for a contour eye gel.

A special biphasic formula which combines a crystal gel containing hydrating and stimulating agents with opalescent filaments enriched with anti-aging vitamins A and E. Smoothes the eyelids and softens and tones the epidermis. Progressively helps to smooth lines and wrinkles and visibly reduces bags and dark shadows. Non-greasy, refreshing and instantly soothing. Helps to relieve congestion and prevent puffiness.

Most of the jargon used here is not normal scientific language and is not readily understood by practicing scientists. So we can only guess at what they are trying to say – and can come up with some bizarre conclusions. The phrase "biphasic formula" may sound like leading-edge technology, but it basically means it is an emulsion of oil and water, just like most other cosmetics. "Crystal gel" is a confusing and contradictory term. A gel is a liquid held together in a solid structure, whereas crystals are completely solid structures. The two seem to be incompatible. The "opalescent filaments" are most likely to be nothing more than opaque, shiny strands of some insoluble material like silk, nylon, carbomer, or some other inert material, with vitamins absorbed onto the surface. The vitamins would have no effect as the filaments would be too large to penetrate the skin – unless they go through like needles or splinters, in which case they would cause severe irritation. The fact that the gel "softens and tones the epidermis" means that it affects only the outer layer of dead skin which is constantly being shed by the body, a process that can be aided by a good rub with a face towel. "Congestion" is a term that refers to the accumulation of an excessive amount of blood, tissue fluid, or lymph in part of the body, as might accompany inflammation. Nasal congestion, for example, is caused by an excessive build up of mucus due to the inflammation of the nasal lining. It is highly unlikely that this eye contour gel would effectively help any type of congestion unless, perhaps, it contains menthol vapors to help you to breathe more easily.

If it did contain a substance that reduced the blood flow to the area around the eyes, it is doubtful that it could be legally sold over the counter.

Your eye gel might feel as though it is working if the water content causes a cold sensation when it evaporates, or if an ingredient like carbomer forms a film that shrinks on drying, or if it contains an astringent which dries the skin. But don't be fooled – the effect is only temporary.

This manufacturer is careful not to make claims that are untrue, by saying that the product "helps" to smooth lines and wrinkles and "visibly" reduces bags and dark shadows. It probably does this by filling in the fine lines. The result is that the light will reflect more evenly off the smoother surface of the skin, but the effect will be minimal – hardly noticeable to the naked eye.

The claim below is not so carefully worded and probably falls foul of the trading standards regulations.

Designed to moisturize and regenerate the delicate area around the eyes. Reduces dark circles and puffiness. Helps to eliminate fine lines and wrinkles.

You cannot "eliminate fine lines and wrinkles" unless you use retinoic acid (a controlled drug available on prescription only), collagen implants, fat transplants, deep skin peels, or a face lift. If this gel did "reduce dark circles and puffiness," it would be classified as a drug and would not be available for general use over the counter.

Some shampoos carry claims to make your hair stronger or more resistant, citing how, for example, results of laboratory tests show that a particular product can make your hair 40 percent stronger, or increase its resistance by 24 percent. This sounds impressive, but what does it mean? Does it mean that it makes your hair less likely to sustain damage from the weather by coating it with a conditioning barrier? Does it mean it helps to stop your hair from falling out? And what does the percentage mean? Forty percent stronger than what? What does more resistant mean? Could it refer to electrical resistance? Will it protect you from a lightning strike?

A COSMETIC OR A DRUG?

Advertisers do have to be careful about the claims they make or they may find that their products become regulated as drugs. In the USA, cosmetics and drugs are clearly defined by the FDA and a product may be classified as a cosmetic, as a drug, or as a cosmetic which is also a drug. A cosmetic is something that when applied, results in a temporary, superficial change. Cosmetics that make a medical claim – such as shampoos that treat dandruff, toothpaste that reduces cavities, sunscreens that prevent sunburn, or preparations that reduce wrinkles – are classified as cosmetics that are also drugs. In this case, the product must be proved to be safe and must comply with the regulations for cosmetics, or drugs, or both, to be freely sold as a cosmetic or as an over-the-counter drug. In order to avoid the product being classified as a drug, advertisers will often use vague terms such as "reveals smoother, fresher skin."

CLAIMS TO BE NATURAL AND HYPOALLERGENIC

Some terms like "natural" and "hypoallergenic" are used liberally by advertisers and, unfortunately, there are no legal, scientific, or accepted dictionary definitions of these terms as they apply to cosmetics. Despite the lack of a definition, it is generally accepted that a hypoallergenic product is formulated to cause fewer allergic responses than a similar, non-hypoallergenic product. The consumer, however, usually believes that hypoallergenic products are much superior to normal products because they have been scientifically formulated to be especially kind to sensitive skin, and that natural products contain mostly natural ingredients (usually extracted from plants), and are free from, or only contain small amounts of artificial chemical additives. This belief is often reinforced by the higher cost of hypoallergenic products and products that claim to be natural.

In the USA, the FDA tried to control the use of "hypoallergenic" and "natural" when used to describe cosmetics and toiletries, so that consumers would not be misled by the manufacturers. It wanted some guarantee that hypoallergenic products had been tested and had been shown to cause fewer allergies, or to be less irritating than standard products. It also wanted a "natural" product to contain substantial quantities of natural ingredients and fewer synthetic chemicals. But the cosmetic manufacturers challenged the FDA through the courts, and the FDA eventually lost the case on the grounds that it had no authority to regulate the way products are advertised. The net result is that, in the USA at least, these words are completely meaningless and misleading. Words like "allergy tested," "non-irritating," "dermatologically tested," and so on, carry no guarantee that the products will not cause skin irritation or allergic reactions. In fact, in the USA, manufacturers can use these words without any supporting evidence whatsoever.

The situation in the UK is much less clear. The British Advertising Standards Authority has no specific regulations regarding these terms, and manufacturers and importers of cosmetics have no common code of practice governing their usage. A recent study carried out by Rohm and Haas, a chemical manufacturer, concluded that, in the EU

The term "hypoallergenic" has no scientific definition and no regulatory guidelines ... It appears that claims such as "for sensitive skin," "hypoallergenic," and "high tolerance formula" should be strictly regulated if not discouraged.

In a recent circular issued by the UK Local Authorities Co-ordinating Body on Food and Trading Standards (LACOTS), it stated that it failed to find "either a legal or accepted dictionary definition" of the term "hypoallergenic" and that, "consultation with representative trade bodies has shown there to be differences in industry understanding and usage" of this term.

There are two pieces of relevant legislation though. The Department of Trade and Industry's *Guide to the Cosmetic Products (Safety) Regulations* states that each product that is manufactured in, or imported into, the EU should have a product information package (PIP). This PIP, which is not usually available to the general public, should contain all of the information about the product that a "competent authority" (i.e., Trading Standards Officers in the UK, or the District Council in Northern Ireland) may require. The PIP should contain evidence for any claims that are made for the product. For example, if a sunscreen is claimed to have a Sun Protection Factor (SFP) of 15 and to protect against both UV-A and UV-B ultraviolet rays, then there should be some laboratory measurements recorded in the PIP to show that these claims are correct, and a product that claims to be hypoallergenic must show that it causes fewer allergies than a comparable, standard product.

The second piece of legislation is the 1968 Trade Descriptions Act, which prohibits manufacturers from making false or misleading claims about their products. If a manufacturer or advertising agency does make such a claim, the Director General of Fair Trading (DGFT) normally asks for a voluntary undertaking to cease these advertisements. The courts only become involved if the false or misleading claims continue to be made. However, manufacturers often make claims that stretch the law to its absolute limit and it may be difficult to show that these claims are misleading. Take the claim by some toothpaste manufacturers that their products can make your teeth whiter. Whiter than what? To show that this statement is misleading, it would have to be proved that it is likely to deceive consumers, and as a result of deceiving them, to affect their behavior. The average consumer may well buy the product believing it would make their teeth whiter but it is unlikely that sufficient numbers of consumers would, after scientifically testing the product on themselves, complain to the DGFT that the product was not working as claimed. Most dissatisfied customers are likely instead to complain to the manufacturer and be happy with a refund and an apologetic letter, or simply buy another brand next time. The law may well be there to protect the consumer but it is often difficult to enforce.

In conclusion, the meaning of terms such as "hypoallergenic" and "natural" are a point of confusion and the evidence must speak for itself. Products on British shelves that claim to be natural sometimes contain less than one percent of natural ingredients (see the sample label in *Chapter 18 – Labels and Legal Matters*). We have found that many hypoallergenic products are not substantially different to the standard version of the same product (other than being much more expensive, of course), and that often they have the exact same ingredients except they contain fewer colorants and fragrances. However, since these ingredients are the most common cause of irritation and allergies, the mere fact that fewer of them have been used may be sufficient to prove the product is hypoallergenic. From a consumer's point of view, a product that contains fewer colorants and fragrances may well be kinder to their skin, but it should not cost more than a comparable, alternative product.

Other terms that often cause confusion are "unscented," "fragrance free," "dermatologically tested," and "allergy tested." There are no legal definitions of these terms and they are often used without any explanation as to their meaning or the outcome of any tests which have been carried out. Many products labelled as being "unscented" do in fact contain small quantities of fragrance chemicals, added by the manufacturer to cover up the unpleasant, natural odors of other ingredients. If you want to avoid fragrance chemicals, ignore the banner on the front and check the list of ingredients on the back of the product for terms that may include "Fragrance," "Flavor," "Parfum," or "Aroma."

What is a "Natural" Substance?

A natural substance is any plant or animal extract, or any rock or mineral obtained from the earth. They are often contaminated with a host of other substances, which must be removed in order to achieve the required degree of purity before they can be used as ingredients in personal care products.

Artificial or synthetic ingredients are made when substances are modified by chemical reactions in industrial processes. It is possible for chemists to make exact copies of natural substances. The synthetic versions are identical in every respect to the original, natural substances: the only differences being the cost and convenience of production. One example is methyl salicylate (oil of wintergreen), an important ingredient in many essential oils extracted from a variety of plants, including plants of the wintergreen family, from which it gets its everyday name. It has soothing and pain-killing properties, and is used in ointments and liniments for rheumatic pains, strained muscles, and minor injuries, and it is used as a fragrance and denaturant in cosmetics and toiletries. Manufacturers find it cheaper and more convenient to synthesize methyl salicylate from raw materials obtained from coal tar and petroleum, than to extract it from plants.

RECIPES FOR HERBAL SHAMPOO AND HAIR RINSE

The following recipes were posted on the Internet. Most of the ingredients are entirely natural and so give the impression that the shampoo and rinse must be completely without harmful effects, and the herbs must be good for your hair.

Herbal Shampoo

6fl.oz (160ml) distilled water
$^1/_2$oz (15g) Soapwort root (Bouncing Bet)
1 tsp (5ml) castor oil
$^1/_4$ tsp (2g) sea salt
15 drops (1ml) Geranium oil
15 drops (1ml) Lavender oil

Herbal Hair Rinse

8oz (220ml) cider vinegar

1oz (28ml) vodka

1oz (28g) dried herbs or 4oz (110g) fresh herbs

1 tsp (5ml) castor oil

A choice of herbs was suggested for dark or light hair, or for treating hair with dandruff. (See *Chapter 9 – Hair Care* for lists of appropriate herbs.)

Comments and Adverse Effects:

- Soapwort (Bouncing Bet or *Saponaria officinalis*) is a common plant found in the USA and throughout Europe. The sap from its roots contain saponins, often in the form of glucosides (meaning that the saponins are attached to sugar molecules). These form lather when agitated with water, but neither saponins nor saponin glucosides are surfactants and cannot, therefore, remove dirt or grease from any surface, including hair. The fact that it produces lather does not mean it can clean your hair and, in this case, the concoction is merely adding to the grease in your hair.
- Saponins from soapwort are mildly poisonous if swallowed, causing mouth, stomach, and intestinal irritation, often with nausea, vomiting, and diarrhea.
- Castor oil (*Ricinus communis*) can cause inflammation, dryness, and cracking of the lips.
- Geranium oils can cause contact dermatitis and skin irritation.
- Lavender oils can cause contact allergies and photosensitivity.
- The hair rinse will contain approximately 2 percent acetic acid from the vinegar. This may cause mild skin irritation and will cause severe eye irritation.
- It will also contain approximately 4 percent alcohol from the vodka. Alcohol causes systemic eczematous contact dermatitis.
- For a list of adverse effects caused by herbs, see *Chapter 9 – Hair Care*.

Another example is vanillin, which occurs naturally in vanilla pods and is an important fragrance and flavoring compound. It has a simple chemical structure and is easily and economically copied by chemists. As well as copying nature, chemists often try to improve on it. One simple modification converts vanillin into ethylvanillin, which has the same odor and flavor but is many thousands of times more potent. In some factories, technicians who add ethylvanillin to a cosmetic or food product, routinely protect themselves by wearing a full environmental suit. Even the tiniest trace of this compound on their skin will leave them smelling like crème anglais for several days!

Does Natural Mean Better?

Many people regard natural substances as being more wholesome or more healthy than artificial chemicals, but this is not necessarily the case. So-called "natural" products may in fact contain more preservatives than their synthetic counterparts, to prevent bacteria from breeding in the more nutritious natural ingredients, and the harm these preservatives can cause may often outweigh the benefits the natural ingredients can bring.

People argue, justifiably, that our bodies are not designed to deal with unnatural chemicals and, therefore, we should not be exposed to them. Three points must be remembered, however. First, the human body is remarkably good at dealing with unwanted chemicals and excreting them harmlessly. Second, many natural substances are extremely harmful – both plants and animals produce some of the most deadly poisons known to Man. Finally, the track record of artificial chemicals in our food and personal care products must speak for itself. These ingredients have caused relatively few serious illnesses. Rather than condemn them out of hand, perhaps we should ask the question: are these chemicals added for my benefit or for the manufacturer's profits? If the answer is the latter, perhaps we should buy another brand.

PROTEINS

Proteins are added to some personal care products for a variety of reasons. They can act as emulsifiers, antistatic agents, film formers, thickeners, and humectants (see the *A–Z of Cosmetic Terms* for explanations of these terms), but they have no biological significance. Contrary to advertisers' claims, proteins cannot be absorbed by hair, skin, or nails and they cannot repair or improve our body tissues. To imagine that these proteins can do what the marketing people suggest is just as ludicrous as trying to repair a crumbling house by throwing bricks and sand at it.

Cosmetics Unmasked

VITAMINS

Vitamins are important nutrients in our diet and are essential to maintain our health. For a number of years now, vitamins have been added to cosmetics and toiletries to "nourish" our skin, hair, and nails. Vitamins A, C, and E are the most commonly used vitamins, with vitamin B added occasionally in the form of cereals such as oat bran or hydrolyzed wheat proteins. Vitamin D_2 (ergocalciferol), and vitamin D_3 (cholecalciferol) are banned from cosmetics in the EU.

> The FDA's *Cosmetics Handbook* states that, where cosmetic ingredients are declared as vitamins, this conveys the misleading impression that these ingredients and products offer a nutritional or health benefit and, therefore, the product in question may be deemed misbranded. For this reason, vitamins are listed in the ingredients under their INCI names, rather than their commonly understood vitamin names. For example, vitamin E would be listed in the ingredients as tocopherol.

Vitamins A, C, and E have antioxidant properties. Vitamin C reacts with oxygen and is often used as an antioxidant in food products. In a similar way it can prevent oxidation of cosmetics. It is a water-soluble vitamin and is not absorbed through the skin. Vitamins A and E are oil-soluble vitamins, which can react with free radicals and destroy them. Cosmetic manufacturers have latched onto these facts and make exaggerated claims that these vitamins will slow down the onset of fine lines and wrinkles, by preventing oxidation of the skin and by inhibiting the action of free radicals. However, these vitamins can only penetrate into the first few layers of the epidermis, and never reach the dermis where the aging process takes place. Therefore, it is highly unlikely that they will have any real effect on the aging process, and any reduction in the appearance of fine lines and wrinkles is almost entirely due to the moisturizing effect of the other ingredients in the formulation.

TYPICAL INGREDIENTS — ACTIVE RENEWAL MOISTURIZING MILK

Ingredients:

Aqua, Glycerin, Sorbitan stearate, Dimethicone, Paraffinum liquidum, Petrolatum, Cetyl palmitate, Cetyl alcohol, Citric acid, Steareth-100, Acrylates/C10-30 Alkylacrylates crosspolymer, Salicylic acid, Glyceryl hydroxy stearate, Sodium stearate, Tetrasodium EDTA, Parfum, Octyl methoxycinnamate, Phenoxyethanol, Methylparaben, Butylparaben, CI 17200.

A more expensive, hypoallergenic version of this product is available. The ingredients are identical with the exception that the Parfum and the CI 17200 colorant have been excluded from the formulation.

Aqua	Water, the main ingredient, adds moisture directly to the skin.
Glycerin*	A humectant to hold water and keep it on the skin.
Sorbitan stearate*	Emulsifier to aid the mixing of the oily ingredients with water.
Dimethicone*	A synthetic silicone polymer which acts as an antifoaming agent and forms a waterproof layer on the skin to prevent water loss by evaporation.
Paraffinum liquidum*	Light, petroleum-derived oil which moisturizes by forming a waterproof barrier.
Petrolatum*	Heavy, petroleum-derived oil which moisturizes by forming a waterproof barrier.
Cetyl palmitate*	Moisturizing ingredient.
Cetyl alcohol*	This ingredient acts as a thickener and has moisturizing properties.
Citric acid*	A beta-hydroxy acid that is used to exfoliate skin (i.e., dissolve the outer layer of skin cells). It also controls acidity in the finished product.
Steareth-100*	Surfactant to aid mixing of ingredients and to aid even spreading of the product.

Acrylates/C10-30 – alkylacrylates crosspolymer	This forms a thin film on the skin, binds the other ingredients together and thickens the product.
Salicylic acid*	A beta-hydroxy acid used to exfoliate skin. It is banned from products intended for use on children under the age of three, with the exception of shampoo.
Glyceryl hydroxy stearate*	A moisturizing ingredient that also acts as an emulsifier.
Sodium stearate	This is essentially soap and is used as a surfactant to aid spreading, and as an opacifier to disguise the watery nature of the main ingredients.
Tetrasodium EDTA	Prevents the calcium and magnesium ions present in hard water from combining with some of the other ingredients.
Parfum	A mixture of fragrance chemicals, often more than 50 in number, many of which are artificial.
Octyl methoxycinnamate*	A UV absorber to protect the skin from the harmful effects of ultraviolet rays. This is needed because the exfoliating ingredients remove the outer layer of skin cells that contain our natural UV-absorbing pigments.
Phenoxyethanol*	Preservative, restricted to 1 percent of the finished product.**
Methylparaben*	Water-soluble preservative, restricted to 0.4 percent of the finished product.**
Butylparaben*	Oil-soluble preservative, restricted to 0.4 percent of the finished product.**
CI 17200*	Red azo dye.

* These ingredients are subject to restrictions or have been linked to harmful or adverse effects.

** Indicates that this ingredient may be used in larger quantities if it is used for another specific purpose other than as a preservative.

What are Pro-Vitamins?

Pro-vitamin is one of the most popular buzz words on the market. It is easy to pronounce and sounds healthy and scientific. Pro-retinol or Pro-retinol-A (a made-up name) sounds even better. Retinol is the chemical name for vitamin A, and so Pro-retinol-A is probably just Pro-vitamin A – which is beta-carotene, a natural colorant found in many roots, including carrots. Cosmetic manufacturers and beauticians will tell you that pro-vitamins nourish the skin, combat free radicals produced in the skin by ultraviolet rays, act as antioxidants, and so on. But this is another myth. The truth is, they add little to the quality of the product and have no discernible biological effect unless you eat them as part of a balanced, healthy diet. Pro-vitamins are, in fact, substances in our diet that are absorbed by the body and converted into vitamins. Panthenol (pro-vitamin B_5), and beta-carotene (pro-vitamin A), are the most common pro-vitamins used in cosmetics.

ACTIVE INGREDIENTS

There is no requirement for cosmetics to list "Active Ingredients," because they do not normally contain ingredients that must be labeled in this way. Only medicinal products or medical devices are required to list the active ingredients that they contain. Conversely there are no regulations to say that manufacturers *cannot* list some of their ingredients as "active ingredients," even when they are not, and manufacturers sometimes do so in order to make their product appear to be better than a competitor's product. For example, we were presented with a face cream which listed rose water as an active ingredient and were asked if this meant that the other ingredients were inactive. The answer is that all the ingredients play some role in the formulation, but none of them would have a therapeutic or medical effect and, therefore, none of them, including the rose water, are "active ingredients" as defined in the EU Medical Devices Directive. Cosmetics, as defined in the EU Cosmetics Products Directive, do not contain active ingredients.

CHOOSING INGREDIENTS

We would all like to believe that manufacturers choose their ingredients because they are the best ingredients available. Nothing could be further from the truth. If you examine the ingredients listed on a shampoo bottle and a conditioner made by the same manufacturer you will often find that many ingredients are common to both. This is not because they are necessarily the best ingredients, but because the manufacturer can maximize profits by bulk-buying one ingredient rather than two, or can make cost savings for other reasons – such as reducing the need for the testing of raw materials. The upside to this is that if you do use a number of products made by the same manufacturer, you are probably exposing yourself to a smaller overall number of cosmetic ingredients, thereby reducing the risk of adverse effects.

On the other hand, if you buy a product that has been manufactured in the USA and compare the ingredients with an identical product manufactured under license in the UK, you will often find that the ingredients are completely different. The two products, despite having different ingredients, will have the same name, same packaging, and even the same television advertisement. The differences are not due to the ingredients being restricted, banned, or unavailable in the UK, but simply to there being cheaper alternatives that do exactly the same job. The same is true of beer: American beer brewed under license in the UK just doesn't taste the same.

3 colorants and fragrances

Relax in a sea of fragrant bubbles

Ease your mind and soak away your troubles

But before you add the colorful gloop

And immerse yourself in the chemical soup

Remember – plain hot water can ease your bones

Without irritating your sensitive zones

The importance of colors and fragrances in the cosmetics industry must not be underestimated. If a shampoo is to be successful in the marketplace, it must smell as though it can clean your hair, and it must disguise the watery, gray color of the main ingredients. But many adverse reactions to cosmetics and toiletries have been linked to colorants and fragrance chemicals and for this reason hypoallergenic products are usually unscented and uncolored. What follows is a detailed look at these ingredients.

COLORANTS

As the name suggests, colorants are pigments or colored chemicals. They are used on their own or mixed with other colorants to impart a certain tint or shade to cosmetics and toiletries. Some are used to color the product to improve its appearance, or to temporarily impart that color or hue to the skin. Other colorants, for example hair dyes, are designed to produce a longer-lasting color change.

The range of colors available to cosmetic manufactures is vast. Colorants can be dyes or lakes. A dye is a natural extract, or a synthetic coal tar or azo dye, that is soluble in water. Because they dissolve in water, they can disperse evenly through cosmetics and toiletries producing clear, colored liquids. They can also absorb into hair and fibers of textiles and paper. Some dyes fade when exposed to bright lights. They can also fade from hair or fabrics if they are leeched out during washing. Lakes are made by combining dyes with metals – usually chromium, aluminum, zirconium, or manganese. They are usually more durable than dyes because they are insoluble in water and are not leeched out during washing. They are often used in make-up because they do not run or stain clothing.

"Interference" colors are rapidly becoming popular, especially with younger people. In the same way that glass prisms, diamonds, and rain drops can produce spectacular rainbows of colors, combinations of solid pigments can cause interference patterns of light that sparkle with gold, red, green, blue, and silver. One such combination, used in eye shadow and lipstick, is black mica – mica, a natural mineral found in volcanic rocks such as granite, coated with black iron oxide, another natural mineral, although both minerals can be produced artificially.

"Active" colors respond to physiological changes in the skin and undergo dramatic color changes. They are mainly used in lipstick and colored lip gloss, and less commonly in eye make-up. Temperature changes, moisture variation, sebum secretions, and changes in acidity, can all cause the pigments to change color. Some people like to believe these active colours can act as a barometer for mood, emotion, or sexual arousal, but they are more likely to indicate the temperature and humidity of the surroundings.

Coal Tar Dyes

At one time the only source of raw materials for the manufacture of artificial dyes was coal tar. This is a chemical soup, obtained when coal is heated strongly in the absence of air, so that it cannot burn. From this sticky, black chemical substance, a large number of useful compounds are obtained, including aniline, cresols, naphthols and phenols – the raw materials for making coal tar dyes. Dyes made using aniline are called aniline dyes or azo dyes. Dyes made from the other extracts were simply called coal tar dyes. Although we now obtain most of these chemicals from petroleum, they still tend to be called coal tar dyes.

Azo Dyes

Azo dyes were first made in the nineteenth century by Sir William Henry Perkin, an English chemist who, after making a synthetic mauve dye from a coal tar extract (aniline), a color reserved by its rarity for kings, emperors, and popes, founded the British aniline or azodye industry and transformed the manufacture of textiles during the Industrial Revolution. These coal tar dyes are still in common use today and find their way into every aspect of our lives, including our food and cosmetics.

Azo Dyes

The following colorants are all synthetic azo dyes:

Acid Red 195	CI 15525	CI 18130
CI 11680	CI 15580	CI 18690
CI 11710	CI 15620	CI 18736
CI 11725	CI 15630	CI 18965
CI 11920	CI 15800 (D&C Red #31)	CI 19140 (FD&C Yellow #5)
CI 12010	CI 15850 (D&C Red #6)	CI 19140:1
CI 12085 (D&C Red #36)	CI 15865	CI 20040
CI 12120	CI 15865:4	CI 20170
CI 12150	CI 15880 (D&C Red #34)	CI 21100
CI 12370	CI 15985 (FD&C Yellow #6)	CI 21108
CI 12420	CI 15985:1	CI 21230
CI 12480	CI 16035 (FD&C Red #40)	CI 24790
CI 12490	CI 16185	CI 26100
CI 13015	CI 16185:1	CI 27290
CI 14270	CI 16230	CI 27755
CI 14700 (FD&C Red #4)	CI 16255	CI 28440
CI 14720	CI 16290	CI 40215

| CI 14815 | CI 17200 | D&C Red #7 |
| CI 15510 (D&C Orange #4) | CI 18050 | D&C Red #39 |

Some people are sensitive to azo and coal tar dyes. Those who are particularly at risk are asthmatics, eczema sufferers, and people who are sensitive to aspirin. The effects of these chemicals are many and varied, ranging from hyperactivity in children to severe headaches. Other reported symptoms include breathing difficulties, asthmatic attacks, itching and watering eyes and nose, blurred vision, skin rashes, swelling (with fluid retention in serious cases), and changes in blood platelets, which control the clotting process after injury.

How Safe are Colorants?

The safety of some colorants has been questioned and these have been restricted by the EU Commission to rinse-off products only. These products include shampoos and conditioners where the colorant is only in contact with the skin for a short time. Non-rinse-off cosmetics such as lipsticks and eye shadow are in contact with the skin for much longer and must, therefore, have no unwanted adverse effects. It is generally assumed that hair dyes do not stick to the skin for long and are safe when absorbed into the hair, which consists almost entirely of dead cells.

In America FD&C colorants have been certified by the FDA for use in any food product, drug, or cosmetic sold in the USA. Colorants that are certified for use in any drugs or cosmetics, but not in food, have the prefix, D&C. The Ext. D&C range of colorants are harmful if swallowed and are certified for use in externally applied drugs and cosmetics only. In addition to FDA-certified colorants, natural colorants (such as annatto from the seed coat of the tropical annatto tree), may be used in any product without FDA certification.

FDA certification requires that a batch of dye be tested for conformity to the FDA's specifications for purity and formulation. This means that the azo dye tartrazine does not automatically become FD&C Yellow #5. If a particular batch of tartrazine is tested and meets the FDA's criteria, it is assigned a certification lot number, indicating to manufacturers that this specific batch of tartrazine is suitable for use and may be listed in the ingredients as FD&C Yellow #5.

Dyes That Are Safe

The following dyes are probably safe. They have no known adverse effects and they are allowed in all products without restriction.

Synthetic Dyes

CI 42051	CI 61565 (D&C Green #6)	CI 74160
CI 42053	CI 61570 (D&C Green #5)	CI 75300
CI 42090 (FD&C Blue #1)	CI 69800	CI 77002
CI 44090	CI 69825 (D&C Blue #9)	CI 77163
CI 47005	CI 73000	CI 77346
CI 58000	CI 73360 (D&C Red #30)	CI 77510
CI 60725	CI 73385	CI 77947

Modified Natural Pigments

CI 75470	CI 75810	CI 77267

Natural Pigments

CI 75100	CI 75125	CI 75135
CI 75120	CI 75130	CI 75170

Natural Minerals or Mineral Extracts

CI 77000	CI 77231	CI 77499
CI 77004	CI 77400	CI 77713
CI 77007	CI 77480	CI 77742
CI 77015	CI 77489	CI 77745
CI 77120	CI 77491	CI 77820
CI 77220	CI 77492	CI 77891

Listing Colors

The EU Commission keeps a list of cosmetic ingredients which includes over 470 hair dyes, colorants, and other substances designed to alter the appearance of cosmetics. A large number of these are named using the color index numbers, e.g., CI 10316. Occasionally the European "E" numbers are used, and other colors are easily spotted as they often include the name of a color. For example, Acid Black 52, Basic Blue 99, D&C Red #33, Direct Blue 86, Disperse Orange 3, HC Blue No 11, Pigment Green 7 and Solvent Green 29 are all obviously colors. Some, however, are known by their full chemical name and are not so easily spotted in a list of ingredients.

There might be 20 shades of eye shadow or lipstick, all slightly different. Some might contain just one of these colors while others might contain two or more in any combination. To save printing several different labels, all the different shades can carry the same label, which shows all the colors that are used in that range of cosmetic. Labeling regulations in the EU allow manufactures to economize by adding something like this at the end of the ingredients:

[+ /- CI 77491, CI 77492, CI 77499, CI 77713, CI 77742, CI 77745].

In the USA the equivalent expression is: "May contain D&C Red #30, D&C Yellow #7, D&C Yellow #10." This means the particular cosmetic might or might not contain some or all of these colors. The problem for you, the consumer, is, you don't know which colors are actually in the cosmetic you are using.

FRAGRANCES

The importance of fragrances should not be underestimated. They are a major factor in attracting customers, many of whom have preconceived ideas about the smells of household items. A disinfectant, for example, must smell as though it can kill microbes, a bar of soap must smell as though it can clean your body, and your foaming bath oil must smell luxurious. Believe it or not, fragrances are not only added to personal care products and household cleaners; they are in everything from writing paper to new cars. Everything you buy must have the correct smell.

ARTIFICIAL RASPBERRY FRAGRANCE

If you have an adverse reaction to a cosmetic or toiletry there is a good chance that colorants or fragrance chemicals are responsible. The following may help to explain why. Many cosmetics come in both a normal and a hypoallergenic form. Commonly, both products have the same ingredients but the hypoallergenic version contains no colorants or fragrance chemicals, and is sold in smaller containers that cost more.

Many artificial flavors and fragrances contain a large number of fragrance chemicals. A hundred or more is quite typical. Notable exceptions to this are artificial raspberry, strawberry, chocolate, pineapple, and celery fragrances. These all contain eight or fewer fragrance chemicals. The recipe below, taken from U.S. Patent No. 3886289, is for artificial raspberry flavor, but it can double up as a raspberry fragrance for use in products such as fruit-scented toilet soap or shower gel. Minor additions or variations to this recipe may be necessary to compensate for any unpleasant odors produced by the other ingredients in the product. If this were the case, the recipe could include a larger number of hazardous, artificial chemicals.

100 Parts	4-(4-Hydroxyphenyl)-2-butanone [1, 5, 6]
30 Parts	3-Hydroxy-2-methyl-4-pyrone (Maltol) [1, 5, 9, 12]
20 Parts	4-Hydroxy-3-methoxybenzaldehyde (Vanillin) [2, 5, 9]
8 Parts	3-Ethoxy-4-hydroxybenzaldehyde (Ethylvanillin) [2, 7, 8]
1 Part	α-Ionone [3, 9]
1 Part	Methyl sulfide [1, 4, 5, 9, 10, 11, 12]
1 Part	2,5-Dimethyl-N-(2-pyrazinyl)pyrrole [9, 12]

The superscript numbers after each ingredient refer to the Risk and Safety Phrases that must be present on laboratory containers of these chemicals, as required by EU legislation. These phrases are:

1   Irritating to eyes, respiratory system, and skin.
2   Harmful if swallowed. Irritating to eyes.
3   May cause sensitization by inhalation and by skin contact.
4   Risk of serious damage to eyes.
5   In case of contact with eyes, rinse immediately with plenty of water and seek medical advice.
6   Wear suitable gloves and eye/face protection.
7   Wear suitable protective clothing, gloves, and eye/face protection.
8   Do not breathe dust.
9   Wear suitable protective clothing.
10   Do not breathe vapor.
11   Keep away from sources of ignition – No smoking.
12   Harmful if swallowed.

When a scent or a mixture of fragrance chemicals are added to a cosmetic or toiletry, this is indicated on the list of ingredients by the word "Fragrance" in the USA, or "Parfum" in the EU. The fragrance may be a natural plant extract or a cocktail of several artificial fragrance chemicals. There are 932 fragrance chemicals listed by the EU Commission, and none of these has to be named separately on the list of ingredients.

A perfumer will use his or her experience, skill and imagination to blend these fragrance chemicals to produce the desired effect. However, they cannot exercise their creative talents with complete freedom, as they must always consider the cost of individual fragrance chemicals – using the less expensive options wherever possible. They must also ensure the fragrance chemicals are compatible with the other ingredients in the product.

Few perfumes contain less than 20 fragrance chemicals and many have more than a hundred. They are used in minute quantities but many of them are known to have irritant, harmful, or toxic properties, so it is no wonder that many adverse reactions to cosmetics are linked to these fragrance chemicals. Have a look at the recipe for raspberry fragrance to see why.

If you have an adverse reaction to a personal care product, try using one that has no added fragrances. Be warned, however, "fragrance free" or "unscented" written on the packaging is no guarantee that the product is free from these ingredients. A small amount of fragrance may be added to cover up the unpleasant smells of the other ingredients.

The Secret of Musk

Musk is a scent secreted from the scent glands of the male Tibetan musk deer, musk ox, civet cat, otter, and several other species. Its name is probably derived from *mushká*, the Sanskrit word for scrotum, which describes the appearance of the musk deer's scent gland. Musk is used as a pheromone to attract and impress females of the same species. Technically, a pheromone is a chemical messenger that has an involuntary biological effect on other members of the species. Pheromones secreted by female moths can attract males from several kilometers away. It is doubtful that humans produce pheromones. Other than making someone move away from you, your natural body odors are unlikely to cause any involuntary behavior in other people!

The odor of musk is not particularly pleasant, but despite this, many females are attracted to it. It also has the effect of heightening and increasing the persistence of scents from flowers. Musk is, therefore, a valued fragrance chemical and is used in many perfumes and deodorants.

Muscone (also spelled muskone) is the active ingredient from the scent gland of the musk deer, while civetone is the main fragrance produced by the civet cat. Manufacturers rely on these animals as the main source of these fragrances. Unfortunately for these animals, and despite the simplicity of their chemical structures, chemists have not yet been able to develop an efficient method for manufacturing these fragrances. Chemically, muscone and civetone are remarkably similar in structure, being based on a ring of 17 carbon atoms rather like a bracelet of beads. It is easy enough to make 17 carbon atoms into a chain, but the problem comes when they try to join the ends together and fasten the bracelet. (These string-of-beads' molecules writhe around like a bucket of worms. Their movement is random and the chance of both ends of the same molecule coming together so that the bracelet can be fastened, is extremely small. The probability that all of the molecules will find their way into this position is zero.) As a result, the synthetic musk can only be produced in minute amounts that cost vastly more than their natural counterparts, which is why manufacturers still have to rely on animals for their main supply.

Musk Substitutes

Nitro-musks are simple molecules that are easily and cheaply made. They are chemically unrelated to muscone or civetone but they have odors that are remarkably similar. They were once widely used as musk substitutes in cheap perfumes and toiletries, but some of these compounds have since been found to be harmful. As a result, three nitro-musks – moskene, musk tibetene, and musk ambrette – have been banned from use in cosmetics in the EU. Nitro-musks are also capable of reacting chemically with other ingredients, forming nitrosamines, which are potent carcinogens, or cancer-causing chemicals.

4 preservatives

The fact of preservatives being used, and their amount, should be stated on the label.
The *Lancet,* 1897

Today EU and FDA labeling regulations allow the names of preservatives to be hidden within the list of ingredients and their quantities not stated.

So far, this book has focused on the adverse effects of cosmetic ingredients, but these are not the only things in cosmetics that can harm you. Dangerous microbes can breed in the products and so it is important to add preservatives to ensure that harmful bacteria are not allowed to thrive and multiply. However, after colorants and fragrances, preservatives are probably the next main cause of adverse reactions to cosmetics and toiletries. It is for this reason that there are regulations and restrictions on the use of most preservatives.

MICROBES AND COSMETICS

Microbe is a common word for micro-organism. It is a general term used to describe any microscopic, single-celled, living organism. It is often extended to include some multi-celled, complex organisms such as mold and fungi, and viruses, which do not have cells.

The most common microbes that can potentially infect personal care products are molds, fungi, yeasts, bacteria, and protozoa. (Viruses rarely infect cosmetics because they can only reproduce inside the cells of other living organisms.) When a microbe infects a product, it feeds on the ingredients to get the energy it needs for reproduction. The rapidly reproducing microbes usually produce a bad smell and may cause some clear products to become cloudy. They also release toxic substances as waste products, to help them digest and absorb food, and to kill other microbes that may be in competition with them. They can also chemically alter ingredients, causing colors and odors to change. The altered substances may be poisonous or harmful.

Microbes enter personal care products during manufacture, when the containers are being filled, and while you are using them at home. There is a danger that microbes in cosmetics and toiletries may be transferred to your body and start an infection. The microbes may feed on your body tissues, causing damage to the tissues, and they often release toxins into your bloodstream. For this reason, virtually all personal care products you buy will contain at least one preservative, and often more, to inhibit the growth of microbes in the product. They may also contain antimicrobials, which control the growth of microbes on your body. Some products are irradiated with gamma rays to kill any microbes that may have entered the product during the manufacture and packaging processes.

MICROBES AND SAFETY STANDARDS

For the purpose of setting acceptable levels of microbial contamination, the EU Commission has divided cosmetics and toiletries into two categories. Category-1 products are those for use on infants under the age of three, for use on or near the eyes, or for use on or near mucous membranes. All other personal care products are classified as Category-2 products. Simply put, when you buy Category-1 products, they must contain 50 times fewer microbes than Category-2 products. Additionally, since microbes are likely to get into personal care products during normal use, there must be sufficient preservatives added to the product, to prevent contamination from rising above these levels.

Three pathogens (disease-causing microbes) that commonly live on the human body are *Candida albicans*, *Pseudomonas aeruginosa*, and *Staphylococcus aureus*.

Normally they do not cause disease or illness because their numbers are controlled by friendly microbes, or by our immune system. If, however, they enter parts of the body where they can breed rapidly, or if our immune system is weakened (for example, during a viral infection such as flu), they may cause illness.

These three pathogens have also been identified as the most likely microbes to enter and contaminate personal care products during normal use. EU regulations require sufficient levels of preservative to be added to kill these microbes – the test being that none of them should be detectable in 0.5 grams (or 0.5 milliliters) of a Category-1 product, or 0.1 grams (or 0.1 milliliters) of a Category-2 product. This means there will be higher levels of preservatives in Category-1 products for babies and sensitive areas of the body, than in the more commonly used Category-2 products. This could imply that baby shampoo is not necessarily more gentle than ordinary shampoo if it contains a higher concentration of preservative than an equivalent formulation for adults.

The importance of keeping our personal care products free from microbes must not be underestimated. Nowhere is this more important than for contact-lens users. During the last decade and a half, *Acanthamoeba*, a single-cell protozoan (member of the amoeba family), has caused eye infections in several contact-lens users. Most of the cases were linked to poor contact-lens hygiene or to using cleaning solutions that did not adequately kill this microbe. As the number of contact-lens users has increased, the number of reported cases of acanthamoeba keratitis has also risen. If caught early, this painful eye disease can be easily treated but some patients have lost eyes to this microbe or have required corneal transplants to correct the damage. To keep this in perspective, during one year in the mid-nineties, there were 70 eyes lost to acanthamoeba in the UK. That same year, 90 eyes were lost to champagne corks.

PRESERVATIVES

Preservatives are chemicals which are added to personal care products to prevent or control the growth of microbes in the product. Several preservatives have dual roles, doubling up as deodorants, antimicrobials and antidandruff agents. By their very nature, preservatives are designed to kill cells or prevent them from multiplying. They are, therefore, potentially harmful cosmetic ingredients, and the vast majority of preservatives have restrictions on their use. Since there are also strict rules concerning levels of microbial infection in personal care products, virtually all products you buy will contain at least one preservative, making it almost impossible to avoid using potentially harmful chemicals on your body.

It's a Fact

Formaldehyde is a cheap and commonly used preservative in products like budget or family shampoo, shower gel, family bubble bath and hand wash. At one time, before refrigeration, it was added to milk to kill the acid-producing bacteria that turned it sour. It failed to kill other, more harmful bacteria, resulting in dangerously contaminated milk which appeared to be fresh and palatable. Formaldehyde's use in milk has long since been banned, and this throws doubt on its effectiveness as a cosmetic preservative. It is also a cancer suspect and is banned from cosmetics in Sweden and Japan. Maybe you should choose another product.

The whole of a product must be protected from microbial contamination. Since many products are emulsions consisting of oily droplets dispersed throughout a watery base, at least one water soluble, and one oil-soluble preservative must be added. In order to ensure all microbes are killed, it is common to find at least two of each type of preservative in a product. Benzoates such as methylparaben, ethylparaben, propylparaben and butylparaben are common preservatives found in a wide range of cosmetics and toiletries, including products for babies. This is a favored range of preservatives because, as you read the list from left to right, they become less soluble in water and more soluble in oils, allowing every part of an emulsion to be protected. (For more information about Benzoates, see p.36.) Methylchloroisothiazolinone and methylisothiazolinone are also commonly found in personal care products.

Mercury compounds are sometimes used as preservatives in eye make-up and eye make-up remover. Despite its ability to penetrate human skin, its neurotoxic effects, and its ability to collect in body tissues, the use of mercury is permitted because it is exceptionally effective at killing *Pseudomonas aeruginosa*, a microbe that can cause severe eye infections and blindness.

There are very few natural preservatives available to cosmetic manufactures, and those that are used, are effective against only a small range of microbes. It is possible to buy cosmetics and toiletries that are preservative-free but they are usually expensive, must be stored in the refrigerator once opened, and discarded after a certain period of use.

ANTIMICROBIALS

Antimicrobials are chemicals that control the growth of microbes on the body. They are used in shampoos, toothpaste, mouthwash, antiseptic lotions, and deodorants, and are added to other cosmetics and toiletries where they may also act as preservatives.

Body odor is caused by bacteria. Washing removes the odor but bacteria are sticky creatures and many survive this ordeal by hiding in the microscopic cracks and crevasses in our skin. They feed on our body secretions and soon multiply, replenishing their numbers and bringing their characteristic odor with them. Antimicrobials either actively kill the bacteria, or reduce their ability to reproduce.

By their very nature antimicrobials are potent chemicals that affect living cells in an adverse way. For this reason many of them are regulated in the EU. Be particularly careful when using aerosol deodorants. The layer of dead cells on the surface of your skin can cope with these chemicals, but the delicate, living cells in your respiratory tract and lungs can suffer severe damage if you regularly inhale them.

ANTIOXIDANTS

Cosmetics and toiletries are not only under attack from microbes, but they can also deteriorate when exposed to bright daylight and oxygen from the air. UV absorbers are added to protect cosmetics from the effect of light, and antioxidants (as the name suggests), protect the product from the detrimental effects of oxygen.

When butter or cooking oil goes rancid we might assume that it had been infected with an unwanted microbe, in a similar way to the microbes that cause bread to go moldy or milk to go sour. However, this is not the case. Fats and oils seldom become infected with bacteria or fungi. Instead they react chemically with oxygen from the air and break down into a variety of smaller molecules, such as butanoic acid, which cause the unpleasant, rancid smell. Since cosmetics are often rich in oily ingredients they are susceptible to becoming rancid. Antioxidants block this chemical reaction and prevent the breakdown of cosmetic ingredients.

Some antioxidants are also used as food additives to preserve the fats and oils present in pre-cooked foods. Both citric acid and lactic acid can improve the efficiency of antioxidants, allowing smaller quantities of these to be used in the product.

BENZOATES – GOOD OR BAD?

In 1909, William Jago wrote in his *Manual of Forensic Chemistry and Chemical Evidence*:

The administration of benzoic acid, either as such or in the form of benzoate of soda [sodium benzoate], is highly objectionable and produces a very serious disturbance of the metabolic functions, attended with injury to digestion and health. There is only one conclusion to be drawn from this data, and that is that in the interests of health both benzoic acid and benzoate of soda should be excluded from food products.

Nearly a century on, benzoic acid, sodium benzoate, and a host of related compounds such as the parabens, are still widely used in foods and cosmetics, including most fizzy drinks consumed by children. They are antimicrobial preservatives. In other words, they are chemicals that kill cells or prevent them from reproducing and infecting the food, toiletry, or cosmetic. They cause gastric irritation, numbing of the mouth, urticaria (nettle rash or hives) and they particularly affect asthma sufferers. This does beg the question why an increasing number of our children suffer from asthma despite the improvement in air quality in recent years.

The parahydroxy benzoates, or parabens, are widely used in cosmetics, including baby products such as moist tissues or wipes, where the chemicals are likely to remain on the baby's skin. We have a collection of labels including one that lists no less than four different parabens and three other antimicrobial preservatives in one product. Surprisingly, the label plays up the fact that this particular toiletry contains mainly natural plant extracts.

Why use so many parabens? Simple – some dissolve in water while others are soluble in oil. Most cosmetics have both watery and oily ingredients blended together in the form of an emulsion, so preservatives must be used in such a way that both parts of the cosmetic are protected. Additionally, EU regulations limit the amount of parabens used to 0.4 percent of the finished product for each paraben used, up to a maximum of 0.8 percent. Manufacturers are required to produce cosmetics and toiletries that meet strict requirements for microbe contamination. Liberal use of preservatives help them to meet these requirements, which are five times more stringent for baby products, necessitating the use of even larger quantities of preservatives.

Asthma and Cosmetic Ingredients

Persulfate bleaches used in hair-care products have been linked to asthma in hairdressers. The ingredients are:

- Ammonium Persulfate
- Potassium Persulfate
- Sodium Persulfate

There is mounting evidence that some food additives can be dangerous to asthmatics, eczema sufferers, and people who are sensitive to aspirin. These people are advised to avoid sulfur dioxide, sulfite, nitrite, benzoate and hydroxybenzoate preservatives; BHA, BHT and gallate antioxidants; flavor enhancers including glutamates such as monosodium glutamate (MSG); and certain azo and coal tar dyes.

Several of these additives are used as cosmetic ingredients but there is no scientific evidence that they are dangerous to asthmatics or linked to asthma. But there is also no scientific evidence that they are safe. Many of these ingredients have restrictions on their use and several have been linked to adverse effects such as contact allergies and dermatitis. These ingredients are easily identified:

- 9 sulfites are commonly used in cosmetics as preservatives. They have names ending with "sulfite," "hydrosulfite," "bisulfite," and "metabisulfite."
- 40 benzoates are used in cosmetics. Many of these are preservatives and they all contain the name "benzoate."

23 hydroxybenzoate preservatives are used and these all end with "paraben." Methylparaben, Ethylparaben, Propylparaben, and Butylparaben are by far the most common. In fact they are so widely used it is difficult to avoid them.

The three commonly used gallate antioxidants are:

- Dodecyl Gallate
- Octyl Gallate
- Propyl Gallate

Finally, BHT and BHA are also commonly used antioxidants.

5 skin care

Tail of newt and cockerel's eye

Placental extract and azo dye

Hubble bubble toil and boil

Pro-vitamins and tea-tree oil

Emulsify into a lotion

Away fine lines with magic potion.

Each year, billions of dollars are spent on products that promise to keep our skin looking young and healthy. For many people, it has become a normal part of the daily cleansing routine and the idea of using these cosmetics is so ingrained they do not even think about whether they need to or not. Do these products work? Are they really necessary? And what can they do for you? This chapter starts by examining the structure of skin, skin types, and color, and why fine lines and wrinkles develop with age. It goes on to look at skin-care preparations such as moisturizing creams, exfoliating products (the so-called alpha-hydroxy acid skin peelers or AHAs), astringents, hair-removal creams, and methods for removing unwanted body hair. Since this is such a vast subject, there is much more about skin care in *Chapter 14 – Sun and Skin*, and *Chapter 16 – Salons and Surgeons*.

WHAT IS SKIN?

Your skin is the largest organ in your body, accounting for about 16 percent of your total body weight, and it has an area of 18,000 square centimeters (2,880 square inches) for an average adult. It is responsible for maintaining the correct body temperature; it senses heat, cold, contact, and pain; it is an excretory organ, discharging waste matter such as urea; it helps to maintain the correct levels of water in your body fluids; it protects you from external dirt, microbes, and chemicals; and it keeps you safe from rain, wind, snow, and sun.

Beneath the two main layers of the skin is the subcutaneous layer, which separates your skin from the underlying muscles. This layer consists mainly of fat cells which help to insulate your body. Above the subcutaneous layer is the dermis, the main layer of skin. The dermis is composed of living cells and contains tiny blood vessels called capillaries, nerve endings that detect temperature and touch, sweat glands that keep you cool, erector muscles that make your hair stand on end, collagen fibers that give your skin its elasticity, hair follicles that supply the growing hairs with food and oxygen, and sebaceous glands that lubricate your hair shafts, hair follicles and skin. When applied to undamaged skin, few cosmetic ingredients can reach the dermis. If they did, they would probably damage the living cells and cause irritation, sensitization, and allergies, and from there they would enter your bloodstream and may cause harm elsewhere in your body.

On top of the dermis is the outer layer of skin, called the epidermis. The epidermis consists of five layers but only one of them, the deepest layer, is distinct. This layer is called the basal layer or stratum germinativum. It consists of living cells that obtain food and oxygen from the dermis, and cells called melanocytes, which contain melanin, a brown pigment that protects you from ultraviolet radiation and gives your skin its color. As the basal cells reproduce, they are pushed upwards toward the surface of the skin, taking about three weeks to reach the surface where they are eventually shed ("desquamated"). During these three weeks the cells gradually die and the substances inside the cell slowly turn to keratin, a tough, fibrous protein which is also found in hair and nails.

By the time the cells reach the horny outer layer of skin that you can see (the "stratum corneum"), they consist mainly of keratin, are flat like paving slabs, and are almost completely dehydrated. This outer layer is usually the only layer you ever hear about. Many cosmetics manufacturers proudly boast that their products can penetrate the stratum corneum – a credible, scientific-sounding phrase that rolls easily off the tongue. Fortunately, you have three more protective layers of skin cells to prevent these chemicals from reaching your living skin cells.

MAINTAINING HEALTHY SKIN

The condition of your skin depends on many factors. Poor diet, illness, and age can all contribute to the loss of collagen from your skin, reducing its elasticity and forming fine lines and wrinkles. This process is accelerated by smoking and by the dehydrating effects of alcohol and of ultraviolet radiation from the sun and sunbeds. Drugs such as heroin, cocaine, marijuana, and hashish, and some prescription drugs can cause loss of skin color and tone, and cause premature aging.

A healthy diet containing fresh fruit and vegetables should provide an adequate intake of proteins, minerals, and vitamins A, B, and C – all of which are essential for healthy skin. Rapid dieting can rob your skin of these essential nutrients and an inadequate intake of liquid (i.e., water) can dehydrate your skin. Lack of exercise will lead to deterioration in muscle condition, directly affecting the tone and firmness of your skin. Stress, tension, and tiredness caused by inadequate sleep, will all take their toll on your skin.

Old Wives' Tales – Herbal Skin Care

Comfrey leaves, feverfew, mint, nettle, and rose petal infusion (rose water) are all said to be good for the skin.

Borage leaves, camomile, elder, fennel leaf infusion, marigold leaves, and marshmallow are all claimed to soften and smooth rough skin.

Elder, lovage, and parsley are said to lighten the color of skin, and remove freckles and minor skin blemishes.

There is no evidence that these herbal treatments work, but then again, there is no evidence that they don't either! Try them but be careful – parsley and camomile can both cause contact allergies and dermatitis. The active ingredient in camomile is Bisabolol, which is often added to cosmetics. It also causes contact allergies and dermatitis.

Hormone changes probably have the most instantly noticeable effect on skin. We all remember the appearance of adolescent spots, zits, and greasy skin during puberty, and changes in skin condition often accompany menstruation, pregnancy, menopause and, sometimes, the use of HRT (hormone replacement therapy) or the contraceptive pill.

It is important to look after your skin by keeping it clean and, if you have dry skin that becomes cracked and sore, by using a suitable moisturizer. A large majority of women use moisturizers regularly and often seek out the more prestigious brands that claim to be hypoallergenic or to keep your skin looking firm and young. It must be said, however, that too much reliance is placed on the wild claims made by cosmetics' manufacturers, and a vast amount of money is wasted on expensive gimmicks containing liposomes, vitamins, and collagen. Many of these products are no better than basic moisturizing creams or lotions that contain just oils and water. Whatever you use, it is important you find one that suits your skin and that you avoid anything that causes even minor irritation. "No pain, no gain" is utter nonsense when it comes to looking after your skin.

Some skin-care products contain keratolytic chemicals that dissolve the outer, horny layer, and sometimes the deeper layers. Manufacturers claim that this revitalizes your skin, or reveals fresher, younger skin – dissolving away fine lines and wrinkles. These chemicals can cause severe skin irritation and can encourage your skin to thicken, locking you into a cycle of using these skin-peeling cosmetics. Hair removal creams and lotions also contain corrosive chemicals that can leave skin irritated and sore, and they have even been reported to cause deep burns, leaving permanent scars.

SKIN TYPES

During the course of your lifetime you are bound to experience dry skin, greasy skin and, if you are lucky, normal skin. Normal or balanced skin is fairly rare, probably reflecting our modern lifestyles of irregular or poor diet, stress, and the tendency to wear skimpier clothing which increases our exposure to the sun. In balanced skin, the epidermis has a creamy color, is fairly thick, and feels smooth and velvety to the touch. It has few irregularities, even under a magnifying glass. There is an even distribution of oil and moisture on the skin, which leaves only a trace of dampness but no grease, when the skin is blotted with dry tissue paper. This skin type becomes drier as it becomes older.

Dry skin is by far the most common skin type, and 80 percent of women will experience dry skin problems at some time in their lives. It is more common in fair-skinned people and fairly rare in dark-skinned races. Dry skin is characterized by a lack of sebum, the skin's natural oil, affecting the skin on the face and hands, and sometimes on other parts of the body, in several ways. The epidermis is often thin and transparent in places, allowing blood vessels to show through. It is usually sensitive, may bruise easily, and often appears powdery or scaly. Dry skin is prone to fine lines in the corners of the eyes and mouth, and to premature wrinkles. Evidence of open pores may be seen under a magnifying glass but no trace of oil or moisture appears on tissue paper used to blot the skin. Oily moisturizing creams may improve the feel of dry skin and make it less sensitive to the wind and weather. Since the sun has a tendency to make dry skin even drier, it is recommended that you use a good quality sunscreen with a suitable SPF (Sun Protection Factor) for your skin type (see *Chapter 14 – Sun and Skin*) whenever you expose your skin to the sun. Many face creams these days contain sunscreens. People with dry skin often have dry hair.

Greasy skin is more common in dark-skinned people and often appears thick and coarse, with an uneven texture caused by larger than average pores. The excessive secretions of sebum often gives the skin a shiny appearance and make it prone to pimples, blackheads, and acne. The excess grease also tends to pick up dust and dirt. When blotted with a dry tissue, obvious grease marks can be seen. Some greasy skin repels make-up, causing it, literally, to slide off. Greasy skin is more tolerant to the effects of the sun and less prone to fine lines and wrinkles, and so looks younger for much longer. It becomes dryer with age. Since the grease can trap dirt and bacteria in the pores, it is important to use a good cleansing agent such as soap and water and, if necessary, to use moisturizing milks rather than greasy moisturizing creams. Some people with greasy skin do not use any moisturizers as nature seems to be providing it for them. People with greasy skin tend to have greasy hair.

People with combination skin have a triangle of greasy skin encompassing their forehead, cheekbones, nose, mouth, and chin, with dry skin on the sides of their face and other parts of the body. Their hair can be dry or greasy.

Dark-skinned races often have greasy skin with a shiny appearance and a smooth or velvety feel, and some individuals are prone to pimples, pustules, or acne. The epidermis is usually thicker than in fair-skinned races and the outer, horny layer sheds more easily. In fair-skinned races the sebaceous glands are generally smaller and most of them empty into hair follicles, but on dark skin, up to 10 percent of the sebaceous glands open directly onto the surface of the skin, making their appearance more obvious. In the absence of strong, tropical sunlight, dark skin tends to stay younger looking for much longer than fair skin. Minor discoloration and skin blemishes are also less obvious on dark skin.

SKIN COLOR

Skin gets its color from melanin – a brown pigment that is made in the melanocytes found in the lower layers of the epidermis; from carotene – the natural yellow pigment of the skin cells; and from the color of blood in tiny blood vessels called capillaries, just below the skin's surface.

Our skin color is inherited from our parents and is determined by a set of genes that control the amount of melanin in our skin. Albinism is a genetic disorder in which melanin production is reduced or absent altogether. Since melanin is also found in hair and eyes, albinos often have light or white skin and hair, and pale or pink eyes. It is a rare condition and affects all races but is most common in the Ibo people of Nigeria.

A melanocyte looks a little like an octopus, with its head in the basal cell layer and its tentacles reaching up into the epidermis. Under the influence of a hormone called melanocyte-stimulating hormone (MSH), the melanocytes produce melanin. The tentacles distribute grains, called melanosomes containing the melanin, into the higher layers of the epidermis. Inside the melanocytes, melanin is formed when an amino acid called tyrosine, is oxidized. This oxidation is often caused by ultraviolet light or by an enzyme called tyrosinase. The main function of the melanin is to absorb harmful ultraviolet rays before they reach the deeper layers of living skin cells.

It's a Fact

Hydroquinone lightens the color of skin by reducing melanin production by inhibiting tyrosianse. Some dark-skinned people use it to bleach their skin in order to disguise their racial origins. This practice is not recommended. Hydroquinone is now banned from skin-lightening products sold in the EU.

Both dark and light-skinned races seem to contain the same number of melanocytes in their basal layer of skin cells but light-skinned people have an enzyme that breaks down the melanin shortly after it is produced, and so very little melanin reaches the outer layer of skin. Ultraviolet rays stimulate the melanocytes to produce extra melanin, resulting in a suntan. If you are one of those people who find it hard to get a tan, you have an efficient enzyme system that breaks down the melanin as rapidly as it is formed.

Melanocyte-stimulating hormone is produced in the pituitary gland. Changes in the levels of this hormone, possibly as a result of injury, illness, or the use of some drugs, can cause changes in the color of skin. Hence we hear horror stories of dark-skinned individuals who have become pale, and have little natural protection from the sun, or white people who become dark skinned.

Blood vessels close to the surface of the skin can give it a red or a blue tint. If we are hot or flushed, the blood vessels become larger and a greater volume of blood flows to the skin, giving it a pink or red hue. On cold days the blood vessels become narrower, slowing down the blood flow. The blood loses its oxygen and picks up carbon dioxide. This deoxygenated blood has a blue or purple color and is not carried away quickly, so our skin may acquire a blue tint. These color changes are more noticeable in light-skinned people.

A number of harmless skin disorders may cause dark or light patches to form on the skin. These can be disguised with make-up, but if the condition worsens, or you have any other symptoms such as reddening or irritation, you should consult your doctor.

AGING SKIN

Every living thing goes through the process of aging. In humans we notice the gradual loss of hair and hair color, the increasing appearance of wrinkles accompanied by a loss of elasticity of the skin, a reduction in muscle tone, and the deterioration in hearing, eyesight, and mental faculties. There have been many theories as to why we age, such as the build-up of toxins in our bodies over the years, the gradual erosion of our tissues by wear and tear and illnesses, and the steady decline in our immune system's ability to fight disease. We now know that aging happens at the cellular level. Inside each cell is a nucleus which contains chromosomes. These are made of long strands of DNA (deoxyribonucleic acid), which are giant molecules that carry the plans for building a new cell to repair or replace tissue, or to allow an individual to grow. The DNA starts this process by making a copy of itself within the cell. When the copy is complete there are two sets of chromosomes which move to opposite sides of the cell. The cell slowly oozes apart, splitting into two separate cells, each with its own set of chromosomes. These two new cells grow and divide again, becoming four cells, and so on as this process is repeated. Once we are fully grown, the cell division slows down, making just enough new cells to replace those that die from time to time, or to replace cells that have been damaged.

Until recently we believed DNA made exact copies of itself, but this is not in fact the case. The new DNA molecules are built on top of the old strands rather like each layer of a house of cards is built on top of the layer below. The house of cards naturally forms a pyramid shape because each layer is slightly shorter than the layer beneath it. They cannot be the same length because there is nothing to support the cards at either end.

It is the same for DNA molecules. When the new molecule is built on top of the old strand, it is a fraction shorter because the ends cannot be supported. So each new generation of DNA is slightly shorter than the previous generation. Luckily, these ends, called telomers, are redundant and do not carry important genetic information so the new cells are fully functional in all respects. Eventually, however, after about a hundred divisions, the redundant telomer ends of the DNA strands become so short they vanish altogether. The next generation which is shorter still means some of the important genetic information at the end of the strand is now missing.

The new cell is faulty and the aging process begins. Fewer skin cells are produced and the outer layer of skin becomes thin and easily damaged, leading to bruising and discoloration. The living cells in the dermis layer produce less collagen fibers – the protein that gives younger skin its elasticity. The quality of hair cells deteriorate, compromising the color, texture, and quantity of our hair. In short, we start to look old.

Life span, grey hair, baldness, and wrinkles run in families. They are inherited from our parents along with the DNA that controls them. Currently there are no drugs or cosmetic chemicals that can correct the faulty DNA and halt the aging process. The best that cosmetics can do for you is to hide the grey with hair dyes and smooth over the fine lines and wrinkles with creams and make-up.

Wrinkles

Fine lines are the first sign of aging skin, usually appearing around the eyes first, then the corners of the mouth. As you age the fine lines become larger and deeper, and turn into wrinkles.

The dermis (the deeper, living layers of skin cells) contains fibers of collagen, a tough, flexible protein, that gives skin its elasticity. Older skin contains fewer collagen fibers in the dermis. If you pinch some skin on the forearm of a young person, it springs back into place as soon it is released. This is because the large number of collagen fibers present in young skin make it very elastic. The same experiment conducted on an elderly person will result in the pinched skin standing up for a few seconds after it is released, only slowly returning to its original position.

Observations of identical twins have demonstrated conclusively that exposure to UV rays and smoking both cause premature loss of collagen from the dermis. Fine lines and wrinkles also run in families, hence the old adage, if you look at your mother-in-law, you can see your wife in 40 years time. (Of course this makes no allowance for the fact that your wife may inherit her father's collagen levels, rather than her mother's.)

Cosmetics cannot permanently remove fine lines and wrinkles. The best they can do is cover them up or moisten and color the skin to make it look younger. Exfoliants can temporarily give skin a younger appearance, but regular use of these so-called skin peelers is not recommended. Retinoic acid can improve the skin's elasticity but this is a potent drug with some serious side effects, and you will not find any cosmetics sold legally in the EU or the USA that contain this ingredient.

Cosmetic surgery is the only certain way to remove fine lines and wrinkles but this is expensive and only lasts between five and ten years. Collagen replacement therapy (CRT) can reduce the appearance of fine lines and wrinkles. Improvements are noticeable immediately and last between two and six months before top-up treatments are required. (See *Chapter 16 – Salons and Surgeons* for more details of CRT and other procedures.)

TAKING CARE OF YOUR SKIN

Now that we know what skin is and why it ages, we can look at the multitude of creams and lotions that promise to keep us looking young and fresh. Cosmetics' manufacturers have coerced us into believing that we all need to use their products all the time by constantly reminding us with drip-feed advertising lines such as "Now contains added moisturizers," or "Refreshes and moisturizes tired skin," or even "New improved formula now contains 65 percent moisturizers." Skin is not healthy unless it is moisturized and we cannot survive without these products – or can we? We have been making our own, natural moisturizers for the last six million years or so. Many people have perfectly healthy skin that needs little more care than keeping it clean and protecting it from too much sun and harsh weather. Try it – see what happens.

Emollients and Moisturizing Creams

These are probably the most basic skin-care products we have, and the benefits of these simple preparations to those who need them should not be underestimated.

Emollients are applied to the skin or mucous membranes to prevent evaporation of water. This has the effect of moisturizing the outer layer of skin cells, making them swell as they absorb water from deeper layers of the skin. This makes the skin feel softer and smoother, and it makes dry or cracked skin more flexible, alleviating any pain or soreness. The appearance of fine lines may also be temporarily reduced. The effects last for six to twelve hours before the cells dry out and shrink again.

Emollients work by forming a thin layer of oil or grease on your skin, trapping water beneath it and acting as a barrier to water vapor, preventing the loss of water by evaporation. Any non-irritating oil will have this effect and cosmetic manufacturers have over a thousand ingredients to choose from, ranging from lanolin (the oily secretions of sheep), to vegetable and petroleum-based oils, and even synthetic silicone oils similar to your furniture polish. The simplest moisturizing substance you can use is petroleum jelly, a purified grease made from crude oil, or a simple vegetable oil such as coconut or olive oil. The problem with these simple emollients, however, is they can block pores and hair follicles, trapping dirt and bacteria that can encourage blackheads and acne.

Emollients do not add moisture to the skin: they simply prevent moisture from being lost. Moisturizing creams include water in the formulation to accelerate the hydration of the dry, outer layer of skin cells.

It's a Fact

If you want to find out how much water your moisturizing cream contains, leave it in the car one frosty night. If it freezes the emulsion will break down and next day it will be a watery mess.

A typical moisturizing cream or lotion will probably be a simple emulsion of an oil and water. This will consist of an oil or grease such as mineral oil (liquid paraffin), vegetable oil, or lanolin, mixed with water and held together with an emulsifier. The product may also include emulsion stabilizers to improve its shelf life, a surfactant (cleaning substance), and a film former to help it spread evenly and remain in place, with colors and fragrances to improve its overall appearance. At least two preservatives are likely to be used, one that is soluble in water and one that is soluble in oil, so that the whole mixture is protected. In an emulsion, the oil is exposed to considerable amounts of oxygen, so an antioxidant may be added to prevent the oil from becoming rancid. Since there is a danger that bacteria may become trapped under the oily layer formed on your skin by the moisturizing cream, an antimicrobial agent may also be included. As the main ingredients – water and oil – are both transparent, the product is likely to have an insipid or weak appearance. Opacifiers will remove the watery appearance and a colorant (like titanium dioxide), will give it a rich, creamy texture. Finally, trivial ingredients such as vitamins, proteins, and UV absorbers may be added for marketing reasons.

TYPICAL INGREDIENTS — NATURAL COLLECTION LIGHT BODY LOTION

Ingredients:

Aqua, Prunis dulcis, Cocos nucifera, Theobroma cacao, Glycerin, Sorbitan Isostearate, Polysorbate 60, Parfum, Triethanolamine, Phenoxyethanol, Carbomer, Methylparaben, Butylparaben, Cetrimonium Bromide.

Aqua	Water – the main ingredient. This adds moisture directly to the skin.
Prunis dulcis**	Sweet almond oil. An oily layer on the skin acts as a barrier to evaporation, thus retaining moisture in the skin.
Cocos nucifera*	Coconut oil. (As above.)
Theobroma cacao*	Cocoa butter. (As above.)
Glycerin*	Humectant. Absorbs water and holds it near the skin, thus preventing further moisture loss.
Sorbitan Isostearate	Synthetic emulsifier to aid the mixing of the oils and water.
Polysorbate 60*	Synthetic emulsifier and surfactant to aid the mixing of the oils and water and to aid even spreading.
Parfum	A mixture of synthetic and natural fragrance chemicals.
Triethanolamine*	Used to control acidity in the product. Restricted to a maximum of 2.5 percent if used in a non-rinse off product such as this.
Phenoxyethanol*	Preservative restricted to a maximum of 1 percent.[+]
Carbomer	Synthetic crosslinked polymer used as a thickening agent.
Methylparaben*	Water-soluble preservative of the benzoate family, restricted to a maximum of 0.4 percent.[+]
Butylparaben*	Oil-soluble preservative of the benzoate family, restricted to a maximum of 0.4 percent.[+]
Cetrimonium Bromide*	Preservative restricted to a maximum of 0.1 percent.[+]

* These ingredients are subject to restrictions or have been linked to harmful or adverse effects.

** People who are allergic to almonds are advised to carry out a patch test before using cosmetics containing sweet almond oil.

+ Indicates that this ingredient may be used in larger quantities if it is used for another specific purpose other than as a preservative.

Moisturizing cream is a water-in-oil emulsion that contains a little water dispersed in oil. It is usually between 70 and 80 percent oil. It is usually applied to the face at night, leaving a continuous oily film which prevents evaporation for several hours, giving the skin plenty of time to hydrate. Moisturizing cream may also be applied before going out in harsh weather conditions. People with greasy skin may prefer to use a moisturizing milk or lotion. These are thinner, oil-in-water emulsions that contain a little oil (20 to 30 percent) dispersed in water.

Hand creams are oil-in-water emulsions that contain non-greasy waxes dissolved in the oily part of the emulsion. They do not leave an oily feeling on your hands and do not leave greasy fingerprints on everything you touch. Barrier creams leave a heavy layer of grease or wax on your hands. They are designed to prevent loss of your natural skin oils when you use strong detergents or other chemicals.

EXFOLIANTS

Exfoliants, also commonly called exfolients, exfoliators, exfoliating agents, or skin peelers, are chemicals that soften or dissolve the outer layer of dead skin cells – the horny or keratinized layer, or "stratum corneum" – allowing this layer to be removed. The belief is that fine lines and wrinkles will be removed along with the outer layer of skin cells. In fact, exfoliants may slightly improve the appearance of fine lines, help to remove discolored or flaking skin, and reduce the incidence of blackheads.

Ingredients such as salicylic acid, alpha- and beta-hydroxy acids, phenols, trichloroacetic acid (TCA), and glycolic acid are potent exfoliants. They have been known to cause severe skin damage when used in concentrations higher than recommended, left on the skin for longer than recommended, or used on parts of the body where the skin is thin. Some people are particularly sensitive to these ingredients and suffer adverse effects despite using them correctly. Because of the potential hazards, you should always be aware of when you are using exfoliating ingredients – and you may be unwittingly using them in cosmetics you use every day such as cleansing lotions or moisturizing creams. Beware such products that claim to renew skin, reveal fresher or younger-looking skin, or dissolve away fine lines or wrinkles.

Abrasive pads and bars of soap containing bran or oatmeal, are also used to exfoliate skin.

Alpha-Hydroxy Acids (AHAs) and Beta-Hydroxy Acids (BHAs)

Alpha- and beta-hydroxy acids are relatively new on the cosmetics scene and are an advertisers dream since the name rolls easily off the tongue and has the ring of frontier technology about it. They are commonly found in fruits or are derived from fruit or milk sugars and are milder forms of the exfoliants used by cosmetic surgeons to remove old and wrinkled skin. Words like "revitalizing," "softening," and "smoothing" are used to encourage you to buy these products, which take the form of cleansing lotions, moisturizing creams, skin conditioners, and even shampoos.

Because the epidermis acts as a waterproof barrier to keep out chemicals and some damaging ultraviolet rays (protecting the more sensitive, living cells deeper in the skin), this layer is less elastic than the deeper, living layers making lines and wrinkles more noticeable. Peeling off this layer can temporarily reduce these natural signs of aging and wear and tear, however, the skin's natural reaction to damage is to produce thicker, tougher skin. This is why manual workers grow calluses on their hands, and hikers and joggers produce thick calluses on their feet. The common reaction to this new, tougher skin is to use more of the exfoliant. Soon you are locked into a cycle of growing new skin and peeling it off.

Alpha- and Beta-Hydroxy Acids

You can easily identify alpha- and beta-hydroxy acids in the list of ingredients under the following names:

Alpha-hydroxy acids – lactic acid, mixed fruit acid, triple fruit acid, tri-alpha hydroxy fruit acids, sugar cane extract, glycolic acid, ammonium glycolate, alpha-hydroxyethanoic acid, ammonium alpha-hydroxyethanoate, alpha-hydroxyoctanoic acid, alpha-hydroxycaprylic acid, hydroxycaprylic acid, alpha hydroxy, and botanical complex and glycomer in crosslinked fatty acids alpha natrium.

Beta-hydroxy acids – salicylic acid, tropic acid, trethocanic acid, and beta-hydroxybutanoic acid.

Both alpha- and beta-hydroxy acids – citric acid and malic acid.

Are AHAs Safe?

AHAs have only been around for about 10 years and the effects of long-term exposure are unknown. The US Food and Drug Administration (FDA) estimate that there have been over 10,000 reports of adverse reactions to cosmetics containing AHAs and BHAs. The symptoms described include itching, burning sensations, severe reddening of the skin, rashes, swelling, blistering and bleeding. They can also lead to exfoliative dermatitis. Without the protection of the outer layer of skin there is a greater sensitivity to sunlight, resulting in sunburn, photoaging (the premature aging of the skin caused by exposure to sun), and an increased risk of sun-related skin cancers. If you experience any of these symptoms, stop using the offending cosmetic immediately.

If you regularly use these cosmetics you should always use a sunscreen with a sun protection factor (SPF) of 15 or higher before exposing your skin to direct sunlight. And don't let children use or play with potent cosmetics such as these. Their skin is much thinner than that of adults and they cannot afford to lose any of its vital protection. To emphasize the potential dangers, one widely used exfoliant, salicylic acid, is banned in the EU from toiletries intended for use by children under the age of three, with the exception of shampoo. Currently, several commonly used exfoliants have not appeared yet on the EU Commission's list of cosmetic ingredients; hence, there are no laws specifically regulating the use of these chemicals in the EU apart from the general law that says a product can only be sold if it is "safe."

In 1997, the Cosmetic Ingredient Review Panel (CIRP), the American cosmetic industry's self-regulatory body for addressing the safety of cosmetic ingredients, concluded that potent AHAs such as lactic acid and glycolic acid, should not exceed 10 percent of the finished product, and the acidity level of the product should not be lower (i.e., more acidic) than pH 3.5. They also recommended the finished product should contain UV absorbers to protect the skin from the harmful effects of ultraviolet radiation. These are only recommendations and have no standing in law. There are some products used in salons that are up to three times stronger than the recommended levels. The CIRP declared them to be safe, providing they are left on the skin for a short time only, then thoroughly rinsed off soon after application, followed by daily use of a good quality sunscreen. Cosmetic surgeons use even stronger acid solutions, containing about 70 percent of trichloroacetic acid (TCA) to achieve deep skin peels. These treatments sometimes cause burns similar to sunburn or discoloration of the skin.

In June 1999, a meeting of top skin specialists concluded that most cosmetics would not live up to the manufactures' claims and remove wrinkles. In fact there is only one controlled drug that can do this – retinoic acid, which has some very undesirable side effects and is banned from cosmetics in both the EU and the USA. Their advice to beat wrinkles is simple. Don't smoke, keep out of the sun, and choose your parents well since fine lines and wrinkles are inherited, along with the rest of your skin.

Anti-aging Creams Do Not Work!

On October 18, 2000, founder and co-chairman of The Body Shop, Anita Roddick, confessed at the Cheltenham Literature Festival that many cosmetics are useless. The following day she repeated her comments on British national television and in the press. She said that moisturizers work, but all other lotions are pap. "There is nothing on God's planet, not one thing, that will take away 30 years of arguing with your husband and 40 years of environmental abuse. Anything that says it can magically take away your wrinkles is a scandalous lie." She added, "In Tahiti the women have skin like velvet and they simply take a lump of lard and rub it into their bodies."

Why would someone who has 1,754 outlets around the world with an annual turnover of $300 million (£200 million) and an estimated personal fortune of $220 million (£150 million) from the sale of her cosmetics, make such a statement – unless she believes it is true!

ASTRINGENTS

Astringents close the pores of the skin, improving its tone and texture, making it feel firmer. They work by reducing the water content of skin cells and can aid the healing of broken or inflamed skin. They can also be used to reduce tear production by inflamed or infected eyes. They frequently sting when applied to recently shaved, exfoliated, sore, or broken skin. Antiperspirants, aftershave lotions, and skin-toning lotions often contain astringents.

Commonly used astringents include sodium chloride (salt), alcohol, aluminum compounds, and some plant extracts such as horsetail and witch hazel. They are used in aftershave lotions to close the pores that have been opened by the shaving lubricant and hot water, producing a smoother-feeling chin. After using a cleansing lotion, which opens the pores to aid cleaning, an astringent should be applied to close them again before other make-up, such as foundation, is applied. This prevents the foundation from becoming trapped in the pores.

Old Wives' Tales – Herbal Astringents

Lemon balm, lavender infusion, mint, rosemary, yarrow, horsetail, nettle, red raspberry leaves, walnut leaves, sage, and witch hazel are all herbs that are said to tone and smooth the skin. Try them; some of them may work, but be careful – witch hazel, rosemary, and lavender have all been linked to allergies and dermatitis, and rosemary and lavender also cause photo-sensitivity.

HAIR REMOVAL

Current fashions and scant clothing designs dictate that body hair is unwanted and must go. Millions of women and a rapidly growing number of men, spend a vast amount of money on products and services to remove hair from places where we no longer want it to be seen. There are several ways to do this. Physical methods include shaving or plucking the hairs. Chemical methods involve the application of strongly alkaline creams called depilatories, which dissolve the unwanted hair at the surface of the skin. These methods are temporary solutions and the hair soon reappears at its normal rate of growth. Electrolysis using needle or tweezer epilators, can permanently remove unwanted body hair, and in 1995, the FDA approved the first laser technique for the permanent removal of unwanted body hair. (See *Chapter 16 – Salons and Surgeons* for details of electrolysis using needle and tweezer epilators, and laser techniques for permanent hair removal.)

Shaving

Shaving remains the most popular method of hair removal for both women and men. Electric razors and wet shaving methods are both widely used by men and women alike. Wet methods involve the application of surfactants to lubricate the skin and soften the hairs, which can then be cut off at the surface of the skin using a sharp blade, or multiple blades, encased in a safety razor. There is some risk of cutting the skin and the surface layer of skin is sometimes removed by the razor, resulting in some discomfort and soreness. Occasionally the shaving foams, gels, or lubricants cause soreness or irritation. Removal of the outer layer of skin cells by the razor allows chemicals in the shaving lubricant to penetrate further into the skin, causing greater irritation. Removal of this layer during wet shaving also removes artificial sun tans.

Electric razors have a thin mesh or a foil, behind which there are rapidly spinning blades. When an electric razor is drawn across the skin, the hairs go through the holes in the mesh and are cut off by the rotating blades. Electric razors can be used on either dry or moistened hair. There is no risk of cutting the skin but, when the blades become blunt, they tug at the hairs and cause discomfort. Wet shaving, especially with a twin blade razor, gives a much closer shave than an electric razor because the hairs are cut off at, or just below the surface of the skin. Since electric razors only cut off the hairs that protrude through the thin mesh, they always leave a short stump of the hair shaft, the length of which matches the thickness of the foil.

Shaving Formulations (Soap, Gel, Foam, and Cream)

Wet shaving involves sliding a sharp blade across the skin, cutting off unwanted hairs that protrude through the skin. The process is made more comfortable and efficient if the hair shafts are softened with water, and a lubricant is applied to the skin to prevent the blade from snagging and cutting the skin.

The thick hair shafts of men's facial hair take between three and five minutes to become fully hydrated and softened. To achieve this, the shaving formulation must produce a watery film that remains on the hairs long enough for the water to soak into the hair shafts. Shaving soap achieves this by forming a tight lather that consists of minute bubbles. Pressurized shaving foam dispensers produce a similar tight lather. Using hot water will speed up the hydration process.

Since large soap molecules are required to make a tight lather, shaving soap often contains sodium stearate and potassium stearate. It is common to find these mixed with a variety of other soaps including tallowates, palm kernelates, and cocoates of sodium and potassium. Fatty acids may be added to promote foaming, and glycerin to prevent it drying too quickly. The soaps double up as a lubricant. The main ingredient in pressurized shaving foams is water, followed by various mixtures of soapy and non-soap detergents, foam boosters such as cocamide DEA, fatty alcohols, oils, emulsifiers, and emulsion stabilizers. Shaving cream is an oil-in-water emulsion containing fatty acids such as stearic acid, emulsifiers, emulsion stabilizers, and a humectant such as sorbitol or glycerin to keep it moist. The oil is the lubricant while the water hydrates the hair. Shaving gels are essentially oil free. They consist mostly of water and contain thickeners, film formers, and humectants. They may also contain surfactants to hasten the wetting process. All of these products contain the usual range of colorants, fragrances, and preservatives.

If, like many people, you shave off unwanted body hair while in the bath or shower, you probably do not need a shaving formulation. The bath or shower water will hydrate and soften the hairs, so all that is required is a lubricant. A film of soapy water or diluted shower gel will do this job perfectly well.

Depilatory Agents

Depilatory chemicals are applied to the skin in the form of creams, lotions, gels, aerosols, or roll-ons. They remove unwanted body hair by dissolving the protein structure of the hair, thus weakening it and allowing it to be rubbed away at skin level. They work at the surface of the skin and do not affect the hair root, so the hair will reappear in two to three weeks' time. Metal sulfides and thioglycolates are the most common depilatories. They are often alkaline and the chemicals are quite toxic, so great care should be taken when using them and they should be kept out of reach of children.

Your hair and skin are made of the same protein – keratin. Any product designed to dissolve the protein in hair can also attack your skin causing soreness, irritation, or more severe inflammation. In severe cases they have been known to cause second-degree burns, or worse. Always test a small area first and never use these products on hair near the eyes or on sensitive parts of the body, or on hairs growing close to mucous membranes, such as the genitals or nose hairs. You should not use depilatories immediately after a hot bath, shower, or sauna. Heat increases the blood flow to your skin and opens your pores, increasing the risk of absorbing the chemicals deeper into the skin, where they are not easily rinsed off.

Depilatories should be in contact with your skin for the shortest possible time and should never be used on broken or damaged skin. Fine hair should be loosened in four to five minutes while coarse hair may take up to 15 minutes. Longer exposure times will increase the risk of skin damage.

Pulling Out the Hairs

Both tweezing and waxing literally tear the hairs out of the skin. This can be painful and result in sore or irritated skin, which may leave it open to infection. Tweezing involves the painstaking plucking of each individual hair using forceps (tweezers). Waxing involves the application of melted or softened wax, which then hardens around the hairs. When the hardened wax is pulled away from the skin the hairs are pulled out with it. Adhesive tape, or cold wax tapes, can be used in place of hot wax. Great care should be taken not to burn yourself with wax that is too hot.

Whether waxing or tweezing, the papilla at the base of the hair root is not usually removed and the hairs return at their normal rate of growth. It will take about a week for the new hair to reach the top of the follicle and appear through the skin. Some people claim that repeated tweezing or waxing will eventually stop the hairs from regrowing.

Waxes are usually petroleum based or natural waxes, such as beeswax, mixed with resins to make them stick to the skin and hair shafts. They should not be used on sore, irritated, sunburnt, or broken skin and they must not be used where there are moles, warts, or varicose veins. They can be used on most parts of the body but they are not recommended for use on the nipples, genitals or eyelashes and they should not be used to remove nose hair or hair growing from the ear canal. Some labels discourage diabetics and people with heart conditions or circulatory disorders from using hot waxes.

As an alternative to hair removal on large areas such the forearms and legs, the appearance of body hair can be reduced by lightening or bleaching the color using a mixture of hydrogen peroxide and dilute ammonia.

6 soaps, shower gels, and cleansing lotions

Soap and education are not as sudden as a massacre but they are more deadly in the long run.

Mark Twain

Keeping clean is very important. This chapter reviews the multitude of toiletries that are designed to help us do this. We start by looking at what soaps and detergents are and how they remove dirt and grime. We then look at some specific cleansing products and consider their relative advantages and disadvantages.

A POTTED HISTORY OF SOAP

The earliest mention of soap in literature dates back to the early 11th century and refers to Savona in Italy, a town that both manufactured and gave its name to soap. It was a small industry supplying soap to a few wealthy individuals, most people making their own at home by boiling animal fats with alkalis made from ashes or from the barilla plant.

In 1787 a method for making soda from salt was discovered but it was not until the Industrial Revolution, when alkalis were manufactured cheaply and on a grand scale, that the soap manufacturing industry took off. The Industrial Revolution in Britain gave rise to increased wages and wealth, and generally to higher standards of living for the population as a whole. The industrial smoke, dirt, and grime which accompanied the growth of factories also made soap a necessity rather than a luxury.

For this reason, in 1853 the Prime Minister, William Gladstone, abolished the excise duty on soap, making it cheaper and more widely used. In the following 50 years, the annual consumption of soap in the UK rose from 90,000 tons to 300,000 tons.

The soap industry became so successful that, between 1900 and 1910 there was a world shortage of animal fat, necessitating a search for new sources of fats and oils. Vegetable oils, especially those from tropical and Mediterranean climates, were previously not used because they produced soaps that were too soft, but advances in technology, especially in the hardening of fats and oils by hydrogenation, meant that these abundant raw materials could be exploited. By the 1950s, detergents too were being manufactured on a large scale from mineral oils obtained from petroleum, opening up the range of ingredients available to the cosmetics and toiletries industry. Today, we can buy bars of soap, bars of detergent, and bars that contain detergents combined with soap.

HOW SOAP IS MADE

All soaps are made by boiling animal or vegetable fats or oils with a strong alkali such as sodium hydroxide (caustic soda) or, less commonly, potassium hydroxide (caustic potash). Fats and oils are composed of glyceryl esters. Any natural fat or oil such as olive oil, contains a mixture of different glyceryl esters. Each molecule of the glyceryl ester is made of one, two, or three fatty acid molecules attached to a molecule of glycerin. When the fats are boiled with strong alkalis, a chemical reaction called saponification (or hydrolysis) takes place in which the fatty acids are separated from the glycerin. Since the fatty acids are liberated into a solution containing a strong alkali, the acids are immediately neutralized by the alkali, forming the sodium (or potassium) salt of the fatty acid, and it is these salts that are the main ingredient in soap.

When the boiling process is complete, the mixture is cooled and common salt is added to "salt out" the soap. The salt causes the soap to become less soluble and it settles out as a white or creamy colored solid. Most of the glycerin is removed and used elsewhere in the cosmetics or food industry. If too much glycerin is left in the soap, it holds onto excessive amounts of water and prevent the soap from hardening, causing the soap to become soft and mushy during use and the bar disappears quickly.

All of the alkali used during manufacture must be carefully removed by rinsing the soap with clean water and by adding controlled amounts of fatty acids, or other acids to neutralize it.

When the correct water, alkali, and glycerin content is achieved, other ingredients are added. Soap has a naturally unpleasant odor, so even unscented soaps contain some fragrance chemicals to disguise this. Colorants are added to improve the appearance and a chelating agent (usually tetrasodium EDTA or pentasodium pentetate), is added to prevent the calcium ions in tap water from reacting with the soap and reducing its cleaning properties. Tetrasodium etidronate is the most commonly used preservative in bars of toilet soap. Since soap usually forms a strong lather, foam boosters are seldom added.

Other ingredients that find their way into soap are deodorants, moisturizing oils, antimicrobials, mild abrasives such as bran or oatmeal, and a range of plant extracts and oils to satisfy the consumer's desire for natural ingredients. Deodorant soap may simply contain strong fragrances, or it may contain antimicrobial ingredients that reduce the growth rate of microbes on the body. Antimicrobials are also added to antiseptic and antibacterial soaps that are useful if you work in an area where infection is a risk, for example if you work with animals or in a hospital, or if you are visiting tropical countries which have hot, humid, climates. A range of oils and emulsifiers are used to reduce the drying effect that soap has on your skin, but these are generally not needed if you have naturally greasy skin.

IS SOAP A COSMETIC?

In the EU all bars of soap are regulated under the EU Cosmetics Directive, but in the USA, a standard bar of soap is not classed as a cosmetic and does not have to carry a list of ingredients on the label. If, however, the manufacturer makes a cosmetic or medicinal claim about their soap (for example, they may state that the soap is a deodorant soap, reduces dandruff or acne, moisturizes your skin, or makes you more beautiful in some way), it is classed as a drug and all of the ingredients must be shown on the label, with the active ingredients listed separately, before the other ingredients.

If a standard bar of soap in the USA had to carry a list of ingredients, it might read something like this: Sodium tallowate, Sodium palm kernelate, Water, Glycerin,

Sodium chloride, Sodium stearate, Disodium phosphate (to control the pH/acidity level of the soap), Fragrance, Tetrasodium EDTA, Tetrasodium etidronate, Colors listed as FD&C or D&C numbers.

TYPICAL INGREDIENTS – TOILET SOAP

Ingredients:

Sodium Tallowate, Sodium Palm Kernelate, Aqua, Parfum, Stearic Acid, Glycerin, Sodium Chloride, Tetrasodium EDTA, Tetrasodium Etidronate, CI 74260, CI 77891.

Sodium Tallowate	Soap – a surfactant made from animal fats.
Sodium Palm Kernelate	Soap – a surfactant made from oils extracted from palm kernels.
Aqua	Water to prevent the soap from becoming too hard and to improve its texture.
Parfum	A mixture of fragrance chemicals, often exceeding 50 in number, many of which are synthetic.
Stearic Acid	A fatty acid obtained from animal or vegetable fats. This improves the texture of the soap, removes residual alkalis used during the manufacturing process, and acts as a mild foam booster.
Glycerin*	A humectant obtained as a by-product from animal and vegetable fats during the soap-making process. Most of the glycerin produced during manufacture should be removed from the soap, otherwise, it absorbs too much water, becomes mushy, and disappears rapidly. However, there must be a small amount of glycerin present in the soap to prevent it from drying out.
Sodium Chloride	Common salt, added during the manufacturing process to aid the separation of the soap from the crude product. It also improves the soap's texture.

Tetrasodium EDTA	Chelating agent used to prevent calcium and magnesium ions present in hard water from combining with the soap and forming soap scum.
Tetrasodium Etidronate*	Preservative. This is currently the most commonly used preservative in bars of toilet soap. It is restricted to 0.2 percent when used in soap.
CI 74260*	Synthetic green dye related to chlorophyll. It is harmful to the eyes and is not allowed in any product that is intended for use on or near the eyes.
CI 77891	Titanium dioxide – a white colorant and opacifier.

* These ingredients are subject to restrictions or have been linked to harmful or adverse effects.

Sodium tallowate and sodium palm kernelate represent mixtures of soaps. Sodium tallowate is a mixture of soaps made from animal tallow, usually beef fat, and sodium palm kernelate is made from the oils extracted from palm trees. In decreasing order, beef tallow would yield mainly sodium oleate, sodium palpitate, and sodium stearate. It would also yield smaller amounts of sodium myristate and sodium linolenate. Sodium palm kernelate would consist of (again in decreasing order), sodium palmitate and sodium oleate, and to a lesser extent, sodium linolenate, sodium stearate and sodium myristate. As you can see, the lists are remarkably similar. This gives the manufacturers some flexibility in the choice of raw materials and it enables them to make soap which is free from animal products but which contains essentially the same ingredients.

HOW SAFE IS SOAP?

The track record for soap is excellent. In fact we rely on soap to remove what we would consider to be more harmful substances from our skin. All soaps hurt if you get them in your eyes, but they seldom do any real damage. Only 70 cases of soreness, irritation, itching, and redness of the skin caused by soap or detergent bars were reported to the FDA during the years 1975 to 1977. Obviously not every complaint was reported but this still works out at less than one person in a million.

If you find a particular brand of soap makes you sore or itch, or even starts your eyes watering and leaves you sneezing, it is highly likely you are reacting to the fragrance chemicals or the colorants. In this case try using an unscented soap that is white or cream in color and avoid deodorant soaps, antiseptic or antibacterial soaps, and any soap that claims to improve your skin in any way. Antibacterial soaps often contain ingredients that should not come into contact with mucous membranes, and therefore you should not use these soaps for genital hygiene unless advised to do so by your doctor – in which case a specific brand, safe for genital use, will be recommended.

Contrary to popular belief, soap on its own cannot kill bacteria. It helps to remove most of the bacteria that clings to the skin or is present in dirt on the skin, but after washing, some residual bacteria will always remain, which will not usually be a threat to your health. People working in the food industry or in hospitals routinely use antibacterial soaps which kill bacteria, but even these cannot kill all of the microbes.

DETERGENTS – AN ALTERNATIVE TO SOAP

Detergents are also called soapless or non-soap detergents. They were first made by a French chemist in 1831, who boiled castor oil with concentrated sulfuric acid and produced a liquid that was remarkably similar to soap. Several similar soapy compounds were obtained using a variety of vegetable oils and sulfuric acid, but it was not until 1916 that a completely synthetic detergent, called Nekal-A, was made from naphthalene, isopropyl alcohol and sulfuric acid – raw materials obtained from petroleum and coal tar. Other synthetic detergents were made in the years that followed but they were not sold commercially until the 1950s. These early detergents were not biodegradable and caused severe pollution in sewers and waterways. Nowadays, detergents are made from petroleum-derived chemicals and oily compounds obtained from fats and oils of animal or vegetable origin. These are biodegradable and cause little visible pollution.

Like soap, detergents are surfactants or cleaning compounds. The most common detergents are anionic detergents. These are made by reacting concentrated sulfuric acid with hydrocarbons (oily compounds) derived from petroleum, or by the action of sulfur trioxide on fatty acid alcohols from either natural fats and oils, or from petroleum. These anionic detergents are everywhere, and are used in everything from shampoo to dishwasher tablets. If a product is used to clean something, it probably contains an anionic detergent. In contrast to soaps, detergents do not make scum – a white or grey, powdery deposit formed when soap chemically reacts with the calcium or magnesium present in hard water.

Detergents often produce less lather than soaps. Lather plays no part in the cleaning process but, since it has an important role in the psychology of soaps and detergents, foam boosters are added to detergent-based toiletries to compensate for this lack of lather.

THE THEORY OF DETERGENCY, OR HOW SOAPS AND DETERGENTS WORK

A text book on the theory of detergency contains more chemical formulae than Einstein's general theory of relativity, but, in fact, it is not that complicated. Imagine you have just eaten a meal of fried chicken and French fries with a sprinkling of salt. Your plate needs to be washed. Holding it under the cold tap will knock off some of the loose fragments and remove all of the salt, but greasy patches will remain and small fragments of your meal will be embedded in the grease.

The water easily removes the salt because it is soluble in water. The grease, however, is insoluble in water and is not removed – it is water-hating and does not want to mix with it. In order to remove the grease, it must be made soluble in water by using a surfactant. Soaps and detergents all have the same basic structure. They are long molecules with two distinctly different ends, looking rather like tadpoles. The tail is rather like the grease on your plate – it is water-hating (hydrophobic). The head is more like the salt – it wants to dissolve in water (it is water-liking or hydrophilic).

When the plate is immersed in the basin with a suitable detergent, one by one, the surfactant molecules approach the greasy deposits and slide their water-hating tails into them. The water-hating greasy molecules and the water-hating surfactant tails get on very well together, and soon the greasy patch is completely covered with surfactant molecules, all buried up to their water-liking heads in grease. Now look at it from the water's point of view. It sees a blob of something that is completely covered with water-liking heads. The water does the obvious thing and tries to dissolve it. The best it can do is break it up into tiny droplets. As it does this, the surfactant molecules completely surround each droplet of grease with their water-liking heads on the surface, and then the water carries them away, leaving the plate perfectly clean. Hot water speeds up the process by making things more soluble and by melting any hardened fats, allowing the surfactants to slide their grease-loving tails into the debris of the meal more easily.

Exactly the same thing happens when you wash your hands or shampoo your hair. Any loose particles of dirt and dust will be rinsed away by the water. Water-soluble substances like salts and urea on your skin will dissolve, but sebum, your skin's natural oil, and any dust embedded in it, will need a surfactant to make it more soluble.

We say that surfactants lower the surface tension of water. This means they help the water to spread over and under the water-repellent deposits such as grease more effectively, allowing the deposits to be easily lifted away from the dirty surfaces.

As mentioned above, lather plays no part in the cleaning process. However, a lack of lather can indicate when the dish water is greasy and needs to be renewed, or that our hair is still greasy after the first wash and needs a second wash with shampoo. But lather plays no part whatsoever in the actual cleaning process.

Soaps naturally produce lots of lather. Anionic detergents, the most common type of surfactants, produce less, and non-ionic surfactants produce little, if any lather. To satisfy our psychological need for lather, foaming agents are sometimes added to toiletries.

Old Wives' Tale – Lemon Juice

It is a myth that lemon juice will cut through grease. A twist of lemon on a greasy meal may make it more palatable, but it will not play any part in the removal of grease or oils during the cleaning process. It is not a surfactant.

SHOWER GEL

Also called body shampoo or body gel, shower gel is a moderately expensive alternative to soap, and is based on a detergent, commonly sodium lauryl sulfate (SLS) or the gentler sodium laureth sulfate. The absence of soap in shower gels means that there will be no soap scum left in the bath or shower.

Shower gel contains essentially the same ingredients as shampoo (see *Chapter 9 – Hair Care*) and many brands can be used on both the body and the hair. It is usually presented as a fairly thick, clear, colored gel rather than an opaque, creamy liquid which is typical of many shampoos. Many brands of shower gel have strong fragrances and added deodorants to control body odor. Emollients are added to moisturize the skin and film formers are added to ensure even spreading and to prevent the gel from being rinsed away too rapidly. Care should be taken when using SLS-based shower gels as this ingredient has been identified as a common cause of vaginal irritation, especially in bath-foaming products.

The marketing of shower gel has a definite gender bias. Inexpensive store brands are usually family shower gels, with colors and fragrances that suit all members of the family. Some brands are definitely aimed at men, having strong colors, masculine fragrances, and boldly designed packages. They even come in larger, man-size containers. Products aimed at women are more likely to have subtle colors and fragrances, and contain a multitude of natural extracts and moisturizers which promise to improve your skin.

CLEANSING LOTIONS AND MAKE-UP REMOVERS

Cleansing lotions and make-up removers have a great deal in common, and several products advertise the fact that they can be used for both purposes. These products generally fall into three groups. Some are based on detergents and are often referred to as 'foaming' cleansers. The second main group are mainly oil-in-water emulsions that act as solvents to remove dirt and grime. The third group of products are the deep cleansing lotions used to remove dirt and blackheads that are trapped in the pores and follicles. They contain water, denatured alcohol, some detergents, and antimicrobials like triclosan.

Foaming cleansers are essentially very thick mixtures of several surfactants and water. There is a vast range of surfactants for manufacturers to choose from and almost any of them can turn up in these products, but by far the most commonly used are anionic detergents such as SLS. We came across one exception to this. In this product, the main ingredients (after water), were four different fatty acids, followed by potassium hydroxide to neutralize their acidity. This seemed strange since fatty acids react with potassium hydroxide to produce soap, and most people use foaming cleansing lotions either because they do want to use soap or because it has an adverse effect on their skin.

After the surfactants, the next most common ingredients are emollients to moisturize the skin. Thereafter follows a multitude of trivial ingredients which add little to the cleaning ability of the product. These include the usual colorants, fragrances, and preservatives, and a host of vitamins, amino acids, and plant extracts added mainly for marketing reasons. Some products also contain mild abrasives to exfoliate the outer layers of skin cells.

The non-foaming cleansing lotions contain water and oils blended together with emulsifiers and emulsion stabilizers. They also contain small amounts of surfactants to aid the even spreading of the product. The oils in the product serve two purposes. They act as emollients to moisturize the skin, and they dissolve any greasy residues left over from moisturizing creams and make-up, and from natural skin secretions. They also help to loosen particles of dirt and grime. The water dissolves salt and urea from the sweat glands and any water soluble cosmetic residues. After the cleansers are applied, they can be rinsed away with water or wiped off with tissues or towels, leaving a moisturizing residue on the skin. Once again, a host of trivial ingredients are added, along with the usual preservatives, antioxidants, colorants, and fragrances.

The vast majority of cleansing products contain a large number of ingredients – 20 to 30 is quite typical, making it more likely that chemical deposits will be left on your skin. It is a good rule of thumb that the more ingredients there are in a product, the more likely it is that one of them will disagree with you. It is also more likely that the product will contain a combination of two or more ingredients that together have an unpredictable adverse effect. And when there are so many ingredients, it is much more difficult to determine which one or which combination of chemicals is responsible for the adverse effect, making it harder to avoid them in the future.

If you use a cleansing product because soap does not agree with you, try using a milder soap or even a baby soap. Choose one that is neither colored nor perfumed and has a slightly acidic pH. Skin is naturally slightly acidic (with a pH level of betweem 5 and 5.6 – men's skin being slightly more acidic than women's). Soap is often mildly alkaline. This conflict can leave your skin feeling dry and sore. You may find that your problems will disappear if you use a soap that has a pH between 5 and 6.

Washing your face with water that is too hot may also cause mild skin irritation simply because the skin on your face is thinner and less tolerant to heat than your hands. The hot water will also open your pores. This is great if you want to clean out all that ingrained dirt, but it also allows cosmetic chemical resides into the pores where they remain. Try using lukewarm water just above body temperature (about 100° Fahrenheit or 40° Celsius). It is also possible that using rough towels or towels that contain fabric conditioner residues may also contribute to sore skin after washing.

HAND WASH AND LIQUID SOAP

Cleansing liquids in pump-action dispensers have become very popular both at home and in the workplace. There are many to choose from but they are all relatively similar in their formulation. They all contain anionic detergents – SLS and sodium laureth sulfate being the most common. Foam boosters are important ingredients and most products are fairly thick, and often contain opacifiers to produce a rich, creamy appearance. Those designed for the bathroom have dainty containers and delicate, often floral fragrances, while those for the kitchen or workplace come in more practical containers and have stronger fragrances that smell as though the product has powerful cleaning properties. They frequently contain antimicrobial agents such as triclosan or formaldehyde, which not only kill microbes on your hands but double up as preservatives. It is not a good idea to wash your face with hand wash containing these antimicrobials.

The advantage of these products is that people may not like using mushy, wet bars of soap, and there is a lower risk of microbes passing from the hands of one person to another.

7 deodorants and antiperspirants

**Be careful with that deodorant spray –
It can take your breath away**

Body odor occurs when bacteria living on our skin break down the natural residues that are secreted by our sweat glands. Strongly spiced foods may also seep out in the sweat, adding to the pungent aroma. Washing with soap and water temporarily removes the offending substances, but they soon return with the unpleasant odors following in their wake. Deodorants and antiperspirants are our next line of defence.

PERSPIRATION

When you becomes too warm or experience a surge of adrenaline, between two to three million sweat glands (properly called sudoriferous glands) secrete water onto the surface of your skin. The water then evaporates, cooling you down. In any watery liquid, water molecules are constantly moving very slowly. In order to fly off as water vapor, they must gain a vast amount of energy. The water molecules in the droplets of sweat get this energy by absorbing heat from your body, thereby cooling you down. You do, in fact, sweat all the time. Each day an average person loses one or two pints of water through sweating. If you participate in energetic sports or hike up a steep hill on a warm day, you can lose anything from four to eight pints of sweat.

If you perspire but evaporation keeps your skin dry, this is called *insensible* perspiration. If a film of water appears on your skin, *sensible* perspiration is taking place. Both types of perspiration produce water containing a little salt and some waste chemicals, such as urea and lactic acid, which help to control the pH of the skin and defend it against some types of bacteria. It is these chemicals that produce the "sweaty" body odor, especially when bacteria start to break them down.

Old Wives' Tales – Herbal Deodorants

Sage, thyme, coriander, and rosemary have all been used as herbal deodorants. They may work but they are no safer than any other deodorant. Thyme and rosemary have been linked to contact allergies and dermatitis, and Linalool, which is extracted from coriander, has been linked to facial psoriasis.

Most of your body, especially your palms, the soles of your feet and your forehead, are covered with eccrine sweat glands, which empty directly onto the surface of your skin. At puberty, a second type of sweat gland develops under your arms and around your genitals. These are called apocrine sweat glands and they empty into the hair follicles of your pubic and underarm hair. Sweat from these glands pick up sebum and protein fragments before flowing out of the follicle and onto the skin. The substances are then broken down by bacteria, resulting in the familiar "underarm" odor.

Deodorants control body odor by killing bacteria on the skin or by restricting their growth. *Antiperspirants* contain aluminum or zinc salts, which reduce the flow of sweat from the glands. *Talcum powder* contains talc, an absorbent mineral which absorbs moisture and lubricates the skin making it feel dry. Most deodorants, antiperspirants, and talcum powders also contain fragrance chemicals to mask the odor.

DEODORANTS

Deodorants reduce or mask unpleasant body odors. They generally work by preventing bacterial growth in warm, damp areas of the body and, at the same time, have a more pleasant smell of their own. They are often used in association with antimicrobials and antiperspirants and come in a variety of forms including aerosols, deodorant sticks and gels, and roll-on deodorant lotions. When using aerosol deodorants, avoid inhaling the spray as this could result in sensitization, breathing difficulties, and lung damage.

TYPICAL INGREDIENTS – DEODORANT STICK (USA)

Ingredients:

Dipropylene glycol, Tripropylene glycol, Water, Sodium stearate, Fragrance, Triclosan, Cetyl alcohol, Sodium chloride, Ext. D&C Violet #2, D&C Green #6.

Dipropylene glycol and Tripropylene glycol	These are solvents and humectants which keep the product soft and moist.
Water	Aid to formulation. Controls the texture and feel of the deodorant stick.
Sodium stearate	Essentially this is soap, a waxy, solid which, when mixed with the solvents, forms a soft, solid stick that spreads easily and evenly over the skin.
Fragrance	A mixture of fragrance chemicals, often exceeding 50 in number, many of which are artificial.
Triclosan*	An antibacterial chemical which acts as both a preservative and deodorant, preventing the growth of bacteria on the body, thus reducing body odor. When used as a preservative, EU regulations restrict it to 0.3 percent of the finished product but it is permitted in greater quantities if used for another stated purpose, such as a deodorant.
Cetyl alcohol*	Assists even spreading of the deodorant stick.
Sodium chloride	Astringent. May help to reduce sweat production.
Ext. D&C Violet #2*	Synthetic coal tar dye.
D&C Green #6*	Synthetic coal tar dye.

* These ingredients are subject to restrictions or have been linked to harmful or adverse effects.

TYPICAL INGREDIENTS – AEROSOL DEODORANT

Ingredients:

Isobutane, Alcohol Denat., Propane, Parfum, Isopropyl myristate.

Isobutane	A liquefied gas used as a propellant.
Alcohol Denat.*	Denatured alcohol. This dries the skin and kills any microbes that may be present on it. It may cause stinging until it evaporates. Since it does not remain on the skin, microbes may reappear relatively quickly. Alcohol can cause systemic eczematous contact dermatitis in some individuals.
Propane	A liquefied gas used as a propellant.
Parfum	A mixture of fragrance chemicals, often more than 50 in number, many of which are artificial.
Isopropyl myristate*	Emollient to moisturize the skin.

* These ingredients have been linked to harmful or adverse effects.

Note that this product contains no antiperspirant or deodorant ingredients and, therefore, relies on the strong fragrance to disguise any unpleasant body odor.

There are a large number of deodorant chemicals to choose from but the two most commonly used are denatured alcohol and triclosan. Alcohol effectively kills most bacteria, then evaporates quickly. But the bacteria often return quickly and frequent applications of the deodorant are required. The alcohol can cause a stinging sensation and has been known to cause sore, red patches on the skin. You can happily use an alcohol-based deodorant for several years, then find it suddenly disagrees with you. If this happens, stop using alcohol-based products on your skin, as the reaction can worsen and turn into systemic, eczematous contact dermatitis.

Triclosan is actually a preservative but it is also an excellent antimicrobial. It has no well-documented adverse effects but, like many chemicals, it is harmful in large amounts. EU regulations restrict it to 0.3 percent of the finished product if it is used as a preservative. In deodorants, however, it may be added in larger quantities.

Deodorants

The following ingredients are deodorants which do not act as antiperspirants:

Ammonium Phenolsulfonate	Phenethyl Alcohol
Cetylpyridinium Chloride	Sodium Phenolsulfonate
Chlorothymol	Triclosan
Cloflucarban	Triethyl Citrate
Dequalinium Acetate	Zinc Gluconate
Dichloro-m-Xylenol	Zinc Glutamate
Dichlorophene	Zinc Lactate
Linalool	Zinc Palmitate
Methylbenzethonium Chloride	Zinc Phenolsulfonate
Phenethyl Acetate	Zinc Ricinoleate

ANTIPERSPIRANTS

As the name suggests, antiperspirants reduce the skin's ability to perspire. They are commonly used to reduce body odor. Sweat, which itself is almost odorless, provides a warm, moist environment in which bacteria breed. These usually have a characteristic odor of their own but body odor is produced when they break down chemicals present in our sweat.

Antiperspirants are usually aluminum compounds, sometimes mixed with zirconium salts. These reduce sweat production by the sweat glands and block the ducts that carry the sweat to the skin. Most aluminum salts are irritants, causing itching, redness, and sometimes a rash. When using aerosol antiperspirants do not inhale the spray, as regular exposure can lead to lung damage. Zirconium salts are harmful by inhalation and are banned from aerosols in both the USA and the EU. Safer alternatives include antiperspirant sticks, gels, and roll-on lotions. You will often find that antiperspirants contain a deodorant and some products contain both antiperspirant and antimicrobial ingredients. Some antiperspirants have been known to discolor clothing.

Antiperspirants

Some anitperspirants are also deodorants

- Aluminum Bromohydrate
- Aluminum Chloride
- Aluminum Chlorohydrate
- Aluminum Chlorohydrex
- Aluminum Chlorohydrex PEG
- Aluminum Chlorohydrex PG
- Aluminum Citrate
- Aluminum Dichlorohydrate
- Aluminum Dichlorohydrex PEG
- Aluminum Dichlorohydrex PG
- Aluminum Sesquichlorohydrate
- Aluminum Sesquichlorohydrex PEG
- Aluminum Sesquichlorohydrex PG
- Aluminum Sulfate
- Aluminum Zirconium Octachlorohydrate
- Aluminum Zirconium Octachlorohydrex Gly
- Aluminum Zirconium Pentachlorohydrate
- Aluminum Zirconium Pentachlorohydrex Gly
- Aluminum Zirconium Tetrachlorohydrate
- Aluminum Zirconium Tetrachlorohydrex Gly
- Aluminum Zirconium Trichlorohydrate
- Aluminum Zirconium Trichlorohydrex Gly
- Ammonium Alum
- Cobalt Acetylmethionate
- Potassium Alum
- Sodium Alum
- Sodium Aluminum Chlorohydroxy Lactate

Do Antiperspirants Cause Breast Cancer?

There is a scaremongering rumor, mainly appearing on the Internet, that aluminum-based antiperspirants are a major cause of breast cancer. The numerous articles that we have discovered are written by people who do not seem to be scientifically or medically qualified, and they offer no scientific, medical, or statistical data to back up their claims. Their reasoning seems to show a lack of understanding of how the human body works, and they ignore all of the medical facts that we do know about breast cancer. In addition to breast cancer, some authors also link aluminum-based antiperspirants to prostate cancer in men and Alzheimer's disease.

All of the medically qualified authors writing on this subject that we found, dismiss the rumor as pure nonsense. The risk factors associated with breast cancer are well known and, unless some solid evidence is produced to say otherwise, it is fair to assume that antiperspirants are not one of them.

In fact there are two pieces of compelling evidence that antiperspirants do *not* contribute to breast cancer. Firstly, the mortality rate from breast cancer in the UK has remained fairly constant throughout the whole of the 20th century, despite antiperspirants not being widely used until the fifties and sixties. Secondly, breast cancer is rare in Japanese women living in Japan, but Japanese women who live in the USA and eat an American diet, have the same incidence of breast cancer as the average American woman. Since antiperspirants are used widely in both the USA and Japan, these cosmetics cannot be a significant risk factor, and diet plays a much greater role. A high-fat, low-fiber diet increases the risk of developing breast cancer.

FEMININE HYGIENE SPRAYS

There are several products that are used for intimate feminine hygiene. For the most part, they are at best unnecessary, and at worst, a cause of irritation. The products include moist tissues, absorbent powders, cleansing solutions and, of course, feminine deodorant sprays, which are essentially deodorants containing antimicrobial ingredients. There have been several reports that these can cause vaginal irritation or aggravate an existing irritation. If irritation occurs while you are using any of these products, stop using them immediately and do not use them if you have an infection or vaginal irritation. Cleanliness is important but the soap and detergents in body shampoos, foaming bath products, or shower gels can all cause or aggravate vaginal irritation.

Feminine deodorant sprays typically contain propellants, which double up as solvents, silicone moisturizers, talc, antimicrobials, and denatured alcohol. A range of antimicrobials are used such as chlorhexidine and its derivatives, various quaternium compounds, and triclosan. Most of these ingredients have no documented adverse effects despite EU restrictions being applied to some of them. Denatured alcohol can cause systemic, eczematous contact dermatitis. The use of moisturizers in these products is mystifying, as these areas should be kept dry to discourage the breeding of microbes.

Vaginal cleansing products seem to contain the same ingredients as a basic shampoo. Sodium laureth sulfate is commonly used as the detergent. Avoid products containing SLS (sodium lauryl sulfate), as this has been linked to vaginal irritation. Triclosan, chlorhexidine, or other antimicrobials are often added to control the growth of microbes on the body. Moist tissues for intimate feminine hygiene are essentially the same as any other moist tissue but they also contain antimicrobials. These often contain denatured alcohol in fairly large amounts.

In the USA, the words "hygiene" or "hygienic" cannot be used on the labeling of feminine care products as this is deemed misleading in that the products do not actually have any cleansing action but merely reduce or mask an odor. These products must contain specific warnings as defined by the FDA, regarding usage of the product and what to do in the case of vaginal irritation or discharge.

Does Talc Cause Cancer of the Ovaries?

It is a well-established fact that inhaling mineral dust, especially asbestos dust, causes lung disease and can result in various forms of cancer, including lung cancer. Talc, an absorbent mineral that is commonly used in a number of cosmetics, especially talcum powders, has recently been highlighted in the media because of the uncertain link between cancer of the ovaries and the use of talc-based powders for genital hygiene. Many articles on this subject have been scaremongering and ill informed, while others misinterpret the scientific data and warn us against using talcum powder and items which may contain traces of talc, such as condoms, tampons, sanitary towels, contraceptive diaphragms, and even rubber gloves.

The link between talc and ovarian cancer was first reported in the 1930s and the anti-talc league misused this fact to start rumors of conspiracies and cover-ups by the cosmetics' manufacturers. Although there have been several articles in the medical literature over the past 60 years, there have been relatively few scientific studies until quite recently.

Between 1984 and 1987 a study was carried out in Boston which involved 235 white American women with ovarian cancer and a control group of 239 women of similar age, race, and residence who were not suffering from any form of cancer. The results showed that 49 percent of the women with ovarian cancer regularly used talc for genital hygiene while only 39 percent of the control group used talc in the same way. The research group concluded that excessive and regular use of talc for genital hygiene may be linked to an increased risk of ovarian cancer but it was unlikely to be the cause of the majority of ovarian cancers.

A similar study in Buffalo, New York involving 499 ovarian cancer patients and a control group of 693 women with other forms of cancer, such as cancer of the colon or stomach, found about the same proportion of each group regularly used talc. This study concluded that there was no link between ovarian cancer and the use of talc for genital hygiene. Critics of this study, however, pointed out that asbestos fibers had been found in some samples of talc and these had been linked to cancer of the stomach, colon, and lungs. They believe that there is a small but significant link between the use of talc and an increased risk of cancer. There have been no studies that have linked the use of talc-based baby powders with ovarian cancer later in life.

In 1994 the FDA decided against a consumer warning on products containing talc because there was insufficient evidence for a causal link between talc and ovarian cancer. Cancer of the ovaries is the fifth most common cause of cancer death in the UK but only about one woman in 12,500 is likely to be affected by it, and using talc is unlikely to significantly increase the risk. Women in the high-risk group for ovarian cancer include those who:

- are over 50 years of age
- have a family history of ovarian, breast, or colon cancer
- are suffering from breast or colon cancer
- have had no children
- have not used the contraceptive pill
- have used fertility drugs for more than three ovulation cycles
- are of Ashkenazi Jewish descent
- live in Western countries.

Some medical experts who have stated opinions on this subject believe that the liberal use of talc should be avoided. If talc does increase the risk of cancer it does so only by a slight degree, but since talc is not essential to health or hygiene, the risk is not worth taking. If you are worried about using talc the answer is simple. Switch to a product that is based on zea mays (cornstarch/cornflour). This is soluble and can be rapidly metabolized to harmless substances in the body.

8 teeth and oral care products

So fair she was to outward view
As many maidens be
Her loveliness was all I knew
Until she smiled at me.

This chapter looks at the structure of teeth and the products we use to keep our teeth and mouth clean.

THE SCIENCE OF TEETH

A child has 20 primary (milk) teeth, which start to erupt about six months after birth and are completely in place by the age of three. They start to be replaced by the permanent (adult) teeth at the age of about six. By the age of 17, the full set of 32 teeth are usually in place, the last four to arrive being the wisdom teeth (third molars), which may appear late or not at all in some individuals.

The tooth is covered by a white or cream-colored substance called enamel. This is the hardest substance made by any living thing. Beneath the enamel is dentine, which is about halfway between the hardness of enamel and bone. In the center of the tooth is a soft mass called the pulp. This is filled with living cells, blood vessels, and nerve endings. The tooth is about three times longer than it looks, about two-thirds of it being the root buried deep inside the jawbone and covered by the gums. The roots are covered with a sensitive, bone-like substance called cementum and the

TYPICAL INGREDIENTS – TOOTHPASTE

Active Ingredients:

Sodium Fluoride 0.24% w/w (1000 ppm F)

Ingredients:

Aqua, Sorbitol, Hydrated silica, PEG-12, Tetrasodium pyrophosphate, Carboxymethyl-cellulose sodium, Sodium lauryl sulfate, Aroma, Cellulose gum, Sodium bicarbonate, Sodium saccharin, Sodium fluoride, CI 77891.

Aqua	Water – the main ingredient.
Sorbitol	Humectant to prevent the toothpaste from drying out when the lid is not replaced.
Hydrated silica	Mild abrasive to polish the teeth.
PEG-12	Thickening agent.
Tetrasodium pyrophosphate	Controls the acidity of the toothpaste.
Carboxymethyl-cellulose sodium	Binding agent. It prevents the other ingredients from separating and it aids dispersal of the toothpaste throughout the mouth, allowing it to be easily rinsed away.
Sodium lauryl sulfate (SLS)*	Anionic detergent to aid removal of food particles and plaque from the teeth.
Aroma	Flavorings which may be natural or artificial.
Cellulose gum	Thickening and binding agent.
Sodium bicarbonate	Mild alkali to help control acidity in the toothpaste and to neutralize excess acidity in the mouth.
Sodium saccharin	Artificial sugar-free sweetener.
Sodium fluoride*	Active ingredient that helps to strengthen teeth and reduce tooth decay. The total fluoride concentration in a cosmetic must not exceed 0.15 percent of the finished product. This product contains 0.24 percent of sodium fluoride, which is only 0.11 percent of

	fluoride (the remaining 0.13 percent being sodium) and, therefore, there is no requirement to declare it separately on the label as an "Active Ingredient." In this case, the amount of fluoride present is also expressed in parts per million by weight of fluoride: 0.15 percent of fluoride equates to 1500 parts per million.
CI 77891	Titanium dioxide, a natural white colorant.

* These ingredients are subject to restrictions or have been linked to harmful or adverse effects.

tooth is held into its socket by periodontal ligaments which act like springs, giving the tooth a small amount of movement and acting like shock absorbers to cushion the impact when biting and chewing.

TOOTHPASTE AND TOOTH DECAY

Toothpaste is a mixture of cleaning agents, antimicrobials, preservatives, and other additives that remove bacteria, plaque, food particles, and minor stains from the teeth, gums, and oral cavity. Dentists recommend brushing your teeth morning and evening, using vertical strokes that move away from the gums, that is, downwards on the upper teeth and upwards on the lower teeth. This action removes plaque but does not push it under the gums where it can cause infections.

Plaque is a sticky mixture of bacteria and food debris. If it is not periodically removed it might cause tooth decay (caries) and gum disease. The bacteria feed on the food particles in the plaque and convert any sugars or carbohydrates into acids which can dissolve the tooth enamel. If the enamel is breached, the acid attacks the dentine and works its way further into the tooth, eventually reaching the soft pulp. The bacteria in plaque also release toxins which attack the gums, making them red and swollen at the margins. This is called gingivitis which, if left untreated, progresses to periodontitis, in which the tooth socket is weakened and the teeth become loose. Gum disease is a progressive disorder and is, therefore, more common in older people – hence the expression "long in the tooth," which describes the receding gums in elderly people. Gum disease causes more teeth to be lost than tooth decay, especially nowadays, since fluoride has been added to our toothpaste for at least 20 years.

The main ingredients in most toothpastes are detergents to remove greasy deposits, abrasives to gently polish the surface of the teeth, humectants to prevent the toothpaste from drying out, thickeners and gelling agents to produce the correct texture of the toothpaste, foaming agents to satisfy the psychological need for lather in a cleansing product, flavorings, and fluoride to strengthen the tooth enamel and help prevent tooth decay. Other additives may include strontium salts to reduce the sensitivity of the teeth to sudden temperature changes, antimicrobials to kill bacteria and reduce the rate at which they reappear, and mild bleaching agents to help whiten the teeth.

The most commonly used abrasives are aluminum hydroxide or hydrated silica, both of which are sufficiently hard to grind away and remove most surface deposits from the teeth, but neither is hard enough to scratch the enamel. They are also compatible with a wide range of other ingredients and flavors. Sodium lauryl sulfate (SLS) is a commonly used detergent in toothpaste, but it does not form a strong lather so a mild foam booster is sometimes added. The foam helps to disperse the toothpaste in the mouth, allowing it to reach most parts of the oral cavity and making it easier to rinse away.

The correct choice of thickeners and gelling agents is important. Sodium carboxymethyl cellulose and PEG derivatives are common choices because they not only thicken the toothpaste but also act as a binding agents and prevent the abrasives from settling out. They also assist in the rinsing of both the mouth and the toothbrush.

Sorbitol is rapidly replacing glycerin as the humectant in toothpaste, mainly because it is cheaper. It prevents water evaporating from the toothpaste if the cap is not replaced. Menthol is often added because it has a refreshing effect in the mouth. Flavors such as mint and spearmint, and spicy flavors such as clove, cinnamon, and aniseed, are the most commonly used because they go well with menthol, whereas other flavors (like fruit flavors) do not. These flavors tend to linger in the mouth and will disguise mild odors on the breath for several minutes after brushing. Sugar-free sweeteners such as sodium saccharine are used to satisfy the modern palate.

Antimicrobials in toothpaste can kill any bacteria the toothbrush cannot reach and they slow down the rate at which the plaque reappears, but their effect is short lived. Claims by manufacturers that they can protect your teeth all day long are far fetched: Toothpaste that contains bleaching agents such as calcium peroxide or strontium peroxide, can whiten your teeth very slightly, but the effect is not earth shattering. Recently in the UK, one manufacturer was admonished for altering the advertising "before" and "after" photographs, making their product appear to have a much greater whitening effect than it actually had. If you want to whiten your teeth, your dentist can coat them with a dental bleaching agent, and then shine a strong ultraviolet light on it to activate the bleach. This can make a noticeable difference to the whiteness of your teeth, especially if they are stained with nicotine or tannin from tea or coffee.

Old Wives' Tales – Herbal Tooth Care

Sage is said to be good for the teeth. It is said to whiten the enamel and strenghen the gums. Try it by all means but there is no scientific evidence to support this.

Clear toothpaste is available that contains extremely fine hydrated silica, which appears transparent in the thick, gel formulation.

TOOTH POLISH

Tooth polish is essentially the same as toothpaste but it is formulated to have a thinner, more fluid consistency and a shiny appearance. The abrasive is often hydrated silica, which is very finely ground; PEG-derived gelling agents are often used to obtain the required appearance.

FLUORIDE

Compounds that contain fluoride are added to toothpastes, mouthwashes, and other oral care products to prevent cavities and dental caries (tooth decay). The fluoride is thought to be absorbed into the minerals in the enamel and the dentine, making them more resistant to acid attack. Some dentists believe it also works by absorption into the surface of the teeth from where it is slowly released. Since fluoride is fairly poisonous, it kills any bacteria that cling to the teeth, including the bacteria responsible for producing the acids that cause cavities.

Children who are brought up in areas where fluoride occurs naturally in the water supply, have 65 percent fewer fillings, and 90 percent fewer extractions than children who live in areas where the fluoride levels in the drinking water are low. This demonstrates that fluoride is incorporated into the mineral structure of the teeth during the development of the child, and gives life-long protection from dental decay. The recommended level of fluoride in the water supply is between 0.7 and 1.2 ppm. Where the levels are lower, fluoride supplements, in the form of tablets or drops, can be given to children. A dentist can directly apply a fluoride solution or gel to a child's teeth, or fluoride can be administered at home in the form of a mouthwash or toothpaste.

In the EU, the level of fluoride in oral care products that are commonly sold as toiletries must not exceed 0.15 percent. This is regarded as a safe level and it is sufficient to protect and strengthen the teeth. Some oral care products, however, contain more than 0.15 percent. In these cases the product may be classified as a medical device or medicinal product and the fluoride must be listed as an "active ingredient" before the main list of ingredients. Most of the brands of toothpaste you buy do not exceed the 0.15 percent limit, but manufacturers commonly list the fluoride as an active ingredient and state its content both as a percentage and in parts per million (0.15 percent equates to 1500 parts per million), although there is no requirement for them to do so. If, for example, the label states that the active ingredient is sodium fluoride and that it contains 0.32 percent w/w (1450 ppm), the manufacturer has not exceeded the allowed limit: 0.32 percent of sodium fluoride is the same as 0.145 percent (1450 ppm) of fluoride, the remaining 0.175 percent being sodium.

Children should not be allowed to use more than a small dab of toothpaste and they should be discouraged from swallowing it, as fluoride is fairly poisonous. Excessive amounts of fluoride, above the recommended levels, may cause fluorosis, a mottling of the tooth enamel. In severe cases the teeth are permanently stained brown.

MOUTHWASH

Mouthwash contains mostly colored and flavored water with some fluoride and oral antimicrobials that kill the bacteria which can cause stale odors from the mouth. Small amounts of thickeners are added to improve the texture, and surfactants are often included to help clean the mouth and to assist in the even spreading of the mouthwash. Strong flavors, usually mint or spicy flavors, temporarily mask odors on the breath.

Can Mouthwash Eliminate Bad Breath?

Many people believe that the use of mouthwash or toothpaste can eliminate bad breath, and that the main cause of bad breath is poor oral hygiene. The truth is that bad breath (halitosis) is often caused by other factors and cannot be cured by a mouthwash or toothpaste alone. Such factors may include smoking, drinking alcohol, eating garlic or other strongly flavored foods, a mouth or dental infection, sinusitis, or certain lung disorders.

9 hair care

**This shampoo cures and mends
Tired hair and split ends.
It has a fragrance you will like
And protects you from a lightning strike.**

The labels on shampoos and conditioners make some pretty amazing claims. If they work as advertised, how come so many people have bad hair days? Of course, the answer is that they do not live up to all these claims and, while they may be good at cleaning and conditioning your hair, they may also be contributing to that bad hair day. To understand how shampoos and conditioners work, you really need to know a little about hair biology. So this chapter guides you through the science of hair and then looks at dandruff and dandruff treatments, shampoos, and conditioners. It then delves into the realm of the salons and hairdressers, looking at hair dyes, perms, and hair straighteners. Of all the hazardous chemicals discussed in this book, those used in some hair-dye formulations are perhaps the most dangerous of all, and a section of this chapter looks specifically at the link between hair dyes and cancer.

WHAT IS HAIR?

If you have a full head of hair, you have about 100,000 hairs growing from your scalp. You also have hairs of varying length, thickness, and color, growing from almost every part of your body – the main exceptions being your lips, palms, and the soles of your feet. Each hair is between 0.0025 and 0.01 cm (0.0001 and 0.0004 inches) in diameter, and grows from a pit called a follicle. These are between 0.25 and 0.30 cm (0.010 and 0.012 inches) deep and reach down to the dermis, or living layer of your skin.

At the bottom of the follicle is the hair root. Inserted into the base of the root is a small piece of the dermis called the papilla, which is filled with minute blood vessels called capillaries. These supply food and oxygen to the hair root. The hair cells grow and multiply, and form a bulb around the root. As they multiply, they are squeezed together and are pushed up through the narrow hair follicle, where the pressure from the sides of the follicle continues to squeeze the cells together, forming a long shaft we call a hair. If you pull out a hair, you can often see a light-colored swelling – the bulb. The root is usually left behind and a new hair will grow from the follicle.

Cells produced from the top of the papilla form the medulla, the thin central core of the hair shaft. The medulla is soft and spongy because the cells are loosely packed, with air spaces between them. Long, stick-shaped cells grow from the sides of the papilla and make up the cortex, which is the main part of the hair shaft that surrounds the central core. Cells that grow from the lower parts of the papilla make up the outer layer, or cuticle. Cuticle cells are flattened by the pressure of the follicle walls, and have the appearance of overlapping scales wrapped around the hair shaft.

As the hair emerges from the root, the materials within the living cells are converted into keratin, a tough, fibrous protein, and when this process is complete – before the hair reaches the surface of the skin – the hair cells die. The keratin proteins are held together by sulfur bridges that give them rigidity. You can imagine these proteins as rope ladders. The ropes represent the protein strands and the rungs are the sulfur bridges which hold the protein strands together. When hair is permed, the sulfur bridges are chemically broken, then rejoined, resulting in a permanent change to the shape of the hair shaft.

The hair shaft is composed entirely of dead cells, which is why we do not feel it when it is cut. The growth rate varies a great deal but, on average, hair grows about 1.25 cm (half an inch) each month. It grows faster between the ages of 15 and 30, and women's hair grows slightly faster than men's. The growth rate is not affected by shaving or cutting the hair, but it can be affected by your state of health.

After a certain time, the hair's growth cycle ends. The follicle starts to shrink and move upwards toward the surface of the skin. Eventually the hair root is pushed out and then the hair falls out or comes out when we comb, brush, or wash our hair. The follicle will grow again, producing a new hair, and the cycle repeats itself. The length of this cycle varies from person to person, and on different parts of the body. The length of the hair depends on the length of the cycle. If the cycle lasts several years, the hair will become very long. However, some individuals never need to cut their hair because their growth cycle is short. Eyelashes have a very short cycle and thus remain a sensible length.

Old Wives' Tales – Herbs to Cure Baldness

Catmint, nettle and southernwood are all said to restore hair and so cure baldness, while the herb horestail is said to strengthen hair, and the regular use of yarrow and marshmallow (the plant, not the candy!) is rumored to prevent hair loss.

Apart from the powerful fragrance of southernwood, there are no adverse effects linked to any of these herbs.

The hair follicles grow at an angle so the hairs naturally lean to one side. There is a small muscle attached to the follicle, called an erector muscle, which can cause the hair to stand up (for example when it is cold, or when you feel threatened or scared). The follicle also produces sebum, a natural oil that lubricates the hair shaft and keeps it in good condition.

While in the womb, babies are covered with a light, downy hair called lanugo. This is replaced shortly before, or soon after birth, by vellus hair – a short, fine, fair hair, which often lasts until puberty. During puberty the vellus hair is replaced by terminal (adult) hair on the head, pubic areas, armpits, and, in some individuals, on the limbs and trunk. The growth of terminal hair is controlled by testosterone, the male sex hormone. Even women produce small amounts of testosterone. Too much testosterone in men can result in the loss of hair from the head but a strong growth of hair on other parts of the body. Around the time of menopause, the level of the female sex hormone estrogen falls, but the tiny amount of testosterone present remains constant, and so causes a growth of hair on the upper lip and chin.

THE COLOR OF HAIR

The color of your hair comes from a pigment called melanin. It is made in cells called melanocytes, which grow at the base of the hair follicle. Red and auburn hair contains red melanin. All other colors of hair come from black melanin. An absence of pigment makes the hair shafts transparent, resulting in white or blonde hair. As we grow older we produce less pigment and the medulla thickens, resulting in a greater air content in the hair shaft. This makes the hair slightly thicker, less flexible and gray in appearance. Melanin fades in bright sunlight and some shades of brown hair can become almost blonde when bleached by the sun.

DANDRUFF

Dandruff, like other visible skin conditions, carries a social stigma because it is incorrectly associated with poor personal hygiene. It causes embarrassment and, if left untreated, can lead to irreversible, premature hair loss (alopecia) and more serious skin conditions.

It is a relatively common, usually harmless condition caused by an excessive shedding of specks or flakes of dead skin cells from the scalp. It is one of the top ten problems for which people seek over-the-counter medical treatment and, surprisingly, it is a condition that medical experts seem unable to agree about, much less to cure. It is usually possible to control dandruff with a medicated or antidandruff shampoo, but the condition returns if the treatment is stopped. If the treatment does not work, this may be because the shedding is caused by a more serious condition such as eczema, psoriasis, or seborrheic dermatitis. Your doctor may be able to treat these conditions with a steroid-based or other medicated scalp treatment.

The outer layer of skin is composed of dead skin cells that are constantly being shed and replaced by cells from deeper down in the epidermis. We normally shed one layer of cells each day, producing particles too small to see. In dandruff sufferers, the growth and shedding of this layer is accelerated, but the reason for this is not known. Greasy skin tends to produce larger, yellower scales than dryer skin, the color coming from the sebum, our skin's natural oil. Dandruff is rarely associated with red, inflamed or sore patches on the scalp, these being indicative of a more serious skin condition.

Children rarely suffer from dandruff. It is most common in adolescents and young adults, and diminishes in middle years although older people can suffer from it, especially stroke victims. Men are more likely to have dandruff than women and people with greasy skin and hair suffer more from it than people with dry skin. For this reason, some medical experts think that the ultimate cause of dandruff is androgens, male sex hormones. Since these hormones serve a very important function, it is unlikely that a treatment based on suppressing them will be ever be available.

Old Wives' Tales – Herbal Dandruff Treatments

Garlic, nettle and southernwood are all said to cure dandruff. None of these herbs has been linked to adverse effects in cosmetics, but then again, dandruff may be preferable to the fragrance of garlic and southernwood in your hair!

Dandruff may be aggravated by excessive use of chemicals on the hair, tight-fitting hats and scarves, cold weather, central heating, infrequent shampooing, and inadequate rinsing. It has also been linked to anxiety, stress, and tension. For many years it was believed that a yeast called *Pityrosporum ovale* was responsible for dandruff, but the use of chemicals to kill the yeast failed to cure the dandruff. This yeast is present in small amounts on everyone's scalp. It is highly possible that although they do not cause dandruff, the flaking, greasy scalp and the warm environment under tight hats and scarves, provide a perfect breeding ground for this yeast. In other words, the yeast is a symptom rather than a cause.

Effective dandruff shampoos contain cytostatic chemicals which reduce the rate of cell growth in the epidermis of the scalp. These include zinc pyrithione and selenium sulfide. Other common antidandruff chemicals are coal tar, sulfur and salicylic acid. The latter is a keratolytic (exfoliant) chemical that loosens the outer layer of dead skin by dissolving the keratin, the protein of which it is made, thus preventing a build up of dead skin cells. Some shampoos also contain anti-yeast or antifungal agents such as Nizoral™ (ketoconazole). Coal-tar shampoos are only available from a pharmacist in the EU and tests have shown that long-term use of products containing crude or refined coal tar may carry a risk of cancer.

Seborrheic dermatitis will not usually respond to normal antidandruff shampoos and it is often associated with further symptoms around the ears, nose, or chest.

Psoriasis usually produces silvery scales from red, inflamed, or irritated patches on the scalp. It also appears on the arms, legs, back, and buttocks.

LOOKING AFTER YOUR HAIR

It is important to keep hair clean and in good condition, but hair is easily damaged by over-washing, overheating with hair dryers, heated rollers or curling tongs, back-combing, over-coloring, or too many perms. Untrained or inexperienced hairdressers can also damage hair by using oxidation hair colors or perming formulations incorrectly. The damage cannot be undone but, eventually, new hair will grow to replace the damaged hair. Meanwhile, a good-quality hair conditioner will improve even seriously damaged hair.

Shampoo

Shampoo is essentially a mixture of detergent and water used to remove dirt and grease from hair. Soap is unsuitable since it leaves behind a dull film of soap scum. Sodium lauryl sulfate (SLS) is the most widely used detergent in shampoos, being found in about 90 percent of them, usually in combination with other detergents.

A typical shampoo will be mostly water, with between 5 and 20 percent of detergent. Shampoo for dry hair contains less detergent than shampoo for greasy hair. Sodium lauryl sulfate does not produce a good lather so the shampoo may also contain sodium laureth sulfate, which produces a stronger foam. A foam booster such as cocamide DEA or cocamidopropyl betaine may also be added in small quantities (usually between 1 and 5 percent depending on the formulation). Lather plays no part in the detergency process but it does keep the detergent and any other active ingredients, such as antidandruff agents, close to the hair and scalp in a concentrated form. It is also used because there is a strong psychological link between lather and perceived cleaning power.

Manufacturers can choose from a wide variety of thickeners, which are added to adjust the texture and pouring properties of the product; colorants and opacifiers are used to give the shampoo a creamy or pearlescent appearance. Oils are often added to counteract the drying effect that detergents have on your hair, and therefore emulsifiers and emulsion stabilizers must also be added. The oils can be anything from natural vegetable oils to synthetic silicone polymers. They also have a conditioning effect, helping to smooth the cuticle layer of the hair shafts. Shampoos, as do almost all other cosmetics, contain natural or artificial fragrances.

It's a Fact

According to the FDA, a shampoo that claims to be an egg shampoo must contain one egg, or the equivalent amount of dried whole egg, in the amount of shampoo that would be used in *one* shampooing of your hair.

Shampoo often contains at least two, and frequently more, preservatives. One must be water soluble to protect the watery part of the shampoo and the other must be oil soluble to preserve the oils in the emulsion. The paraben family, formaldehyde, glyoxal, and the methylchloroisothiazolinone/methylisothiazolinone mixture are all commonly found in shampoos.

All-in-one conditioning shampoos contain oils to condition the hair, film formers to distribute the oils, and antistatic agents such as cationic surfactants or silicone polymers (methicone and dimethicone derivatives). They usually contain only a small amount of detergent otherwise the conditioning ingredients might be washed away.

Medicated shampoos, usually for dandruff treatment, contain a variety of ingredients but zinc pyrithione is probably the most common, followed by coal tar; the latter is banned from cosmetics in the EU and is only available on prescription or from a pharmacist. (See *Dandruff* on p.90 for full details of antidandruff agents.) Insecticidal shampoos for treating head lice or fleas, contain insecticides based on organophosphates. These are highly toxic if swallowed and must not be used by children without adult supervision.

Antichlorine shampoos are available to protect dyed hair from the bleaching effect of the chlorine in swimming pools. Once the color has faded, however, these shampoos are unlikely to restore it. Swimming pools often contain chemicals that slowly liberate chlorine to maintain a constant but low concentration of chlorine in the water. These chemicals soak into the hair shafts and may not be completely rinsed away by showering. Chlorine is then slowly released into the hair shaft, where it attacks the dyes. A mild reducing agent, such as sodium thiosulfate, sodium sulfite or sodium nitrite, harmlessly destroys both the chlorine and the chlorine-liberating compounds before they bleach the hair dyes. It is important to use this type of shampoo as soon as possible after swimming and give it time to soak into the hair shaft in order for it to work effectively.

Baby shampoos are milder than adult shampoos because they contain lower concentrations of detergents and they often use less irritating ingredients. As a rule of thumb, sodium laureth sulfate is a fairly low irritation detergent, followed by ammonium laureth sulfate. Sodium lauryl sulfate (SLS) is a slightly stronger irritant, with ammonium lauryl sulfate being slightly worse still. The bottom line is, any detergent will make your eyes sting. The more detergent there is, the more your eyes will sting and so shampoos for greasy hair will be stronger irritants than shampoos for dry hair.

If you find that a brand of shampoo does not agree with you or makes your scalp itch, change your brand immediately *before* your scalp becomes sore. If you persist in using this product your scalp condition may deteriorate to dandruff or worse. The irritation is likely to be caused by colorants, fragrance chemicals, or preservatives in the shampoo, so try a brand that contains different preservatives, has a different color, and has little or no scent.

Conditioners

Conditioners are applied to the hair after shampooing to improve its sheen, feel, and controlability. They are usually rinse-off preparations, but recently many non-rinse-off conditioners have come onto the market. They generally contain water emulsified with an oily substance, emulsifiers, non-ionic and cationic surfactants, antistatic agents, thickeners, preservatives, colorants, and fragrances. Other additives include vitamins, proteins, amino acids, antifoaming agents, and various plant extracts, few of which are essential to the function of the conditioner.

Nature intended hair to be covered with a thin film of water-repellent grease. That is why it provided us with sebaceous glands which secrete sebum, our natural oil. This oily film keeps our hair in good condition, giving it a glossy sheen, smooth texture, and bounce. Shampoos remove too much of this oil and leave us with dry, lifeless, flyaway hair. After a few days the oils return and the condition of the hair improves. Most of us can't wait that long so we apply conditioners that, amongst other things, leaves a film of oil on our hair. At one time lanolin or a related substance was commonly used, since it is closely related to our own sebum, but this has gradually been replaced by a host of less natural oily compounds.

The outer layer of hair, the cuticle, is covered with flattened cells rather like the scales on a fish or the feathers on a bird. Shampooing, brushing, blow-drying, back-combing, and even wind and weather, can cause these scales to stand out – rather like a bird with its feathers ruffled. Cationic surfactants present in the conditioner help to keep the oily compounds mixed with the water, help the conditioner to be spread evenly over the hair, and encourage the scales to lay flat against the hair shaft, making the hair easier to comb and less likely to suffer further damage. Even serious cuticle damage caused by excessive chemical treatments such as coloring or perming, or overheating with curling tongs and heated rollers, can be masked by using a suitable conditioner.

Antistatic agents prevent the build up of static electricity when the hair is brushed, combed, or rubbed during dressing. Static electricity causes hairs to repel each other, and you to have bad hair days!

Contrary to popular belief, even greasy hair benefits from the use of a conditioner; however the hair becomes greasy again quite quickly and requires more frequent shampooing. Shampoos and conditioners for greasy hair often contain citrus fragrances such as lemon because there is a strong psychological association between lemon juice and the removal of grease. But that is the only effect – it does not actually reduce the oiliness from your hair.

If you are concerned about having these artificial chemicals on your hair, try abandoning your conditioner for a few weeks and use a good quality, mild shampoo for dry hair, or a baby shampoo. You may find your natural oils quickly return to your hair and do a better job than any artificial conditioner made in a test-tube.

Can Shampoos Strengthen Your Hair?

Many shampoos and conditioners carry claims that they can strengthen your hair, especially if it has been damaged by perming or color treatments. They imply that the keratin or vitamins, or other ingredients added to the shampoo or conditioner, can penetrate into the hair shaft and repair the damage, or strengthen brittle hair making it more resistant (resistant to just what though, they do not say). They even go so far as to state that tests show this can happen.

If you dip a paintbrush into a pot of paint, it will come out covered in paint. In the same way, if you cover a strand of hair in a shampoo or conditioner containing a protein (such as keratin), the test will no doubt show the presence of the protein on the hair. But this does not mean the protein penetrates into the shaft – even if it did, it does not prove the protein could repair the hair. It is hard enough to get a small molecule of hair dye to penetrate the hair shaft, let alone a protein molecule which is two to three hundred times larger! Do not be fooled by these claims. They are purely gimmicks and no amount of added keratin, amino acids, vitamins, or whatever can penetrate into the hair shaft in order to repair your hair, make it stronger, or more resistant.

COLORING YOUR HAIR

Hair dyes bring with them a host of problems. There are four types of hair dyes: progressive hair dyes, which gradually darken your hair; temporary hair dyes, which wash out as soon as you next shampoo your hair; semi-permanent hair dyes, which last between five and ten washings; and permanent hair dyes, which last until the roots grow out and look unsightly.

Progressive Hair Dyes

These contain lead acetate or bismuth citrate. They are used to cover up gray hairs that are a natural result of the aging process, but the darkening process is slow and it is not immediately obvious that the hair is being colored. They work by reacting chemically with the sulfur in your hair proteins, forming sulfides of lead or bismuth, which are black, insoluble solids. Lead acetate and bismuth citrate are very poisonous ingredients, so progressive hair dyes must be stored well out of the reach of children. There is no evidence that any lead or bismuth is absorbed through the skin when used correctly but you should make sure they are never used on broken or damaged skin, and always wash your hands thoroughly after using them.

Temporary and Semi-permanent Hair Dyes

Temporary hair dyes wash out as soon as the hair is shampooed. They are water-soluble dyes, applied shortly after shampooing the hair. These dyes contain film formers which form a thin, colored layer on the hair shaft. They do not penetrate into the hair and can be easily washed out. They are used for one-off occasions such as parties or theatrical make-up. Be warned, however. If your hair has already been permanently colored or tinted, the temporary hair dye may not wash out so easily as the structure of your hair will have been altered and so may allow the temporary dye to penetrate the hair shaft. Make sure the temporary dye will wash out by testing it on a small lock of hair, so that you don't have to put up with pink hair for six weeks after the party.

Semi-permanent hair dyes consist of small molecules that are not very soluble in water and can penetrate the surface of the hair shaft. They are applied as an emulsion, the dye being soluble in the oil part of the emulsion. This is massaged into the hair in the form of a foam, which holds the dye against the hair long enough for it to penetrate the hair shaft. After the dye has soaked into the hair, the unwanted emulsion can be washed out. Semi-permanent hair dyes last for between five and ten washings. They are not good at covering gray hair but they do give even results on younger hair and can be easily applied at home.

Permanent Hair Dyes

Permanent hair dyes are also known as oxidation hair dyes. They give even results and cover gray hair very effectively. Permanent hair dye consists of two parts, a chemical, which is not yet a dye, and an oxidizing agent, usually hydrogen peroxide, which converts this chemical into a dye. These chemicals are mixed together shortly before the dye is applied to the hair. The mixture is left on the hair for 20 to 30 minutes before being rinsed out. The idea is that the smaller chemical molecules can penetrate deeper into your hair shaft where they are joined together, forming the hair dye – a larger molecule which becomes trapped deep inside the hair shaft from where it cannot be washed out. A number of things may cause permanent hair dyes to fade including some shampoos, chlorine in swimming pools or sunlight, but generally the colors do not need to be re-applied until the roots grow out and become noticeable. Great care must be taken as hydrogen peroxide is highly corrosive and can cause damage to skin and eyes.

Some people are worried by these dyes because they do not understand the chemical reactions that take place. There are horror stories of people who develop allergies to them and cannot remove them from their hair. Generally speaking, these hair colors are safe but their long-term use is not advised. Lengthy exposure to chemicals can cause adverse effects, although some experts believe that the length of time your hair is colored is not as important as the frequency of the color applications. Most of the dye is trapped in the hair shaft where it can do no harm. The only time you are at risk is when the dye is applied and comes into contact with your scalp. Therefore the more often you have your hair colored, the more often you are exposed to the dye.

Old Wives' Tales – Herbal Hair Colors

Camomile, marigold flowers, mullein flowers, and lemon juice are all said to lighten the color of hair, while rosemary, sage, and vinegar will all darken or deepen hair color. Henna (*Lawsonia inermis* or Lawsone) is a red-brown dye used to color hair.

These herbal hair colors may work, but if you think shampoo stings, try getting lemon juice or vinegar in your eyes. Both rosemary and camomile have been linked to contact allergies and dermatitis.

Some of the dyes used are known to be harmful. In fact, some of them are allowed to be used only in oxidation hair dyes as they are considered to be too harmful to apply to the skin on other parts of the body.

Home kits for oxidation hair dyes are available and generally give good results, but the final color may not turn out the same as the color shown on the packaging. This may be due to printing errors on the packaging but it is more likely to be caused by the natural color of your hair showing through the dye and contributing to the final color. Professional hairdressers often mix their own colors and can compensate for this. They also keep client records so that the exact color can be reproduced in the future.

Most hair dyes contain several colorants, blended together to achieve the desired shade. Washing, the action of chlorine in swimming pools and the bleaching effect of sunlight may cause some of the colorants to fade at a greater rate than others, causing the shade of your hair to gradually change.

Coloring Your Eyelashes

Never use permanent hair dyes to color your eyebrows or eyelashes. If these chemicals get into your eyes they can cause blindness. There are no permanent eyelash or eyebrow colors that have been approved by the FDA. In fact, the FDA prohibits the use of hair dyes for eyelash or eyebrow tinting or dyeing, even in beauty salons or other establishments. The first cosmetic product to be seized by the FDA after the 1938 Food, Drug and Cosmetic Act was passed, was a permanent eyelash and eyebrow color called 'Lash Lure.' The ban was prompted by the death of one woman and the permanent blinding of another. Despite these dangers and prohibitions, some people still use permanent hair dyes in this way and some salons still offer permanent eyelash and eyebrow coloring using oxidation hair dyes. This is particularly common in the summer months during the swimming season when other types of eye make-up wash off in the pool.

An alternative method to using hair dyes on eyebrows originated in the Far East and is now offered by some salons in the West. This involves injecting vegetable dyes under the skin above and below the eyebrows, effectively tattooing the color into place. This, of course, is permanent and irreversible, and there has been no health or safety validation of this technique by the regulating authorities.

HAIR DYES AND CANCER

Temporary and semi-permanent hair dyes often contain azo dyes or coal tar dyes, which have been demonstrated to cause cancer in some laboratory animals and allergic reactions in some individuals. Chemicals used in permanent hair dyes have also been linked to cancer. The *Index of Cosmetic Ingredients* lists over a dozen such chemicals in addition to several others which cause a variety of other adverse effects.

There have been many arguments over the safety of hair dyes and some manufacturers have voluntarily stopped using them in their products. In the USA, the FDA has the power to prohibit the sale of any cosmetic that is found to be harmful – except hair dyes. This dates back to the 1938 Food, Drug and Cosmetics Act, when it was known that coal tar dyes in hair-coloring products caused allergic reactions in some people. Fearing that the FDA would have powers to ban the sale of hair dyes, the manufacturers successfully lobbied for an exemption for their products. Hair dyes do, however, have to carry a warning label stating that these products can cause allergic reactions in some individuals. One specific ingredient requires the following warning:

Warning – Contains an ingredient that can penetrate your skin and has been determined to cause cancer in laboratory animals.

No such warning is required on products sold in the EU, and for those in the EU who are interested, the offending ingredient is called 4-methoxy-m-phenylenediamine, also known as 2,4-diaminoanisole or 4-MMPD.

The problem with cancer-causing chemicals (carcinogens) is that the cancer appears after long term, low-level exposure. This is worrying since nearly 40 percent of adults, including men, color their hair. You can minimize the risk by reducing the number of times you color your hair – older people who use colors to cover up gray hair will be exposed to less of these chemicals during their lifetime than younger people who color their hair as a fashion statement or for a different look. The younger you are when you start to color your hair, the greater the risk, because the exposure time is much longer.

When using these products, check the ingredients carefully and do a patch test before using them. You can do this easily by placing a small amount of dye on the skin behind your ear. Leave it there for two days. If you develop soreness, itching, or any other symptoms, do not use that dye. Try other dyes, carrying out a patch test each time until you find one that suits you. In the USA, labels on hair-dye products that contain non-approved coal tar dyes which are known to cause adverse reactions, are required to instruct you to carry out a patch test and describe how you should do it. The following mandatory wording must be present:

Caution – This product contains ingredients which may cause skin irritation on certain individuals and a preliminary test according to accompanying directions should first be made. This product must not be used for dyeing the eyelashes or eyebrows; to do so may cause blindness.

Salons are also required to carry out a patch test before coloring your hair. Of course, not all salons will do this and no such requirements exist in the EU. A patch test also only tests for allergies. It will not prevent the development of cancer.

HAIR PERMS AND HAIR STRAIGHTENERS

Hair perms are chemical treatments that permanently change the shape of the hair shaft. They are used to make straight hair curly, or to straighten curly or frizzy hair, in which case they are called hair straighteners. Whether hair is straight or curly depends on the cross-section of the hair. Round hairs tend to be straight while oval shapes are usually curly. Perms and straighteners work in exactly the same way.

The protein fibers in hair are held together by sulfur bridges (disulfide bonds). These give hair its rigidity. During a perm an alkaline chemical, called a reducing agent, breaks these sulfur bridges and allows the protein strands to be pulled away from each other. The hair is formed into a new shape, using hair rollers or some other device which puts the hair under some tension, to separate the protein fibers. Then a second chemical, an oxidizing agent, is applied, which causes the sulfur bridges to reform, locking the fibers into the new position. The oxidizing agent is usually hydrogen peroxide, which may lighten the color of the hair slightly. It reforms most, but not all, of the sulfur bridges, leaving the hair shafts slightly weaker than they were before the perm. This is why perms can damage hair. If you perm your hair too frequently, you will destroy too many disulfide bonds and your hair will be permanently damaged until new hair grows to replace it. The damage cannot be reversed but a good quality conditioner will improve your hair's texture and appearance. Qualified hairdressers seldom wreck your hair during a perm.

There are home-perming kits available that are often successful, but the main problems with these perms arise from uneven application of the chemicals and resetting the hair at the wrong tension.

10 baby products

Please little baby do not cry
Our shampoo is gentle on your eye.
So sorry about your asthmatic cough
But the benzoates stop it going off.

There is a daunting range of toiletries designed specifically for babies, and the advertisers would have us believe that we are less than adequate as parents if we do not buy them and plaster our children in creams and lotions from the day they are born. They even suggest that we should use them ourselves to keep our skin baby-soft. This chapter explains why you should not use adult toiletries and cosmetics on babies, what to look out for when choosing a baby product, and at what age you can switch from baby products to family or adult products.

WHAT'S SO SPECIAL ABOUT BABY PRODUCTS?

You can buy new-born baby products, regular baby products, and products for young children, and when you read the ingredients they look much the same as the standard family toiletries. So why do you need to pay more for a baby product? The answer is simple. EU regulations define toiletries for children under the age of three as Category-1 products. This means they must contain at least 50 times fewer microbes than cosmetics and toiletries for children over the age of three and adults, and they must contain sufficient preservatives to maintain these lower levels. These rules are necessary because microbes pose a much greater risk to young children than to older children or adults. New-born babies have not yet developed an immune system. They rely on physical barriers such as skin and mucous membranes, and on antibodies and immunoglobulins passed from the mother while in the womb, and later from her breast milk. It is essential that babies are not exposed to unnecessary microbes during this crucial period of development. (See *Chapter 4 – Preservatives* for full details of Category-1 and Category-2 products.)

WHICH BABY PRODUCT DO I CHOOSE?

If you feel you must use a cosmetic or toiletry on your baby, then you should avoid using products that contain potentially irritating or harmful chemicals. Baby skin is much thinner and more sensitive than adult skin. Generally speaking, baby products are gentler than normal toiletries. This is achieved in several ways. Baby shampoo almost always contains sodium laureth sulfate, which is considered to be one of the least irritating detergents available. It is certainly much less of an irritant than sodium lauryl sulfate (SLS) – the most commonly used detergent in the majority of shampoos, shower gels, foaming bath products, and cleansing products for adults. If you find a baby product that contains SLS put it back on the shelf and choose one that contains sodium laureth sulfate.

Colorants and fragrance chemicals are major causes of adverse effects. Most baby products are only lightly perfumed and subtly colored. If the product has a strong fragrance or a bright color, choose another brand. There is no law that requires all babies to have that familiar baby-lotion smell – if you can find unscented and uncolored baby products they may be worth considering, providing the other ingredients are OK.

So what should the other ingredients be? That is a hard question to answer. In an ideal world, the products should not contain any of the ingredients listed in this book (i.e., those having adverse effects). In practice this is almost impossible. Baby products contain the same wide range of preservatives as any other product and most preservatives have restrictions applied to the amount that can be used, presumably because larger quantities are considered to be potentially harmful. Choose a product that contains just one preservative rather than a list of three or four. In fact, it is best to choose the product that has the smallest possible list of ingredients. The longer the list, the greater the chance that your baby will have an adverse reaction to one of them, or to a combination of two or more ingredients which, on their own, are normally harmless.

WHEN CAN I START TO USE STANDARD PRODUCTS?

As a rule of thumb you can start to use regular toiletries when your child turns three. Your child will now have a functional immune system and can easily cope with normal levels of microbes in standard products. Relatively few cosmetic ingredients have age restrictions placed on their use, and almost all such restrictions lapse at the age of three. One exception is hydroquinone, which is used in local skin-lightening products and some oxidation hair colors; this should not be used by children under the age of 12 (from February 29, 2000 its use in skin-lightening products sold in the EU was prohibited completely). Having said that, there is no reason why you should not continue to use baby soap and shampoo for a few more years. If you do switch to regular products, start with fairly simple ones. As already said, avoid brightly colored or highly perfumed toiletries and go for products with short, simple lists of ingredients. If you stick to simple products your child will be less likely to suffer any adverse effects.

WHAT ARE THE DANGER SIGNS?

Very young babies cannot tell you that they are itching and they will not have sufficiently developed motor skills or co-ordination to scratch. The best they can do is cry. Look out for red or discolored patches, raised patches, a rash or flaking skin, or any other skin condition that does not seem normal. If the problem is on your baby's head it may be caused by the shampoo you are using, but since you are most likely to wash your baby's hair in the bath, the problem may occur on other parts of the body as well. Of course the condition may be unrelated to toiletries. Cradle cap – characterized by flaking, yellow scales on the scalp – is surprisingly common and easily treated at home. If the standard cradle-cap treatments (available over the counter), do not clear up the problem in a week or so, consult your doctor. It may be a more serious condition like seborrheic dermatitis, which can also appear on the face, neck, behind the ears, and in the diaper (nappy) area.

If the baby's skin does become sore in the diaper area, it is likely to be the start of diaper rash – a reaction to chemicals contained in the urine and feces. The best treatment is to prevent diaper rash in the first place. The area must be kept as dry as possible and regular changing is essential. A waterproof layer of an emollient such as petroleum jelly will help to keep these chemicals away from the skin. If the skin starts to look red or sore, it is tempting to think that you should use more of the emollient, but it is possible that the emollient itself is the cause of the problem. If the condition worsens when you apply more cream, stop using it and try another product. If the condition does not improve, seek medical advice.

It is worth remembering that diaper rash may be the first sign that your baby has sensitive skin and may have more problems with cosmetics and toiletries in the future. Keep a close eye on your child's skin and be ready to swap toiletries if a persistent problem occurs. Sensitive skin may also burn easily, so make certain your child is adequately protected from the sun. Do not expose your baby to strong sunshine before the age of six months. After that, limit the exposure time to short periods at first, and avoid the noonday sun when it is at its strongest. Even when your child's skin is tanned, continue using a good sunscreen, with an SPF of at least 15. Make sure the sunscreen is suitable for children too.

WHAT ELSE SHOULD I KNOW?

There are several cosmetic ingredients that are banned from products intended for use on children under the age of three, and several more that are not recommended for use on infants. These are listed below. None of these ingredients should be used in baby products so there should be no problem, providing you stick to products designed specifically for babies and infants.

Banned Ingredients for Babies

EU regulations state that the following ingredients must not be used in products for children under the age of three:

- Boric Acid
- Calcium Salicylate*
- Magnesium Salicylate*
- MEA-Salicylate*
- Potassium Salicylate*
- Salicylic Acid*
- Sodium Salicylate*

* May be used in shampoo for children under the age of three.

The use of hydroquinone in skin lighteners was prohibited in the EU from February 29, 2000. Before that date, skin lighteners containing this ingredient had to carry a warning that they were not to be used on children under the age of 12.

Don't be tempted to color or perm a child's hair. These products contain harsh chemicals that are likely to irritate the child's skin. Several hair dyes and perms contain chemicals that are banned from use in children's products or are not recommended for use on children.

Baby powders that contain talc are harmful if inhaled. Don't use talc anywhere near the baby's mouth or nose, and make sure that neither you nor your baby accidentally inhales the dust.

You don't really need to buy all-over body wash for your baby. This is the child's equivalent of shower gel or body shampoo, but soap has an excellent safety record and a good brand or a well-known store brand of baby soap is probably even safer. Why expose your child to a cocktail of detergents, foam boosters, thickeners, preservatives, colorants, and fragrances when you can use something as simple as soap?

Consider washing your baby's hair with a mild baby shampoo, then foregoing the conditioner. Your child's hair is unlikely to need conditioning and is probably far better off without being constantly coated with the chemical residues of the surfactants, oils, antistatic agents, preservatives, and so on. A conditioner will make your child's hair more greasy, requiring you to wash it more often – resulting in even more exposure to cosmetic chemicals.

When you are out and about, moist tissue wipes are a godsend when your baby needs changing, but you should not use them at home. These wipes are full of chemicals like alcohol, preservatives, fragrances, surfactants, moisturizers, and antimicrobials and constant exposure to these ingredients may cause skin problems, if not now, then later in the child's life. Soap and warm water, using suitable disposable tissues or a towel, is probably much safer in the long run than relying on chemical wipes that are not rinsed off.

Some colorants are not allowed to be used in products that remain on the skin for any length of time. They can, however, be used in products like shampoo and shower gel that are rinsed away soon after application. You may well ask, if it is not safe for these colorants to be in contact with skin for more than a few minutes at the most, then why should they be applied to my child's skin (or my own) at all? The colorants you may wish to avoid are listed below.

Harmful Colorants

The following dyes are harmful or irritant by prolonged contact with the skin. EU regulations state that they are allowed only in products that are rinsed off immediately after use:

CI 10006	CI 20040	CI 45220	CI 11725
CI 20470	CI 50325	CI 12120	CI 21100
CI 51319	CI 12370	CI 27290	CI 60724
CI 12420	CI 28440	CI 61585	CI 12480
CI 40215	CI 62045	CI 12700	CI 42080
CI 73900	CI 15620	CI 42100	CI 73915
CI 18130	CI 42170	CI 74100	CI 18690
CI 42520	CI 74180	CI 18736	CI 45100
CI 18820	CI 45190		

Finally, keep all cosmetics and toiletries out of reach of young children. There are several more general safety tips in *Chapter 13 – Common Sense and Cosmetic Safety.*

ARE BABY PRODUCTS BETTER FOR ME?

Yes, if you don't mind smelling like a baby! Generally speaking, products for babies are milder than those for adults. They usually have fewer ingredients, less color and fragrance, and contain fewer microbes. If you find that some standard toiletries don't agree with you, baby products may be the answer. The downside is that they have lower levels of microbial contamination only because they tend to have higher levels of preservatives than an equivalent formulation for adults. These preservatives may be the cause of the problems in the first place (see *Chapter 4 – Preservatives*). The bars of soap may also be irritatingly small, and may work out more expensive to buy.

FACE PAINTS – TOYS OR COSMETICS?

Children's face paints are not explicitly mentioned in either the FDA's *Cosmetic Safety Handbook* or in the EU Cosmetics Directive. The UK Department of Trade and Industry's *A Guide to the Cosmetic Products (Safety) Regulations* gives an illustrative list of products that are covered by these regulations, and the nearest it gets to children's face paints is, "Products for making up and removing make-up from the face and eyes." This does not adequately define face paints as cosmetics. Inspection of the toy-shop shelves' clearly shows that manufacturers interpret the rules in different ways. Some brands of face paints are not labelled and do not list the colorants or ingredients on or inside the package. Other brands clearly list all the ingredients using their INCI names, following the labeling laws of the EU.

In the absence of firm guidance, common sense must prevail. The law is very simple. Retailers cannot sell products that are unsafe and, in the EU, toys must comply with the 1995 EU Toy Safety Regulations. This may not be fully reassuring to a concerned parent, so you might be well advised not to buy products that are inadequately labeled. But having a list of ingredients on the box is still no guarantee that the product is safe. Restrictions have been placed on the use of a large number of colorants. Some colors must not be used in products that remain on the skin for any length of time, while others must not be used in products applied near the eyes or mucous membranes. The restricted colorants are listed below. Do not buy face paints containing these colorants – they are certain to be used near the eyes, and there is not a child alive who will not transfer the paint from their face to the mucous membrane of their mouth.

Colorants That May Cause Eye Damage

EU regulations state that the following colorants are not allowed to be used in any product intended for use on or near the eyes:

CI 10316 (Ext. D&C Yellow #7)
CI 15510 (D&C Orange #4)
CI 26100 (D&C Red #17)
CI 45405
CI 74260

See also *Chapter 11 – Make-up* for a list of colorants banned by the FDA from use in eye products.

More Harmful Colorants

EU regulations state that the following colorants are banned from products that are intended for use on or near the mucous membranes of the eyelids, mouth, nose, respiratory tract, or genitals:

Acid Blue 1	CI 20170
Acid Green 1	CI 21108
Acid Orange 24	CI 21230
Acid Red 195	CI 24790
Acid Violet 43	CI 42045
Basic Blue 26	CI 42510
Basic Violet 14	CI 42735
CI10020	CI 44045
CI 11680	CI 47000
CI 11710	CI 50420
CI 12010	CI 59040 (D&C Green #8)
CI 15800 (D&C Red #31)	CI 60730 (Ext. D&C Violet #2)
CI 16230	CI71105

Even if the colorants used have no restrictions placed on them, many of them will be azo dyes or coal tar dyes, which have known or suspected adverse effects. For this reason it is advisable to remove the face paint after a few hours. Do not let your children wear face paint all day, and certainly do not let them sleep in it. Follow the manufacturer's instructions for removing the paint and make sure none is transferred into the mouth or eyes while doing so. Soap and water should be enough, but if you use a make-up remover, make sure it is suitable for children. You should supervise children while the face paint is being applied and when it is being removed.

Having emphasized the dangers, it must be said that there have been no well-publicized reports of children coming to grief with these products, and face paints generally have a good safety record. However, we seldom hear about the silent but significant number of people who suffer minor skin irritation or soreness after using these products, or other cosmetics.

Theatrical make-up is another gray area not explicitly mentioned in the safety regulations. Professional face painters at fairs, theme parks, and exhibitions sometimes use it on children. Again, it is probably perfectly safe, but don't let your child wear it all day.

Not Suitable for Children

There are a number of ingredients that are not recommended for children under the age of three. These are:

Exfoliants containing the following Alpha- and Beta-Hydroxy Acids:

Alpha-Hydroxy and Botanical Complexes	L-Alpha Hydroxy Acids
Alpha-Hydroxy Ethanoic Acid	Lactic Acid
Alpha-Hydroxy Octanoic Acid	Malic Acid
Ammonium Glycolate	Mixed Fruit Acids
Beta-Hydroxy Complex	Sugar Cane Extract
Beta-Hydroxybutanoic Acid	Tethocanic Acid
Citric Acid	Tropic Acid
Glycolic Acid	
Glycomer in Crosslinked Fatty Acids	
Alpha Natrium	

Depilatories containing:

Hydroxide*

Sulfide*

Thioglycolic Acid*

Thioglycolate*

Oral care products containing Fluoride or Strontium compounds:

Children should only use a small, pea-size portion of toothpaste containing the following fluorides and should be discouraged from swallowing it or any other oral care product containing fluoride:

Fluoride

Fluorosilicate

Monofluorophosphate

Hydrofluoride

Dihydrofluoride

Oral care products containing Strontium acetate* or Strontium chloride* are not recommended for frequent use by young children

Other products:

Progressive hair dyes containing Lead acetate* should not be used on children

* EU regulations require products which contain these ingredients to carry warnings stating that they are not recommended for frequent use by children under the age of three, or that they must be kept out of the reach of children.

11 make-up

Mirror, mirror on the wall
Who is the fairest of them all?

Manufacturers convince us to use their shampoos, conditioners, deodorants, and skincare products by constantly telling us they will improve the health and condition of our skin and hair. The make-up market, on the other hand, is driven by fashion and by the desire of people to make themselves more attractive by highlighting their good features and disguising the blemishes. Young people often use make-up, hair color and clothing to mimic their role models and to identify with a social group. Make-up will be used without encouragement from the manufacturers, who will simply focus their energies on convincing people that their red lipstick is better than another brand because it is hypoallergenic, non-smudging, contains 65 percent moisturizers, is long-lasting, or easy to clean off.

A visit to a make-up factory is usually enough to put most people off from wearing make-up for as long as the memory remains of the large, foul-smelling vats of greasy, molten gunge, or of the giant slabs of the pungent, brightly colored, congealed, waxy lard. This chapter looks at what exactly this stuff is made of.

EYE LINER

Eye liners are decorative cosmetics used to highlight or accentuate the eyes. They may come in the form of colored, water-based paints which are applied with a fine brush, as cakes of pressed talc and magnesium stearate, consolidated with oily ingredients, or thick, waxy creams in the form of a pencil. They are used to draw a thin line on the upper eyelid, just above the line of the eyelashes. They may also be drawn on the lower eyelid, below the lower eyelashes.

TYPICAL INGREDIENTS – EYELINER

Ingredients:

Aqua, Isopropyl alcohol, Ammonium acrylates copolymer, Magnesium aluminum silicate, PEG-75, Stearic acid, Hydroxypropyl methylcellulose, Propylene glycol, Triethanolamine, Methylparaben, Ethylparaben, Sodium laureth sulfate, BHA, [+/- CI 77491, CI 77492, CI 77499, CI 77891].

Aqua	Water – the main ingredient.
Isopropyl alcohol	Solvent which dissolves the other ingredients, aids application and reduces drying time.
Ammonium acrylates copolymer	Film former which forms a thin film on the skin and binds the other ingredients to the skin, thus preventing smudging.
Magnesium aluminum silicate	Thickener giving solidity to the eyeliner.
PEG-75*	Thickener, also aids even spreading.
Stearic acid	Emulsifier to aid the mixing of, and prevent the separation of the other ingredients.
Hydroxypropyl methylcellulose*	Thickener.
Propylene glycol*	Humectant which prevents the product from drying out.
Triethanolamine*	Controls acidity in the eyeliner. It is limited to 2.5 percent of the finished product.
Methylparaben*	Water-soluble preservative, limited to 0.4 percent of the finished product.[+]
Ethylparaben*	Water-soluble preservative, limited to 0.4 percent of the finished product.[+]
Sodium laureth sulfate*	Surfactant, aids even spreading.

BHA*	Antioxidant, preventing deterioration of the product through exposure to oxygen in the air.

The product may contain some or all of the following colors in varying proportions. They are all purified forms of natural minerals:

CI 77491	Iron oxide – Red form.
CI 77492	Iron oxide – Yellow form.
CI 77499	Iron oxide – Black form.
CI 77891	Titanium dioxide – White.

* These ingredients are subject to restrictions or have been linked to harmful or adverse effects.

+ Indicates that this ingredient may be used in larger quantities if it is used for another specified purpose other than as a preservative.

Eye liners may contain natural or petroleum-derived waxes softened with solvents or oils, or they may be water based, containing surfactants, film formers, emulsifiers, and thickeners. They all contain colorants, antioxidants, and preservatives. Since they are to be used near the eyes, eye liners are Category-1 cosmetics and subject to stringent regulations concerning the level of microbial infection in the product. They must, therefore, contain sufficient levels of preservatives to comply with the regulations (see *Chapter 4 – Preservatives* for further details).

EYE SHADOW

Eye shadow is used to enhance the appearance of the eyes. It is commonly available in the form of creams, powders, cakes, and gels. The creams usually contain either natural waxes such as beeswax or carnauba wax, or petroleum-based waxes such as ozokerite or ceresin, mixed in an oily emulsion. Powders and cakes are based on talc, kaolin, and magnesium stearate. Gels are water-based suspensions of insoluble pigments (lakes), thickened with methylcellulose or crosslinked polymers (carbomers).

All of these products contain surfactants to aid spreading, film formers to give an even, unbroken coat, and pH controllers to prevent skin oils or tears from altering the colors. Preservatives and antioxidants are added to increase the shelf life of the product. Some manufacturers add silicone polymers (methicones) to make the eye shadow run resistant. Proteins, vitamins, and pro-vitamins may be added for marketing reasons, but these add little to the effectiveness of the product or to the health of the skin.

MASCARA

Mascara is applied to the eyelashes to both thicken and darken them. This frames the eyes making them appear larger and more alluring. As you age, your eyelashes become thinner and lighter in color, and mascara has the effect of making the eyes appear more youthful.

Liquid mascara is convenient to use, but cake mascara is gaining in popularity again. Modern mascaras contain a number of ingredients to stop them from running or becoming brittle and flaking into your eyes. They usually come in dark colors, mainly black, brown, or deep blue. Liquid mascara is water based, sometimes with some alcohol added to help dissolve the ingredients. Waxes such as beeswax, carnauba wax or microcrystalline wax (cera microcristallina), reinforced with proteins, fibers of nylon or rayon, or synthetic polymers or resins, add thickness to the lashes and render the mascara waterproof and smudge resistant. Vegetable oils are added to prevent the mascara from drying out and becoming brittle, and surfactants and film formers are included to help it spread easily and evenly. The usual range of antioxidants and preservatives are added too. Cake mascaras contain similar ingredients but are often made in a soap base.

Mascara is a Category-1 cosmetic and subject to strict microbe contamination standards. It is important that no microbes are allowed to breed in your mascara. If you get an eye infection such as conjunctivitis (red eye), throw away all eye make-up you are using at the time, and don't use any eye make-up until the infection clears up. Never share eye make-up, and never dilute it, especially by spitting into your cake of mascara.

TYPICAL INGREDIENTS – MASCARA

Ingredients:

Aqua, PVP, PVP/Hexadecene Copolymer, PEG-75, Carnauba, Cera alba, Magnesium aluminum silicate, Oleic acid, Cetyl alcohol, Cera microcristallina, Butylene glycol, PEG-20 Methyl glucose sesquistearate, Phenoxyethanol, Sodium phosphate, Disodium phosphate, Butylparaben, Ethylparaben, Methylparaben, Propylparaben, BHA, [+/- CI 77007, CI 77491, CI 77492, CI 77499, CI 77891].

Aqua	Water – the main ingredient.
PVP* and PVP/Hexadecene	Film formers which form a thick film on the eyelashes,
Copolymer*	binds the other ingredients together, and prevents smudging.
PEG-75*	Thickener, and aids even spreading.
Carnauba*	Plant-derived wax. Texture modifier.
Cera alba*	Beeswax. Texture modifier.
Magnesium aluminum silicate	Thickener giving solidity to the mascara.
Oleic acid*	Emulsifier to bind the other ingredients together.
Cetyl alcohol*	Emulsifier to bind the other ingredients together.
Cera microcristallina	Petroleum-derived wax. Texture modifier.
Butylene glycol	Humectant. Prevents the complete drying of the mascara, keeping it flexible and preventing it from flaking.
PEG-20 Methyl glucose sesquistearate*	Emulsifier to bind the other ingredients together.
Phenoxyethanol*	Preservative (limited to 1 percent of the finished product). +
Sodium phosphate	Controls acidity in the mascara.
Disodium phosphate	Controls acidity in the mascara.
Butylparaben,* Ethylparaben,* Methylparaben,* and Propylparaben*	Paraben preservatives are limited to a total maximum amount of 0.8 percent and individually to 0.4 per cent. +
BHA*	Antioxidant, preventing deterioration of the product through exposure to oxygen in the air.

The product may contain some or all of the following colors in varying proportions. They are all purified forms of natural minerals:

CI 77007, CI 77491, CI 77492, CI 77499 and CI 77891.

* These ingredients are subject to restrictions or have been linked to harmful or adverse effects.

+ Indicates that this ingredient may be used in larger quantities if it is used for another specified purpose other than as a preservative.

FOUNDATION

Foundation, as the name suggests, forms a base over which other make-up is applied. It comes in a variety of forms such as powders, cakes, or creams, having a subtle color designed to tone in with the skin and to give an even hue to the whole of your face. It can cover up minor skin blemishes such as freckles, or skin that had been darkened or reddened by the sun. If a cream foundation leaves a sheen or glossy appearance, talc-based powders can be applied to dull the finish. Foundation, like any make-up, should not be applied to broken, sore, inflamed, or infected skin. Medicated foundation creams are now available, however, to disguise acnegenic skin.

Foundation creams are often water based and contain thickeners, film formers, oils and waxes, emulsifiers to keep the oils and water evenly mixed, surfactants to aid the even spreading of the cream, and, of course, the inevitable preservatives, antioxidants, and colorants.

Your skin secretes a cocktail of chemicals and, during the day, the pH (acidity level) of your skin changes. These acids can change the color of your make-up, so, like much other colored make-up, your foundation will probably contain ingredients that counteract this acid and maintain a constant pH on your skin. These pH controlling chemicals are called buffers. Oily sebum secretions can also discolor make-up, so absorbents are sometimes added to foundation creams to prevent darkening or discoloration caused by your body's sebum.

POWDERS

Loose powders and pressed powders (cakes) are used to reduce the gloss of oily skin or foundation and form the base of blushers (rouge) highlighters and shaders. They are basically mixtures of minerals: mainly talc and kaolin with magnesium and calcium or zinc stearate to aid adhesion. Pressed powders contain a higher proportion of stearates to bind the powder together than do loose powders. Pigments such as zinc oxide or titanium dioxide increase the covering power, and chalk enhances the matt finish. Pigments (or lakes) are added in varying amounts to obtain a range of colors from neutral to strong tones. Since microbes cannot feed on minerals such as talc and kaolin, the level of preservatives found in powders is often lower than in other cosmetics. However, manufacturers often add proteins, amino acids, vitamins, and other additives for marketing reasons, which may require the level of preservatives to be increased.

Inhaling mineral dust is harmful and can cause breathing difficulties, allergies, or more serious lung diseases.

LIPSTICK AND LIP GLOSS

Lipsticks can be purchased in the form of waxy sticks, pencils, creams, liquid paints, and gels. They are used cosmetically to highlight the lips, or can be applied as a medical treatment for damaged, infected, or inflamed lips.

Waxy lipsticks contain natural waxes such as beeswax or carnauba wax, or waxes such as ozokerite, ceresin or microcrystalline wax (cera microcristallina), which are derived from petroleum. The waxes are softened with mineral or vegetable oils, or with petroleum jelly. Film formers are added to help the product spread evenly over the lips and remain in place. Colorants and preservatives are added, and since there is such a high concentration of waxes and oils, antioxidants are frequently added as well. Moisturizers such as lanolin, PEG derivatives or silicone (methicone or dimethicone) derivatives are added to keep the lips moist, and some lipsticks contain UV absorbers to protect the lips from the sun.

Cream lipsticks contain essentially the same ingredients but the proportion of wax is much lower. Lip pencils, on the other hand, have more wax and less of the oily ingredients used to soften the wax.

TYPICAL INGREDIENTS – LIPSTICK

Ingredients:

Ricinus communis, Ozokerite, Cera alba, Aceylated lanolin alcohol, Cetyl acetate, Cera microcristallina, Stearalkonium bentonite, Carnauba, Butylparaben, Propylene glycol, Lanolin, Propyl gallate, Citric acid, Aqua, Benzophenone-3, [+/- Titanium dioxide, Mica, CI 15850, CI 15880, CI 19140, CI 45410, CI 77007, CI 77491, CI 77492, CI 77499, CI 77510.]

Ricinus communis*	Castor oil to soften the waxes.
Ozokerite	Wax derived from petroleum (also spelled ozocerite).
Cera alba*	Beeswax.
Aceylated lanolin alcohol	Emulsifier to aid mixing of ingredients.
Cetyl acetate	Moisturizer and solvent.
Cera microcristallina	Hard, petroleum-derived wax which also acts as an emulsion stabilizer and binding agent to prevent the ingredients from separating.
Stearalkonium bentonite	Viscosity adjuster derived from bentonite clay, which controls the thickness of the lipstick.
Carnauba	Plant-derived wax which aids the formation of a thin film on the lips.
Propylene glycol*	Humectant to prevent the lipstick from drying out. Also acts as a solvent and has moisturizing properties.
Lanolin*	Moisturizer.
Propyl gallate*	Antioxidant.
Butylparaben*	Preservative. Restricted to 0.4 percent of the product.[+]
Citric acid	Controls acidity and improves the antioxidant properties of propyl gallate.
Aqua	Water – adds moisture to the lipstick.
Benzophenone-3*	UV absorber, also called oxybenzone. It prevents the fading of the colorants and protects the lips from UV rays in sunlight.

The product may contain some or all of the following colors in varying proportions: CI 15850* (red azo dye), CI 15880*(red azo dye), CI 19140* (yellow azo dye), CI 45410 (syntheic red dye), CI 77510 (Prussian blue made from iron salts and cyanide).

The remaining colorants are all purified forms of natural minerals:
Titanium dioxide (CI 77891) (white), Mica (black/silver sparkles), CI 77007 (blue), CI 77491 (brick-red), CI 77492 (yellow), CI 77499 (black).

* These ingredients are subject to restrictions or have been linked to harmful or adverse effects.

+ Indicates that this ingredient may be used in larger quantities if it is used for another specified purpose other than as a preservative.

Water-based lipsticks contain mainly water, thickened with methylcellulose or natural gums. Colorants, together with the usual range of preservatives and film formers, are added and sometimes a little alcohol is added to speed up drying.

It's a Fact

Many manufacturers advertise the fact that their "New Improved" make-up "Now contains 65 percent moisturizers." This is hardly surprising since oily and waxy ingredients form the bulk of many types of make-up, especially lipstick. These ingredients form a waterproof film on your skin, which prevents evaporation of water and keeps your skin and lips moisturized.

Lip gloss is usually a non-greasy gel that gives a shine to the lips. It contains an oil-in-water emulsion or a mineral oil made into a gel by mixing it with bentonite clay. It is usually neutral or only lightly colored, and contains the usual range of film formers and preservatives. Lip gloss is sometimes used over a lipstick to enhance its gloss.

Lip balm and chapsticks form a greasy film over the lips to moisten them if they are dry or chapped. They usually contain a UV absorber to prevent further damage from the sun, and may contain some medication. They are usually uncolored or very lightly colored.

Since lipstick is used near the mucous membrane of the mouth, it is a Category-1 cosmetic and subject to strict EU regulations concerning levels of microbial contamination.

Colorants That May Be Harmful To Eyes

The following colorants and lakes of these colorants have been certified by the FDA for use in all cosmetics except for products that are intended for use on or near the eyes.

D&C Red #6 (CI 15850)	D&C Red #27 (CI 45410)	FD&C Green #3 (CI 42053)
D&C Red #7 (CI 15850)	D&C Red # 28 (CI 45410)	FD&C Yellow #5 (CI 19140)
D&C Red #21	D&C Red #30 (CI 73360)	FD&C Yellow #6 (CI 15985)
D&C Red #22	D&C Yellow #10	

The following colorants and lakes of these colorants have been certified by the FDA for use in all externally applied cosmetics except for products that are intended for use on or near the eyes.

D&C Blue #4	D&C Orange #11	D&C Yellow #7 (CI 45350:1)
D&C Brown #1	D&C Red #17 (CI 26100)	D&C Yellow #8 (CI 45350)
D&C Green #6 (CI 61565)	D&C Red #31 (CI 15800)	D&C Yellow #11
D&C Green #8 (CI 59040)	D&C Red #33	Ext. D&C Violet #2 (CI 60730)
D&C Orange #4 (CI 15510)	D&C Red #34 (CI 15880)	Ext. D&C Yellow #7 (CI 10316)
D&C Orange #5	D&C Red #36 (CI 12085)	FD&C Red #4 (CI 14700)
D&C Orange #10	D&C Violet #2	

The following colorants and lakes of these colorants are subject to additional restrictions:

D&C Green #8	- limited to 0.01 percent of the finished product
D&C Orange #5	- limited to 5 percent of the finished lip product
D&C Red #33	- limited to 3 percent of the finished lip product
D&C Red #36	- limited to 3 percent of the finished lip product

12 nail care

If you eat a box of jelly for three days in a row,
You can be assured that it won't help your nails grow.
Neither will it make them less inclined to break;
The best that it can do for you is cause a belly ache.

The state of our nails reveals a great deal about our lifestyles, habits, personalities, and health. Well-manicured nails suggest a measure of wealth. Clean, unbroken nails are more likely to be found in professional workers than in manual workers or dish-washing veterans. Chewed nails suggest bad habits, stress, or a nervous disorder, and nails that are stained yellow are typical of someone who smokes. For this reason we spend a great deal of money on manicures and nail cosmetics. What follows is a scientific description of our nails, some basic guidance on how to look after them, and a review of the cosmetic products we use to pamper our nails.

WHAT ARE NAILS?

Like hair and skin, nails (correctly called onyx) are composed of the tough, fibrous protein called keratin. The main part of the nail is called the nail plate. This is attached to the underlying skin, which is called the nail bed. Around the edges of the nail, the skin forms a nail fold which wraps around, and overlaps, the edges of the nail. The cuticle is a thin flap of skin that covers the nail fold and is attached to the nail plate. Its job is to prevent dirt and microbes from going under the nail fold where they may start an infection.

How Fast do Nails Grow?

On average your nails grow 0.5 mm (0.02 inches) each week, but this can vary from as little as 0.05 mm (0.002 inches) to as much as 1.2 mm (0.15 inches) per week. Children's nails grow faster than those of adults, and elderly people's grow even more slowly. Nails grow faster in the summer and in warmer climates, and fingernails grow faster than toenails – probably relecting the lower temperature of the feet, resulting in slower blood circulation and therefore less nourishment and oxygen reaching the toes. Nails grow faster on the middle fingers and slower on the thumbs and take, on average, five to seven months to grow out completely. Toenails take twice as long as this.

The nail grows from the germinal matrix at the beginning of the nail. The cells start as living, jelly-like structures, which gradually die and turn their cell contents into keratin. The lunula, the pale-colored half moon, is a midway stage between the living cells in the germinal matrix and the dead cells in the nail plate. The nail plate has no nerves and no blood supply, so it has no sensation of pain. When it grows out from the nail bed to form the free edge, we can file and trim it because it has no nerves. The lunula and the nail bed, however, are rich in nerve endings and quite sensitive to touch and pain.

LOOKING AFTER YOUR NAILS

Nails are constantly under attack. They can become chipped and dirty while working, chewed, or stained while smoking. Nails can become brittle or split through poor diet or illness, or they can become seriously discolored through nail infections caused by bacteria or fungi. Long nails are more likely to catch on things and be damaged or lifted from the nail plate. Repeated damage can result in the loss of a nail.

There are a number of cosmetic products that can improve the appearance of your nails and there are a number of simple remedies for cleaning off dirt and stains. If you suspect discoloration may be caused by an infection or illness, you should seek medical advice and not use nail make-up until your doctor tells you it is safe to do so.

Old Wives' Tales – Jelly is Good for Your Nails

This, alas, is not true. The proteins in gelatin may be similar to the proteins in your nails, but once you have digested them, they will be broken down to amino acids and used in any part of your body where needed. The amino acids do not know you want them to go to your nails.

Removing Stains from Nails

Stains on nails may be caused by nicotine from cigarettes, remnants of nail polish, hair dye, or chemicals. The stains can usually be removed by gently wiping the nails with a mixture of one teaspoon of domestic bleach in ten teaspoons of water. A cotton bud is ideal for this but do not allow the bleach to stay on the nails for too long, and try to avoid getting it on the surrounding cuticle or skin. Afterwards, rinse your nails thoroughly and apply an oily moisturizing cream. For more severe stains that do not respond to bleach you can try buffing the nails, but this removes the outer layer and makes them thinner and weaker.

Colored nail polish will hide the stains, but if all else fails, you will have to wait until the nail grows out and takes the stain with it. Never use bleach to try to remove marks such as bruises or discoloration caused by infections, as these are under the nail plate. Bruises, and some other marks under the nail, will eventually fade or grow out. Meanwhile they can be disguised with colored nail polish.

Old Wives' Tales – Herbal Nail Care

Horsetail infusion in water is said to remove white specks from fingernails.

Dirty marks and stains under the free edge of the fingernails can be removed with nail bleach, which can be purchased as a cream containing a variety of buffing agents, bleaching agents, and white colorants, or you can make up your own bleach as described above. Stains caused by processing fruits or vegetables can often be removed by digging the nails into a slice of lemon. Pencils containing white pigments such as titanium dioxide or zinc oxide in a soap base can also disguise stains under the free edge.

NAIL POLISH

Nail polish, also called nail varnish or nail enamel, is usually an acrylic polymer or another resin, dissolved in a solvent, with colors added. These may be reinforced with strands of nylon or other fibers, and plasticizers are added to allow a little flexibility to prevent cracking. Surfactants and film formers allow the polish to spread easily and evenly, and to stick to the nail. Proteins and vitamins added to nail cosmetics are not absorbed by the nail, and do not therefore have a therapeutic effect either on the nail plate, the nail fold, or on the cuticle.

Nail polish is painted onto the nails and allowed to harden as the solvent evaporates. Since fingers are usually warmer than toes, nail polish often dries faster on fingernails. Shaking the nail polish before it is applied is often recommended, but this can produce small bubbles in the polish that can spoil the finish. Rolling the bottle between your palms prevent bubbles forming, and the warmth of your hands will thin the polish, allowing an even coat to be painted on. Make sure your nails are dry and free from oily residues from hand or moisturizing creams, as nail polish will not stick to greasy or wet nails.

Nails have natural furrows and ridges. It is not advisable to buff these off before applying nail polish as it makes the nails thinner and more likely to split. This will lock you into a cycle of using more nail products such as nail hardeners and nail strengtheners. A clear nail polish can be applied before the colored polish. This will act as a base coat, filling in the furrows and ridges and preventing the pigments in the nail polish from soaking into and staining the nail plate.

NAIL POLISH REMOVER

Nail polish remover is a solvent that dissolves the nail polish. Acetone, ethyl acetate, butyl acetate and amyl acetate are commonly used solvents, but these will also remove the natural oils from the nail and surrounding skin. If you use these solvents, follow it with an oil-based hand cream. Nail polish removers based on oil-in-water emulsions take a little longer to dissolve the polish but they are less damaging to the nails.

NAIL BUFFERS

Nail buffers contain an abrasive powder such as iron oxide (jeweller's rouge), kaolin, talc, and stannic acid. These grind away the surface of the nail to produce a shine and the polishing action stimulates blood flow to the nail bed, improving the pink color of the nails but making them thinner and weaker, and more likely to split.

NAIL LENGTHENERS, STRENGTHENERS, AND HARDENERS

Nail lengtheners are products that help the free edge of the nail to grow without being chewed, chipped, split, or otherwise damaged. Nail strengtheners are similar to nail polishes but are formulated to produce a thicker, reinforced coating. They may be clear or colored. Nail hardeners contain formaldehyde resins. They stick to the nails and form a very hard film. Many people are allergic to formaldehyde resins or are sensitive to formaldehyde. It is also a cancer suspect, so it is essential not to allow the resin to touch the surrounding nail fold or cuticle. In the EU, regulations require the label on nail hardeners containing formaldehyde to warn you to protect your cuticle with grease or oil before using the product.

ARTIFICIAL NAILS

Artificial nails are made of plastic and are glued onto the nail plate. These can greatly improve the appearance of damaged or discolored nails and will prevent nails from being chewed. As the nail grows a small gap appears at the end of the nail. This can be filled in with an acrylic or gel-based nail strengthener. The artificial nails must be regularly inspected for signs of lifting. If water gets in between the nail plate and the artificial nail, bacteria will breed and the water will soften the nail plate, allowing the bacteria to eat their way through to the nail bed.

Artificial nails can be removed by softening the glue with a solvent. Acetonitrile-based solvents should be avoided because they are extremely poisonous; they are banned from sale in the EU.

CUTICLE SOFTENERS

Before the cuticle is pushed back during a manicure, a cuticle softener is applied to both loosen and soften the cuticle. A cuticle softener usually contains water to soften the skin, surfactants to speed up the wetting and softening process, and oils to moisturize the skin and nail. Emulsifiers and emulsion stabilizers are often added, allowing the oily ingredients and water to mix. Preservatives are added to kill microbes that get into the softener, and antimicrobials control any microbes on your skin or nails, preventing them from starting an infection under the nail fold. The usual collection of fragrances and colors are added, and often unnecessary additives, such as vitamins, plant extracts, amino acids, and proteins are included in the ingredients. Some cuticle softeners contain exfoliants such as alpha- or beta-hydroxy acids. These dissolve the proteins in skin and soften the cuticle more effectively.

Cuticle solvents can be used as an alternative to cuticle softeners. These are solutions containing a strong alkali such as sodium, or potassium hydroxide, which dissolves the cuticle. Great care must be taken with cuticle solvents, as they are highly corrosive substances.

13 common sense and cosmetic safety

If sense is so common, why don't more people have it?

The responsibility for cosmetic safety falls into four areas. The regulating authorities set the ground rules for the safe production and sale of cosmetics and toiletries, and they police the industry, taking action whenever the rules are infringed or new problems arise. Reputable manufactures follow these rules and work to the highest possible standards to ensure the consumers' safety. The retailers, hairdressers, and beauticians make sure the products are safely stored, used correctly, and sold hygienically and they are available to give professional advice when needed. Finally, you are responsible for the safe keeping and use of cosmetics and toiletries in your home. And it is here that many problems start. What follows is a list of common-sense precautions that will make your bathroom cabinet safer.

FOLLOW THE INSTRUCTIONS

Always read the labels and follow the instructions. Never over-apply the cosmetic, especially potent products like hair removers, skin lighteners, hair dyes, and hair-perm formulations, and if you develop an irritation, itching, soreness, or any other symptoms, stop using that product immediately and try another brand.

TYPICAL INGREDIENTS – FAMILY BUBBLE BATH

Ingredients:

Aqua, Sodium laureth sulfate, Parfum, Cocamidopropyl betaine, PEG-90M, Tetrasodium EDTA, Formaldehyde, Citric acid, Benzophenone-4, [+/- CI 15985, CI 17200, CI 42090, CI 47005]

This is a brightly colored product sold in large, clear plastic bottles.

Aqua	Water – the main ingredient.
Sodium laureth sulfate*	Surfactant used to create a foam.
Parfum	A mixture of fragrance chemicals, often more than 50 in number, many of which are artificial.
Cocamidopropyl betaine*	A surfactant and foam booster to create a large quantity of stable foam.
PEG-90M*	A thickening agent to disguise the watery nature of the other ingredients.
Tetrasodium EDTA	Chelating agent to remove calcium and magnesium ions from hard water, which would otherwise impede the formation of foam.
Formaldehyde*	An inexpensive preservative. It is limited to 0.2 percent of the finished product. It is a cancer suspect and is banned from cosmetics in Sweden and Japan.
Citric acid*	This controls the acidity of the product.
Benzophenone-4*	This is a UV absorber which prevents daylight from fading the brightly colored dyes in this product. It is an unnecessary ingredient used to protect unnecessary colorants, none of which improves the quality of the bubbles.

This product may contain some of the following colorants:

CI 15985*	Red azo dye.
CI 17200*	Red azo dye.
CI 42090*	Blue coal tar dye.
CI 47005*	Yellow coal tar dye.

* These ingredients are subject to restrictions or have been linked to harmful or adverse effects.

Soaking in a bath containing foaming bath oils or bubble-bath formulations is a common source of skin and urinary tract irritation. Follow the instructions carefully and do not add more than the specified quantity of the foaming agent to the bath. There is a hidden risk with family bubble-bath products. Many of these are supplied as brightly colored liquids in large containers. These tend to fade in daylight so UV absorbers (like benzophenone-3 or benzophenone-4), are frequently added to preserve the color. It could be argued that these are unnecessary ingredients added to preserve unnecessary colorants, since neither the colorants nor the UV absorbers will improve the quality of the bubbles. Annex VII of the EU Cosmetics Directive gives a list of permitted and provisionally permitted UV filters that cosmetic products may contain. It also states that,

Other UV filters used in cosmetic products solely for the purpose of protecting the product against UV rays are not included in this list.

This suggests that, providing the product is not intended to be applied to the skin to protect it from the harmful effects of UV rays, manufacturers are free to use a wide range of ingredients, including ingredients that are not on the list of permitted UV filters, to preserve their products. Are you happy to pour these chemicals, which are not on the permitted list, into the bath and allow your children to play in them?

If there is a "Best before" date on the product, do not use it after this date has expired. These dates are compulsory in the EU if the product is expected to deteriorate within 30 months of manufacture. If there is a date printed on the packet, this is a clear indication from the manufacturer that they have carried out tests on the product and expect to it deteriorate during storage and use. FDA rules do not require a date on products sold in the USA, and they even advise consumers that any dates that are printed on containers should be taken as rules of thumb and treated as rough guides only. But reputable manufacturers *do* have the consumers' interests at heart (or at least, they don't want to be sued), so you should make use of these "best guess" dates and not use a product if the expiry date has passed.

DOS AND DON'TS

If a product develops a bad smell, or its color changes, or a clear liquid becomes cloudy, it is a strong indication that mold, fungi, or bacteria are breeding in the preparation and you should dispose of it immediately. Oxygen attacks fatty or oily substances, giving the product a rancid smell and, once again, you should throw it away immediately if this happens.

You can reduce the risk of microbial infection and oxidation by following a few simple rules:

- **Never share cosmetics**. Manufacturers add preservatives to kill any microbes that get into the product during manufacture and any that could infect the product during normal use, but if two or more people are adding microbes to the cosmetic there may be insufficient preservative to deal with them all. Sharing cosmetics is also a good way to transfer bacteria from one person to another.
- **Make sure your hands are clean** when using cosmetics and toiletries. Dirty hands will introduce bacteria to the cosmetic, and from there germs will be passed on, to infect other parts of your body.
- **Never spit into your mascara**. Bacteria will breed in it and you will transfer it to your eyes.
- Similarly, **never clean grit from your contact lenses or moisten them by licking them** or putting them in your mouth. Always use a quality contact-lens cleaning solution, then rinse the lenses in sterile water or saline solution before putting them back into your eyes. Make sure your lens cleaning solution can kill acanthamoeba – a common amoeba (or single-celled protozoan), that causes acanthamoeba keratitis, a painful and disabling eye disease.
- **If you dilute cosmetics** for any reason, either to get the last drop of shampoo out of the bottle or to reconstitute something that has dried up, **use it immediately and throw the rest away**. The levels of added preservative are adequate to kill microbes during normal use, but if you reduce this level by diluting it, the preservatives will be unable to kill the microbes effectively, allowing them to breed rapidly. This is especially true if the product

contains nutritious ingredients such as amino acids, proteins, vitamins, or plant extracts.

- **Always store cosmetics and toiletries with the lid on**. If you leave the container open to the air, microbes and oxygen will get in faster than the preservatives and antioxidants can deal with them.
- **Store cosmetics in a cool, dark place**, never on the bathroom windowsill and definately not in a hot car. Light will damage the preservatives, making them less effective at killing microbes, and the heat will encourage growth of bacteria, mold, and fungi. Storing cosmetics in a dark cupboard also keeps them out of the sight of children.
- **Never use cosmetics on broken, sore, or infected skin**. If you do, microbes will be transferred into the product or, worse still, from the cosmetic into your body. Creams, especially moisturizing creams, provide a warm, damp environment on your body in which some bacteria can breed rapidly.
- **If you discover you have an eye infection** such as conjunctivitis (red eye), **throw away all eye cosmetics you were using at the time**. It is possible you got the infection from the cosmetic in the first place and, even if you didn't, it is highly likely you have infected the product, which may then re-infect you some time in the future.
- **Make sure there is no dust or dirt on the outside of the container** when you use it. This is easily transferred onto your hands, then into the cosmetic and onto other parts of your body.
- **During a home or salon manicure, make certain your hands, your nails, and any implements you use, are clean** before you push back the cuticles. Parts of the cuticle, including any dirt and microbes that are on the cuticle, may become lodged under the nail fold, resulting in an infection. This can, in some cases, travel to the nail bed where there is a risk of nail loss. (See *Chapter 12 – Nail Care*.)
- **Never buy a product that has a broken seal**, even if it's on the discount shelf. Rather than ask for a tester, some shoppers like to open the bottles to check the fragrance before they buy it and then leave the rejects on the shelf. There is a small risk of microbial contamination from the nose of the person or people who have smelled it.

AEROSOL SAFETY

Many cosmetics come with their own special problems. Aerosols and pump-action sprays create a mist of fine droplets in the air. Inhaling this mist will put chemicals into your lungs that were never intended to be there. This can lead to breathing disorders and lung disease. Never use aerosols and sprays in the same room as young children or babies. Their lungs are much more susceptible to damage than yours. You are probably safer using roll-on, stick, or gel deodorants and antiperspirants, and hair sprays can be replaced with mousse.

Another problem with aerosols is the propellants are often highly flammable. Never use them near a source of ignition and never smoke while using them. If you have a hairstyle with a lot of volume, flammable gases can be trapped in your hair for several minutes after you have used the sprays.

It's a Fact

A typical 150 ml aerosol deodorant that contains mainly alcohol and propellants, will release about 3.8 MegaJoules of energy if it all burns. This is sufficient energy to lift a 170 pound (12 stone or 76 kg) person over 5000 meters into the air. Of course most of this energy will be wasted as heat, light, and sound in the explosion, which will be used to burn and tear flesh rather than to propel the victim into the air. Warn your teenagers.

ARTIFICIAL NAILS

Artificial nails that are not properly stuck down can lead to bacterial or fungal infections that could result in the loss of your fingernail. If there is a gap between the artificial nail and your fingernail, water and air will get in, providing ideal breeding conditions for microbes, which can attack the proteins in your fingernail already softened by the water trapped against it. If you get a fungal infection under your fingernail it will be unsightly and almost impossible to cure.

Getting artificial nails off again is another problem. Solvents for artificial nail glue can be toxic. Acetonitrile was a common solvent at one time but is so toxic it can be fatal if swallowed, and it is now banned in the EU. Make sure adolescent daughters use artificial nails properly, and it is probably best if you take charge of the remover.

SKIN PEELERS AND AHAs

Skin peelers (exfoliants) are potent products and should be used with caution. They contain keratolytic acids that literally dissolve and remove the outer layer of your skin cells. This exposes more sensitive, deeper layers and effectively makes your skin thinner. This means that you will have less protection from the sun's ultraviolet rays, and that cosmetic chemicals for use on the outside of your body may now be able to penetrate your skin and permeate your bloodstream. If you use skin peelers, cover up against the sun. Use a strong sunscreen with a sun protection factor (SPF) of at least 15 (better still, around 25) and make sure you wear a sun hat. Don't apply other make-up immediately after using a skin peeler.

You may be using skin-peeling cosmetics without being aware of it. Watch out for phrases like "exposes fresher skin" or "dissolves away wrinkles" and check the ingredients for alpha- and beta-hydroxy acids. (See *Chapter 5 – Skin Care* for more details about these.) If any cosmetic makes you sore or leaves your skin itching or sensitive, stop using it. Try writing to the manufacturer and complain about the product – after all, how else are they to know their product is causing problems if you don't tell them?

HIDDEN DANGERS

The reason why so many ingredients are restricted is because they are harmful in large quantities. For example the EU legislation says that the preservative triclosan is restricted to 0.3 percent of the finished product, but if it is used for another stated purpose it can be used in larger quantities. This suggests that when it is used as a preservative in a product such as mouthwash, it is considered dangerous if it exceeds that level, but is not so dangerous when used in larger quantities as an anti-microbial in deodorants. Sunscreens containing oxybenzone, a UV filter, must clearly state "Contains Oxybenzone" on the label, but brightly colored bubble bath containing the same substance to stop the color from fading, does not have to make such a declaration, even though children, who have lower tolerance levels to such things to start with, soak their whole bodies in it. So even if there are no warnings, it is worth checking the ingredients for chemicals you wish to avoid. There are some who believe that if a chemical is found to be harmful in large doses, then no one can really say what the safe level is, and that perhaps there can be no safe level at all.

PROBLEMS WITH MASCARA

Mascara is generally safe if you use it correctly, but you should always wash it off before going to sleep. It can flake into your eye where it can scratch your cornea, cause irritation, soreness, and infection. Never apply mascara in a moving car, train, subway (tube), or airplane. Any sudden movement of the vehicle could cause you to scratch your eyeball, or worse. Certainly never apply any make-up if you are driving a car – not only is it dangerous, it is against the law.

COSMETICS AND CHILDREN

Many cosmetics and toiletries warn you not to use them on children under the age of three. Even if this warning is absent you should never use any product on young children unless the label says it is safe to do so. There are many cosmetic ingredients that are irritating to the eyes and skin, and children have much more sensitive skin than adults. In the EU there are regulations defining the number and type of microbes that are allowed to be present in cosmetics and toiletries. This level is 50-times lower in young children's products than in products intended for older children and adults. This means that if you use an adult product on young children, you may be exposing them to a level of bacteria 50-times higher than is safe for them.

Even if the label doesn't say so, always keep all cosmetics and toiletries out of the reach of young children. They are bound to find the colors and smells irresistible and children like to investigate and copy. If they have watched you using lipstick, you can be certain it will go into their mouths. Children love to make up. If they do so, make sure they are supervised and that the cosmetics are suitable for young children. Do not let them wear the make-up for longer than necessary, and check the make-up remover is suitable for children. Eye make-up and eye make-up remover sometimes contains mercury compounds as preservatives. Check the ingredients carefully and never use products that contain mercury on young children. Watch out for Thimerosal or names that start with Phenyl mercuric, e.g. Phenyl mercuric acetate.

BUYER BEWARE

If you are going abroad for your holidays, buy your cosmetics and toiletries from reputable dealers at home or in Western countries. Never buy them in Third World countries or parts of the world where the standards of hygiene and quality control are lower than you are used to. Even if you buy a top brand-name cosmetic in a Hong Kong market say, whether in an airport or a large department store, there is a good chance that it is a pirate copy and, if this is the case, you can be certain it does not contain the ingredients described on the label. You can be equally certain the forgers have not gone to the expense of ensuring that all microbes and toxic contaminants, such as 1,4-dioxane, have been carefully eliminated from the raw materials. And don't buy their sunscreens. If they are pirate copies, you cannot guarantee they will give you the level of protection indicated by the SPF (sun protection factor) on the label.

Manufacturers in Third World and non-Western countries sometimes use dangerous ingredients. In July 1996 the Texas Department of Health issued a warning that it had found high levels of mercury in two face creams manufactured in Mexico. Tourists visiting Mexico purchased these creams, which were also found on sale in flea markets and small stores in New Mexico, Arizona, and even Washington. The cosmetics contained up to 10 percent by weight of mercury in the form of a highly toxic white pigment called calomel, the common name for mercurous chloride. The manufacturers were not concealing this ingredient in their product – despite being written in Spanish, it was clearly named as calomel in the list of ingredients.

The use of mercury preservatives in cosmetics is highly restricted and the level of mercury in these Mexican products was a thousand times higher than the levels allowed by the FDA. Although no one was reported to have suffered any serious health problems after using these products, more than 230 people contacted their state health departments to report they had used these cosmetics. Blood samples taken from 113 of them showed that 89 percent had elevated levels of mercury in their bodies.

Nor is the cost of a cosmetic any guarantee of its quality. If you check the ingredients of a supermarket brand of shampoo against a famous brand-name product, there will be a remarkable degree of similarity. The supermarket or drugstore brands are cheaper because they have fewer overheads. They do not have to pay for the expensive advertising to sell you an image. They can make huge economies in the manufacture of vast amounts of the products and they also have enormous buying power, which reduces their costs. Advertisers spend millions on coercing us to buy expensive brands that are no better, and often no different, to the drugstore and supermarket brands. Sometimes they are even made in the same factory. Why spend more on a cosmetic or toiletry than you have to?

COSMETIC CONTAMINANTS

Contaminated cosmetics and toiletries are more common than we would like to believe, and some of the contaminants pose a real threat to our health. They enter the products in a number of ways, often in microscopic quantities, but even at these minute concentrations there is a risk of adverse effects. The three most notorious contaminants are 1,4-dioxane, nitrosamines, and the so called "gender benders" (endocrine disrupter chemicals or EDCs). These are described in some detail below. Less worrying, perhaps, but no less important are pesticide residues from the plethora of plant extracts that are added to cosmetics to satisfy our insatiable desire for more "natural" products. Many of these residues are known to be harmful and some are known to be EDCs.

Gender Benders

This is the popular name for a group of chemicals known as endocrine disrupter chemicals (EDCs), or hormone disrupter compounds (HDCs). The endocrine system produces a range of hormones – chemicals which control the way our bodies grow and function. They also determine what sex we are. EDCs are chemicals which have molecules with similar shapes to hormone molecules. When they enter the body they are mistaken for hormones and can trigger those functions that are normally controlled by our own hormones. Hormones are fairly potent chemicals so we only produce a small amount of them. It is because of this that the endocrine system can be disrupted by extremely small quantities of EDC contaminants.

The name, "gender bender", was coined after it was discovered that one of the main effects of EDCs was their ability to mimic female sex hormones. One such EDC is a substance called DDE – a chemical which results from the slow biodegradation of the pesticide DDT. DDT was once widely used in an attempt to eradicate the anopheles mosquito which carried malaria. Indeed it was the aim of the World Health Organization to spray every part of the globe in order to completely eliminate this disease. It did not work. The mosquito become resistant to DDT and survived. Unfortunately, so did the DDT. It is remarkably resistant to biodegradation and is only slowly broken down to DDE, which remains in the environment today, decades after the large-scale use of DDT was banned.

DDE is a strongly feminizing EDC. Along with other chemical pollutants in the environment it is responsible for reduced sperm counts and malformed male genitalia in almost every species of animal in the world, including mammals, reptiles, birds, fish, and amphibians. And Man is no exception. Human sperm counts are falling too. At one time we thought the fashion for tight-fitting underwear, which reduced heat loss from the testes, led to higher temperatures that killed sperm. We now know EDCs are responsible.

Over 45 gender benders have been identified, and the list includes pesticides and partly degraded pesticides; chemicals that leech out of plastic containers into cosmetics and food; detergents, surfactants, and antioxidants used in cleaning products, cosmetics, toiletries, spermicides, and food; and pollutants that are generally at large in the environment, such as PCBs (polychlorinated biphenyls), industrial and domestic effluent – containing detergents, and garbage – containing plastics. Some of the more common EDCs are detailed below.

Nonylphenol is a widely used surfactant found in cleaning products, cosmetics, and spermicides. It is a potent EDC and it accumulates in tissues where it can build up to dangerous levels. BHA (butylated hydroxy anisole or E320) is an antioxidant widely used in cosmetics, toiletries, and processed foods. It is a suspected EDC. Bisphenol-A is another EDC that can contaminate food and cosmetics. It is used in the plastic lining of food cans and in the manufacture of polycarbonate bottles.

PVC is a hard plastic used as a building material to make cladding, drain pipes, gutters, doors, and windows. When chemicals called phthalates are added to PVC they act as plasticizers and the PVC becomes soft and pliable. In this state it is used for making packaging and containers for food, cosmetics, and toiletries, and for making soft toys and teething rings for young children. The phthalate plasticizers are added in large quantities, typically making up between 30 and 40 percent of the total weight of the PVC so there is a real and documented danger of these chemicals leaking out of the plastic container and into the food or cosmetic, or the child's mouth.

The range of phthalates commonly used to soften PVC is under investigation for EDC activity. Dibutyl phthalate, di-2-ethylhexyl phthalate, di-isopropyl phthalate, and benzyl butyl phthalate are all commonly used plasticizers, but none of these is actually used as a cosmetic ingredient.

To reassure the public, the EU Scientific Committee on Food had set a tolerable daily intake (TDI) of these chemicals of 0.5 milligrams per kilogram of body weight for the first three, and 1 milligram per kilogram of body weight for the fourth. This is 0.5 or 1 part per million (ppm) of body tissue – which may sound low but we must remember two things. First, some EDCs can accumulate in body tissue, so the levels can build up over time. Second, we are being exposed to a large number of these chemicals. They are in the food we eat, the water we drink, the cosmetics and toiletries we apply to our skin, and even in the detergent residues on the plates we eat from. If we only have one-twentieth of our TDI for each gender bender, but are exposed to 20 or more of these chemicals each day, then we will easily reach or exceed the tolerable daily intake.

Dioxane (1,4-Dioxane)

This compound is a known carcinogen (cancer-causing agent), causing systemic cancer in rodents when painted on their skin, and liver and nasal cancer when fed to test animals. It is known that this compound is readily absorbed through human skin although much of it is thought to evaporate quickly.

1,4-Dioxane is accidentally formed as an undesirable by-product in the manufacture of some cosmetic ingredients, when two molecules of ethylene oxide combine together in an unwanted chemical reaction. It must be carefully removed by vacuum stripping before the ingredient is used. Ethylene oxide is used in the manufacture of some non-ionic surfactants, emulsifiers, and film formers. These can often be recognized by the inclusion of PEG, polyethylene glycol, polyoxyethylene, -eth, or -oxynol in the name of the ingredient.

One study tested 54 cosmetic ingredients which were ethoxylated using ethylene oxide. All of them were found to be contaminated with 1,4-dioxane in levels up to and exceeding 100 ppm. The levels were significantly lower in the finished product, presumably because the manufacturer carefully removed the dioxane before using the ingredients. However, a study reported in the *International Journal of Dermatology* in 1991, found that of finished cosmetics tested, 40 percent contained high levels of dioxane, up to 85 ppm. When the study was restricted to only those cosmetics and toiletries that contained ethylene oxide derivatives, 48 percent of them contained dioxane in varying amounts between 7.3 and 85.9 ppm. Admittedly the study was carried out in the Far East where standards are lower and there is a greater chance of cosmetic piracy. In the EU and USA, reputable manufacturers rigorously test the ingredients before they are used.

No one really knows what the safe level of dioxane is, but when it comes down to a life-threatening disease like cancer, there are many people who believe that there can be no safe level of any carcinogenic chemical.

Nitrosamines

Also called N-nitroso- compounds, nitrosamines are potent carcinogens which are known to penetrate human skin. They are not used as cosmetic ingredients but, like dioxane, they can be accidentally formed during the manufacture of individual ingredients or by the interaction of two, otherwise harmless, ingredients in the finished product. It has even been reported that chemicals secreted by our skin can react with cosmetic ingredients to form nitrosamines.

In 1977, a study of 29 cosmetics found that 27 of them were contaminated with nitrosamines in concentrations ranging from 10 parts per billion (ppb) to 50 parts per million (ppm). Between 1978 and 1980 the FDA analyzed more than 300 cosmetics and found that 7 percent of them contained less than 30 ppb of nitrosamines, 26 percent contained between 30 ppb and 2 ppm, and 7 percent contained between 2 ppm and 150 ppm of nitrosamines. On April 10, 1979 the FDA published a public notice in the Federal Register, stating that cosmetics containing nitrosamines may be considered adulterated and subject to enforcement action. Twelve years later, in a follow-up study in 1991–1992, 65 percent of the cosmetics tested contained up to 3 ppm of nitrosamines, suggesting a deterioration of manufacturing standards.

If nitrosamines are accidentally formed in the manufacturing process, they must be carefully removed from the ingredient before it is added to a personal care product. Reputable cosmetics' manufacturers know which ingredients are likely to be contaminated with nitrosamines, and they routinely test them to make sure they meet the stringent purity regulations. These regulations require any nitrosamine contamination to be reduced so as not to exceed a prescribed limit. Since many scientists agree that there is no safe level of nitrosamines, perhaps the regulations should require their complete elimination, although that would be time consuming, expensive, and difficult to achieve. However, you should avoid buying expensive brands of cosmetics cheaply in discount stores, market stalls or in foreign countries where standards are lower. There is a greater chance that these products are pirate copies and the criminals who make them are unlikely to observe the Western safety regulations.

Nitrosamines are formed when ingredients called secondary amines, react with ingredients called nitrosating agents. Primary and tertiary amines, given the right conditions, can also be nitrosated. Several ingredients, including sodium nitrite – a corrosion inhibitor – some nitrated hair dyes, and preservatives such as 2-bromo-2-nitropropan-1,3-diol (BNPD or Bronopol) and 5-bromo-5-nitro-1,3-dioxane (Bronidox C), are known to be nitrosating agents, and reputable manufacturers will not use these ingredients when the product contains the amines mentioned above.

Nitrosamines are not just a cosmetic problem. Nitrites are frequently used as food preservatives, especially in cured meats such as salami, pastrami, ham, and bacon. Amino acids, the building blocks of proteins, are amines. These can react with the nitrite preservative, especially when in contact with a hot metal during cooking, producing low levels of nitrosamines. There was a great deal written about this problem in the 1970s, but it has not proved to be a major health issue. It is reasonable to conclude, therefore, that providing cosmetics' manufacturers follow the rules and maintain high standards of purity and safety, it is unlikely that nitrosamines in cosmetics will cause any problems. Of course you may undo all of this good work if, for example, you mix together two different brands of shampoo and unwittingly allow nitrosating preservatives from one, to react with secondary amines in the other.

A FINAL WORD

After reading this, you may get the impression that all cosmetics are hazardous to your health, but you must remember that the track record of the vast majority of cosmetics and toiletries speaks for itself. Statistically, you are unlikely to suffer any serious health risks from your cosmetics, but you may well find something that you don't like. At this point, the advice from the experts is contradictory. Some will tell you to find something that suits you and stick with it, while others warn you not to expose yourself to the same chemicals day in and day out, because to do so increases the risks of sensitization, allergy, and possibly cancer. In fact, the problem is often solved by the manufacturers themselves. As soon as you find something you like, the manufacturer either changes it to a "new improved formula" or they stop making it altogether!

14 sun and skin

He hands out life and beauty with his gaze
Then claws it back with his UV rays.

The world market for sunscreens is estimated to be worth $4 billion annually, and it continues to grow as consumers become increasingly aware of the dangers caused by sun exposure such as sunburn, premature skin aging and skin cancer. Sunscreens and brightly colored sunblocks have become so widely used, they are now regarded as sports-fashion accessories, and products have been carefully crafted to meet this market. There is a daunting choice of sunscreens with sun-protection factors (SFPs) to suit every combination of skin type and holiday destination. Everyone knows they should choose the right product and that it should protect against both UV-A and UV-B rays, but few people know what it all means. A recent report suggested that too many people were spending too much time in the sun, wrongly believing their sunscreen would completely protect them. This chapter attempts to set out the facts about sun, suntans, and sunscreens, and to dispel some myths that people hold dear.

SUN AND SKIN CANCER

The incidence of melanoma (skin cancer caused by exposure to the sun) has risen dramatically since the 1960s. This has been attributed to an increased exposure to the sun's harmful rays, whether it be due to increased personal wealth and leisure time allowing us to travel to sunny holiday destinations; to the fashion that dictates we wear more revealing clothing to show off our sun-bronzed skin; or to the thinning of the protective ozone layer caused by pollution. Here are some alarming facts about skin cancer in the USA:

- 7000 Americans die of skin cancer each year: 2000 women, 5000 men. That is one person every hour.
- In American women aged 25–29, melanoma is the most common cancer. It is the second most common cancer in women aged 30–34.
- One in every five Americans alive today will get skin cancer during their lifetime.
- African-Americans can also develop sun-related melanoma, but the incidence is 20 to 40 times lower than in white Americans, depending on the level of pigmentation of the skin.
- The rise in melanoma is alarming: in 1938, one in 1500 Americans developed skin cancer. This rose to one in 105 in 1991 and one in 75 in the year 2000. This is an increase of 2000 percent since 1930.
- 40,000 new cases of melanoma were reported in 1997, a 5 percent increase on 1996's figures.
- Each time you suffer sunburn, you double the likelihood of developing skin cancer.
- However, if a melanoma is detected early, before it grows deep into the dermis, the survival rate is 90 percent.

Despite these appalling statistics:

- 60 percent of Americans still actively seek a suntan – the skin's first indication of sun damage.
- About 75 to 80 percent of the average person's lifetime exposure to the sun takes place before the age of 18. The cancer may develop many years on, even if you reduce your exposure to the sun after this age.
- Less than 30 percent of Americans apply sunscreen regularly while on vacation.
- Less than 20 percent of Americans wear sunscreen year round.

Skin cancer is also an issue in Australia where there has been a public health campaign to encourage the correct use of sunscreens, and it is an increasing risk in the UK as an ever-growing number of British tourists take advantage of cheap package holidays to sunshine destinations.

ULTRAVIOLET RAYS

The sun bathes the Earth in warmth and light and breathes life into the planet. Every creature and plant living in daylight depends on it. We cannot exist without it. But it also bombards us with deadly radiation. Most of this is absorbed high in the upper atmosphere and by the ozone layer, and never reaches us on the ground, but some of it gets through. It is called ultraviolet radiation (UV) and it can burn skin, bleach hair, and cause skin cancer. But it also darkens our skin, which many of us believe is desirable, attractive, and healthy. How true is this?

Ultraviolet rays are similar to light rays but they carry much more energy and are invisible to our eyes. Both light and sound travel in waves. We can hear a wide range of sound waves but we cannot hear a dog whistle because its pitch is too high and beyond the range of our hearing. In a similar way, our eyes can see a range of light waves which represent all the colors of the rainbow, but ultraviolet rays are like the pitch of the dog whistle – the frequency is higher than our eyes can see. They are not the highest frequency waves: X-rays and gamma rays from radioactive materials have higher frequencies still, and we all know how harmful they are.

Ultraviolet-A (UV-A) is composed of rays just beyond the limit of our vision and is present in both sunlight and sunbed lamps. It can penetrate both the ozone layer and light clouds, and is responsible for tanning. Too much UV-A can cause the skin to become red and burn. It can pass through the epidermis into the dermis where it damages skin tissue, causing it to dry out, lose its elasticity, and age prematurely. UV-A is also responsible for some forms of skin cancer, including melanoma.

UV-B has a higher frequency than UV-A and much of it is absorbed by the ozone layer. It is much more damaging than UV-A, causing skin to burn fairly quickly and contributing little to the tanning process. It is strongly connected to skin cancer and premature aging. Some sunbeds produce small amounts of UV-B.

UV-C has the highest frequency of all and falls just short of X-rays. It is mostly absorbed by the ozone layer, but significant amounts of UV-C reach the ground when the sun is strongest between the hours of 10:00 am and 2:00 pm. It causes severe skin damage and burns. It is used to kill microbes in some sterilization processes. Few sunbeds produce any UV-C.

The UV Index or Sun Index

The UV index is a scale from 1 to 10 that indicates the intensity of the ultraviolet radiation from the sun. It is often announced on local weather forecasts or is available at some hotels and resorts. The sunburn time given is for an average, fair-skinned person.

- 0–2 (Minimal) – Minimal danger from the sun's UV radiation. Fair-skinned people can stay in the noonday sun for up to an hour without burning.
- 3–4 (Low) – Low risk of harm to the skin from the sun's radiation. Burn time is 30–60 minutes at noon.
- 5–6 (Moderate) – Some risk of skin damage. Unprotected exposure to the sun can result in sunburn in only 20–30 minutes.
- 7–9 (High) – High risk of harm from unprotected exposure to the sun. Time in the sun should be limited between 10:00 am and 4:00 pm, as burn time is as little as 13–20 minutes.
- 10 (Very High) – Very high risk of skin damage from unprotected exposure to the sun. Sunbathing between 10:00 am and 4:00 pm is not recommended as burn time may be less than 13 minutes without protection.

PROTECTING YOURSELF FROM THE SUN

Protection against the sun brings up many issues and misconceptions. The sun produces UV-A, UV-B, and UV-C rays. The ozone layer stops most of the UV- B and UV-C, but UV-A is with us summer and winter. It can even penetrate a light cloud cover causing tanning, sunburn, premature skin aging (wrinkles) and, in the long term, skin cancer. Experts advise that you should protect yourself from the sun all year round. In the summer, avoid the sun between 10:00 am and 2:00 pm when it is at its most intense and use a suitable sunscreen, which you should apply before you go into the sun and re-apply frequently – at least every 60 to 80 minutes. Make sure your sunscreen will protect you from both UV-A, and UV-B. It will normally announce this on the label if it does.

Very few sunscreens claim to protect against UV-C but some protection is given by UV-B absorbers, especially if the product has a high sun-protection factor. UV-C is best avoided by covering up during the noonday hours.

Choose a sunscreen with a high sun-protection factor (SPF). The SPF for a sun-screen indicates the level of protection it offers you. If your skin is fair and likely to burn in 20 minutes, a sunscreen with an SPF of 10 will let you stay in the sun for ten times as long before you burn. In other words it will protect you for 20 times 10 minutes – 200 minutes, or three hours and twenty minutes. During this time you should re-apply the sunscreen every 60 to 80 minutes, or you will not get the expected level of protection. Applying a factor 10 sunscreen three times will not give the same protection as a factor 30 sunscreen. No matter how many times you apply it, it will only let you stay in the sun for 10 times your unprotected burn time.

Many people believe that they will not get a tan if they use a sunscreen with a high SPF. This is not true. It may take longer for your tan to develop but it will stop you from burning while you are tanning. Some products contain tan boosters that speed up the tanning process, but the "added tan" will give you no extra protection against the sun's UV rays. However long it takes for you to tan, you should avoid sunburn at all costs. You do not need to go red in order to get a suntan. Reddening is a sure sign you are burning and the problem is, you do not know you are burning until it is too late. The reddening and burning sensation can take up to six hours to appear after you finish sunbathing, and you often don't notice it until you go to bed and the sheets feel like sandpaper.

Some people like to start their tan before they go on holiday, especially if they are self-conscious about showing their winter-white skin on a beach crowded with well-bronzed sun-worshipers. Sunbeds are ideal for this or you could try some early summer sunbathing in the back yard, but don't underestimate the burning power of the sun during May or early June. And this pre-holiday tan is no substitute for a suitable sunscreen. It only has an SPF of about 2 to 4, which will give you little protection from the intensity of the sun you are likely to encounter on holiday.

Sunbed Warning

Sunbeds produce mainly UV-A rays that penetrate far deeper into the skin than UV-B. Many experts consider the regular use of sunbeds to be a health risk.

There is a common misconception that you cannot burn if you already have a suntan, and many people with a light, sunbed tan go into the sun with too little protection. Even if you have a good suntan, you will still suffer skin damage and sunburn if you do not use a good-quality sunscreen with an SPF adequate to protect you. If you do intend to spend all day in the sun you should use a sunscreen with an SPF of at least 25, and you will need a greater level of protection on your face where your skin is thinner. Likewise, an artificial tan gives you no protection from the sun whatsoever.

Sitting in the shade is no guarantee of protection. Sand reflects 25 percent of the UV rays, paved courtyards reflect 45 percent, and white-painted buildings and glass reflect even more. Grass and water, however, reflect only 3 percent of the sun's UV radiation. Tightly woven fabrics like cotton, polycotton, and linen offer the best protection. Loosely woven fabrics and see-through materials let through sufficient UV rays to cause sunburn.

CHOOSING A SUNSCREEN

Exposure to UV rays from the sun or from sunbeds stimulates melanocytes in the basal layer of the epidermis (outer layer of skin cells) to produce larger amounts of melanin, a brown pigment, to act as a natural barrier against the harmful effects of UV rays. The pigment is formed when the amino acid, tyrosine, is converted into melanin. But the melanin produced by sunbathing only has a sun-protection factor (SPF) of between 2 and 6, depending on the intensity of the tan. If you intend to spend a long time in the sun, you will need much more protection or your skin will burn and you will increase the risk of developing skin cancer. It is important to choose a good quality sunscreen with an SPF that is high enough to protect your skin type, even if you already have a suntan. If you live in a sunny part of the world and regularly expose yourself to the sun, your tan will not protect you from premature skin aging or skin cancer. You must use additional protection. Better still, cover yourself up.

Your choice of sunscreen should be based on your skin type, described in the table below. Generally speaking, if you have fair skin (Types I and II), which has not seen the sun for several months, you must use a sunscreen with an SPF of 35 to 50. People with darker skins (Types III and IV) can use a lower SPF depending on the intensity of the sun and the time of day spent in the sun (see *UV Index*, p.146). Even dark-skinned people (Types V and VI) who work in offices will suffer from sunburn if they do not protect themselves for the first week of their holiday. Whatever color your skin is, topless sunbathing will require an even higher level of protection than shown in the table.

Whatever SPF you need, make sure your sunscreen will protect you from UV-A and UV-B. If you intend swimming, you should choose one that is resistant to water since ultraviolet rays can penetrate about three feet (one meter) of water. If your holiday takes you to parts of the world that have an insect problem look for one that contains a mosquito repellent such as diethyl toluamide (DEET).

Obviously the fragrance and feel of the sunscreen is an important consideration, but don't buy an unsuitable product based on its image. Most men would not feel comfortable on a crowded beach with a small, pink bottle of rose-scented suntan lotion. For this reason, manufacturers are increasingly formulating sunscreen fragrances and packaging designed to appeal to men; however, if it is not going to protect you adequately, choose another brand. There are plenty of sunscreens that are unisex.

Skin Type	Description of Skin	SPF requried at start of holiday	SPF required after first week of holiday
I	Red or blond hair, blue-green eyes, very light skin. Burns easily. Does not tan. Limited exposure times recommended.	35–50: reapply every 30–40 minutes	25–35: reapply every 30–40 minutes
II	Light to medium skin color, hair and eyes. Often burns. Slight tan. Limited exposure time recommended.	35–50: reapply every 30–40 minutes	15–30: reapply every 30–40 minutes
III	Medium to olive skin. Medium to dark eyes. Medium brown hair. Moderate burns if not protected. Usually tans.	25:30: reapply every 40–60 minutes	15:25: reapply every 60–80 minutes

IV	Dark olive to light brown skin. Dark hair and eye color. Mild burns if not protected. Strong suntan always.	15–20: reapply every 60–80 minutes	8–15: reapply every 60–90 minutes
V	Brown skin, black hair and dark eye color. Strong, persistent, brown tan. Seldom burns.	8–15: reapply every 60–90 minutes	5–8: reapply every few hours
VI	Dark brown or black skin and hair. Dark eyes. Tolerant to the sun and rarely burns.	5–8: reapply every 1–2 hours	2–5: reapply every few hours
Babies – new-born to 6 months	Do not expose to the sun. Keep skin covered and in the shade.		
Infants – 6 months to 5 years	Keep exposure times short. Use a stronger SPF than recommended for the child's skin type.		

Note: The figures shown in this table should be used as a rough guide only. Some sunscreen manufacturers recommend much lower levels of protection than shown in the table, while some medical advice, help groups, and cancer research charities advise the use of higher SPFs than shown above. The best advice is that it is better to be overprotected than underprotected.

TYPES OF SUNSCREENS

The most common sunscreens, also called sunblocks or suntan lotions, are preparations that are rubbed onto the skin. They prevent harmful ultraviolet rays from reaching the skin or reduce their intensity to a level that is safe for your skin type. They fall into two main groups: chemical sunscreens and physical sunscreens.

Chemical Sunscreens

These contain UV absorbers that absorb the ultraviolet rays and reduce their energy, allowing a tan to form while reducing the risk of burning. They are formulated in light oils or oily emulsions that generally do not stain clothing. Many products have a neutral appearance but some leave a glossy sheen on the skin. The energy absorbed by the UV absorbing chemicals slowly breaks them down so that chemical sunscreens must be reapplied every 60 to 90 minutes to maintain the correct level of protection.

There is a wide range of chemical sunscreens to choose from but many of them use one or more of the three most common UV-absorbing ingredients. PABA (para-amino benzoic acid), and PABA derivatives, make up the first group. Some of these have been linked to skin irritation and sensitivity. The second group is the benzophenone family, which includes oxybenzone. These are common ingredients in sunscreens and many moisturizing and skincare creams, but some of them do not appear on the EU lists of permitted or provisionally permitted UV absorbers. The third (and most commonly used) group of UV absorbers are cinnamates; some of these have been reported to produce a stinging effect, especially if washed into the eyes by sweat. If you experience any skin irritation, choose a brand with a different UV absorbing ingredient, but be careful – a stinging sensation or irritation may be an adverse effect of an ingredient, or it could also be an early indication of sunburn.

Physical Sunscreens

Physical sunscreans contain reflective materials that reflect the ultraviolet rays away from the skin, so that tanning is very slow or does not happen at all. They are applied as conspicuous, thick white or colored coatings, and are often messy, tending to rub off and mark clothing and other items they encounter. These products generally have a high SPF and are particularly useful on lips and noses. They are popular for use in sporting activities such as cricket, skiing, and mountaineering.

Reflective materials in physical sunscreens include finely ground zinc oxide, titanium dioxide, talc, or kaolin in a greasy or oily emulsion base. Since they reflect the sun's rays rather than absorb them, they are not usually degraded by the energy of the rays and do not need to be reapplied as frequently as chemical sunscreens. Many reflective formulations include UV absorbers to increase their effectiveness, and vivid colors to comply with fashions.

Other Sunscreens

Oral sunscreens in the form of tablets, were once popular but they have now been banned by the FDA and are not licensed as a drug in the UK, hence pharmacists do not sell them. Since they are based on natural dyes found in a variety of living things, including carrots and flamingo feathers, they are available as a "dietary supplement" from some health-food shops and are widely advertised on the internet. They color the skin yellow and give no protection from the sun.

The best sunscreens of all are tightly woven fabrics like cotton or linen, which prevent the sun's rays from reaching the skin altogether.

Some sunscreens contain tanning agents such as bronzers, tanning accelerators (tan boosters), and tan extenders. These increase the rate of tanning or the intensity of the tan. Some formulations give the tan an artificial color making it obvious that tanning agents have been used. These are described on p.155.

THE SCIENCE OF SUNSCREENS

UV absorbers in chemical sunscreens are usually complex organic compounds that contain a number of special chemical bonds that allow the substance's electrons to absorb the energy from UV rays easily, and then to release this energy gradually in the form of heat, which is harmlessly lost to the surrounding air.

When chemicals absorb energy in this way they become more chemically reactive and may break down or react with other chemicals to form new substances. It is essential that UV absorbers in sunscreens should not produce toxic chemicals from these unwanted reactions. Before they are allowed to be used in sunscreens, they must be rigorously tested to make sure this does not happen. (See *A–Z of Cosmetic Terms – Phototoxin.*) As an additional precaution it is probably a good idea not to apply sunscreens on top of other cosmetics such as moisturizing creams. The ingredients in the other cosmetics may interact in an unpredictable and undesirable way with the energetic UV absorbers.

This steady degradation of the sunscreen chemicals, and their gradual removal by rubbing against clothing or towels, is the reason why sunscreen should be reapplied at regular intervals while you are in the sun.

New Technology Sunscreens

A product called Sol-Gel, a recent development from the Hebrew University in Israel, promises to solve the problem of allergies and adverse reactions to sunscreen ingredients. The researchers have discovered a way to encapsulate the UV-absorbing chemicals in microscopic glass bubbles. These glass bubbles are tiny – about one-thousandth of a millimeter in diameter. They are applied in an inert lotion and are smooth enough to be rubbed into the skin without scratching it. Since the active ingredients never come into contact with the skin there is little risk of skin reactions. In some respects, the pursuit of this kind of technology is an acknowledgment by the manufacturers that cosmetic ingredients and UV absorbers do cause adverse effects.

DEALING WITH SUNBURN

Treatment for sunburn is controversial and doctors often disagree on what to do about it. There are two levels of sunburn. If you go red and your skin feels hot and painful, and sometimes swelling occurs, you have first-degree burns, which can be treated by home remedies. First you should drink plenty of fluids, but not diuretics like tea, coffee, alcohol, or soft drinks that contain caffeine. Diluted fruit juices or water are best. Cool showers will reduce the pain and soothing creams can help. Some experts advise against the use of pain-killing formulations that contain "-caine" ingredients – like Benzocaine, Novocain (procaine) or, worst of all, Lidocaine (lignocaine). These are local anesthetics that can cause sensitization. The sunburn reduces your skin's ability to act as a barrier to chemicals and the "-caines" can penetrate deep into the dermis and, from there, into the bloodstream where the sensitization starts. In the worst imaginable situation you may find yourself in the emergency room where a doctor injects a "-caine" before stitching you up. If you have previously become sensitized to the "-caines" you could have a serious reaction and even suffer anaphylactic shock.

If your sunburn starts to blister you have second-degree burns. If the burn area is small, it can be treated in a similar way to a first-degree burn, but there is a risk of bacterial infection so the burn should be covered with a sterile dressing. If a second-degree burn covers more than one percent of your body (that's about the same area as your hand), you should consult a doctor immediately. You should also consult a doctor if an infant suffers any type of sunburn, however slight, if your sunburn seems worse than a second-degree burn, or if you feel seriously unwell, develop a fever, sweat profusely then stop sweating, or become weak, faint, delirious, or unconscious. This could indicate a more serious, life-threatening condition such as heat stroke or sunstroke.

Old Wives' Tales – Herbal Sunburn Treatment

An infusion of salad burnet leaves in water is said to take the sting out of sunburn. It may work but be careful – sunburnt skin is not a good barrier and so may allow substances to be absorbed through it. Make sure the herbs are clean and free from pesticide residues.

TANNING AGENTS

There are four types of tanning agent: bronzers, extenders, accelerators or boosters, and tanning pills.

Bronzers

A bronzer is a colored lotion that temporarily stains the skin. It may be applied as part of the sunscreen or as a separate product. It washes off with soap and water and offers no protection from the sun. Some are designed to withstand a wash by absorbing into the outermost layer of skin cells. This layer is shed fairly quickly and will be lost if exfoliating cosmetics or abrasive cleansing pads are used. To prolong the bronzers' effect it is recommended to shave your legs and use exfoliants before applying them.

Tan Extenders

Extenders are chemicals that are applied as lotions or in sunscreen products. The chemicals darken as they react with proteins in the skin. They can produce a good fake tan but sometimes the color is disappointing. The fake tan cannot be washed off but it will fade in time. Dihydroxyacetone (DHA) is the most commonly used tan extender but this is known to cause contact allergies in some people. Fake tans from tan extenders offer no protection from ultraviolet rays.

Tanning Accelerators or Boosters

Tanning accelerators have not been approved by the FDA. The most common tan booster is tyrosine, an amino acid that is used by the body to produce melanin, the skin's natural pigment. It is assumed that increasing the levels of tyrosine in the skin will increase the rate of production of melanin. However, there is no scientific evidence that tyrosine can penetrate the skin and be converted into melanin. In fact some animal studies have demonstrated that ingesting tyrosine or applying it to the skin has no effect on the production of melanin. So where does the tan come from? Copper compounds and other tanning aids such as DHA are usually added to enhance changes in skin color, and give the tan a bronze tone. The tan obtained from this type of product is persistent and cannot be washed off, but it is mainly artificial and gives little protection from the sun.

5-Methoxypsoralen, which can be made synthetically and also occurs naturally in bergamot oil, stimulates the production of melanin by the melanocytes. It achieves this by making your skin more sensitive to sunlight. There has been some concern that 5-methoxypsoralen may be linked to skin cancer and some variants can cause pigmentation disorders. As a result, several psoralen derivatives have been banned from cosmetics in the EU.

Tanning Pills

Tanning pills have been banned by the FDA and are not licensed medicines in the UK. Consequently, they cannot be purchased from a pharmacist, but they are widely available on the Internet. They contain carotene (which is related to vitamin A), or canthaxanthin – both of which are found as natural pigments in plants (e.g., carrots). Canthaxanthin is found in mushrooms, marine animals, and tropical bird feathers. Flamingo feathers get their color from the canthaxanthin present in the small water animals they feed on. Some tanning pills also contain tyrosine. Tans obtained from tanning pills offer no protection from the sun.

Carotene and canthaxanthin are safe if they are taken in moderation as part of a balanced diet but large quantities are needed if they are to alter the skin's color. Carotene is normally present in skin cells and gives skin a yellow hue. It is a free radical scavenger that collects and destroys free radicals (highly reactive, damaging particles, formed during some chemical reactions and when ultraviolet rays strike skin cells). This property is thought to reduce the aging effect of sunlight on the skin. When taken in huge excess for about two weeks, these colorants eventually build up in the layer of subcutaneous fat and show through the skin, making it appear yellow and jaundiced. It colors all parts of the body except the eyes, and even gives a red color to the feces and other body waste. Canthaxanthin can be deposited as crystals in the eyes, and there is one reported case of a woman who died from aplastic anemia, which was attributed to her use of tanning pills.

Tyrosine taken orally will be absorbed into the bloodstream and used by any cell in the body. The chances of it being used specifically by the melanocytes to produce melanin is very small indeed.

FREE RADICALS

Strong sunlight can cause premature aging of skin. The sun's ultraviolet rays generate free radicals in the skin and it is thought that these cause the breakdown of the collagen which gives skin its elasticity. Free radicals also play a vital role in the conversion of the amino acid tyrosine to melanin, the skin's natural brown pigment.

Cosmetics' manufacturers have exaggerated the role of free radicals in the formation of fine lines and wrinkles, and have convinced consumers that they will remain wrinkle free if they buy products that contain free radical inhibitors (free radical scavengers) such as vitamins A and E. These are compounds that react with the free radicals and destroy them. However, since these free radical inhibitors are not absorbed deep into the skin's dermis where the free radicals are thought to be doing the damage, they are unlikely to have much effect. If they did, they would probably prevent you from tanning.

A free radical is an atom or molecule that possesses an unpaired electron, which makes the molecule extremely reactive, usually in a destructive way. Free radicals play an important role in a number of natural chemical processes in living systems, but the free radicals that are produced by these reactions are carefully contained in an environment where they can do no harm. Free radicals that appear in the wrong place can be extremely destructive, often starting a chain reaction that can damage many thousands of molecules before they decay.

The action of free radicals can, however, be advantageous. For example, during photosynthesis, the green pigment in plants absorbs the sun's energy and free radicals are generated inside the chloroplasts of leaf cells. Certain weed killers, such as paraquat, allow the free radicals to escape from the chloroplasts and destroy the leaf cells. Once sprayed, the plant turns brown and withers within a few hours of the sun falling on the leaves. Another example is the use of gamma rays to irradiate and sterilize medical equipment, food products, or personal care items. When the gamma rays strike water molecules, free radicals are generated that kill any microbes present. (See *A–Z of Cosmetic Terms – Irradiation*.)

15 medical matters

Many women believe they are allergic to cosmetic products when they are in fact suffering from irritation [caused by chemicals in the products they use] ... The study showed that 42% of women believe they have sensitive skin...

(Study by the chemical company, Rohm and Haas, reported in the journal *Manufacturing Chemist*, July 1999.)

Cosmetics have been linked to a large number of health and skin problems. The main culprits responsible are usually the fragrance and color chemicals but other ingredients such as preservatives, UV absorbers, and any number of other ingredients, whether natural or artificial, may also play a part. People with a history of eczema, psoriasis, asthma, or a similar condition often believe they were born with it and are stuck with it forever, or they attribute it to an unavoidable agent in the modern environment. Only recently are we becoming aware of the part played by a host of artificial chemicals in our food, washing powders, and cosmetics.

If you suspect a cosmetic or toiletry is causing an adverse reaction, you should stop using it immediately and wait until the condition clears up before trying an alternative product – preferably one not containing the ingredients you suspect may be causing the problem. Try using a hypoallergenic product, but take care to check the ingredients carefully to ensure it does not contain any perfume, color, or other ingredient you think may be responsible. Of course, if the condition does not clear up when you stop using the suspected cosmetic, or if the condition gets worse, you should always seek medical help.

This chapter deals with the main medical conditions that can be triggered by the use of cosmetics and toiletries, and other conditions which have been linked to ingredients that are used in cosmetics, such as cancer. When a problem is linked to a cosmetic, people commonly assume that they are allergic to the substance concerned, which is not always the case. Most people do not know the difference between a simple case of contact dermatitis and a full-blown allergic reaction, nor do they know the difference between an allergy and sensitive skin. These terms are clarified below.

ALLERGIES AND SENSITIVE SKIN

The words allergy, sensitivity, and hypersensitivity are often misunderstood and misused when describing a reaction to some cosmetics and toiletries.

Sensitive Skin

Your skin is an effective barrier to most things but some substances can penetrate this barrier and cause irritation. The thinner your skin, the less effective it is at keeping out these irritants. Skin varies in thickness on different parts of your body. It is thickest on the palms of your hands and the soles of your feet and thinnest on your eyelids. Elderly people and young children in particular, have thinner and more sensitive skin. A corrosive or irritating chemical such as a strong acid or the juice from chillies, will cause more immediate irritation on thin or cracked skin than on thick skin. If your skin responds quickly to irritating cosmetic ingredients, it would be fair to say you have sensitive skin. Itchiness, red blotches, and sometimes a rash (urticaria) may occur but these symptoms rapidly subside when the affected area is washed or soothing lotions are applied. If you know you are sensitive to a particular cosmetic it is best to try another brand with significantly different ingredients.

Allergies

An allergic reaction is quite different and occurs when your body's immune system is triggered into action by a substance that does not normally affect most other people. The first time you encounter this substance, you become sensitized to it but experience no symptoms. The allergic reaction occurs on the second or subsequent exposure to the substance, which is now called an allergen.

During an allergic reaction, certain cells in your body release a hormone called histamine in excessive quantities, which causes the familiar symptoms of an allergy. Normally histamine is produced in small amounts and controls the supply of digestive juices in the stomach, causes smooth muscles to contract or tighten, and starts the healing process for tissues that have been damaged by injury or infection. Most tissue cells contain histamine. When the cells are damaged, the histamine leaks out and causes tiny blood vessels in the surrounding tissues to enlarge – increasing the supply of blood and other body fluids to the damaged area. This provides greater quantities of blood-clotting agents to seal any wounds, and it increases the number of antibodies and white blood cells to fend off any microbes that have invaded the damaged tissue.

Your immune system normally looks for foreign proteins, such as those on the surface of harmful bacteria or viruses, and destroys them. This process takes a few days to work and during this time you may have the symptoms of an illness. Once the invading microbes have been eliminated, you recover and your immune system remembers what the foreign proteins look like and immediately attack them when they next appear. This is why you only get some diseases once.

Sometimes the lymphocyte cells in your immune system mistakenly identify a relatively harmless substance as an invading foreign protein and start the process of destroying it. That substance, which may be a harmless cosmetic ingredient or something as simple as grass pollen, becomes an allergen. The lymphocyte cells produce a special type of antibody, called an IgE antibody, specifically designed to recognize the allergen. These antibodies attach themselves to what are known as mast cells which contain histamine and then bide their time, waiting for their next encounter with the allergen. The mast cells are found in the stomach lining, skin, lungs, and airways of the nose and throat. As soon as the antibodies come into contact with the allergen, they signal the mast cells to release the histamine and the symptoms of the allergy appear immediately. Symptoms include itchiness, swellings on the skin, rashes, sneezing, excessive mucus secretions, and muscle cramps. In serious allergic reactions several organs may be affected and medical intervention may be required. Generally the symptoms are mild and subside fairly quickly, and recovery can be hastened by taking antihistamine drugs.

Simple cosmetic allergies of this type can be avoided by not using the offending product. It may be possible to identify the individual cosmetic ingredient by trial and error, or by consulting your doctor and arranging a patch test.

Cosmetic Ingredients that Can Cause Allergies

Over 80 cosmetic ingredients have been linked to allergic reactions in some individuals; the most commonly used of these are listed below:

2,4-Diaminophenol (and HCl)	Glyceryl Stearate
2-Bromo-2-nitropropane-1,3-diol	Isopropanolamine
BHA	m-Phenylenediamine (and Sulfate)
BHT	Methylchloroisothiazolinone
Cocamide DEA	Methylisothiazolinone
Cocamide MEA	Myristyl Alcohol
Cocamide MIPA	Oleamidopropyl Dimethylamine
Cocamidopropyl Betaine	Phenoxyethanol
DEA-Oleth-10 Phosphate	Propyl Gallate
Dihydroxyacetone (DHA)	Propylene Glycol
Glyceryl Oleate	Stearyl Alcohol

Hypersensitivity

Like allergies, hypersensitivity is an abnormal immune response to an allergen. There are four types of hypersensitivity. Type I is called immediate or anaphylactic hypersensitivity, and is generally the same as the allergic reaction described above. Anaphylactic shock is a rare and life threatening Type I hypersensitivity reaction that occurs in people who develop an extreme sensitivity to an allergen. In Types II and III, the immune system not only attacks the allergen but also destroys some of the body's own tissues and can lead to an auto-immune disorder, such as rheumatoid arthritis. Type IV hypersensitivity can lead to inflammation and cause a series of skin disorders including contact dermatitis (dermatitis caused by chemicals touching the skin). As with allergies, avoidance of the offending ingredient is the best treatment for hypersensitivity to cosmetics.

It must be said that, although some allergic or hypersensitivity reactions can be extremely serious or life threatening, the number of cases caused by cosmetics and toiletries is extremely small – less than one in a million. Unfortunately, however, these rare events can become headline news and can spawn unwarranted fears and bad publicity for perfectly safe products.

DERMATITIS

Dermatitis is an inflammation of the skin that is related to eczema. It may be caused by an allergy or a reaction to something that comes into contact with the skin, or there may be no easily identifiable cause. The three main types of dermatitis are contact dermatitis, seborrheic dermatitis and photodermatitis. Exfoliative dermatitis is a less common, life-threatening complication of some serious illnesses, or it can be the result of worsening psoriasis or eczema, or a serious allergic reaction to a particular drug.

Contact Dermatitis

Contact dermatitis appears as a rash in the area that has come into contact with the offending substance. The rash is usually itchy and it may also flake or blister. It may be the result of an allergic reaction to a substance, or the substance may have a direct toxic effect on the skin. The most common causative substances are chemicals, metals, and plants such as poison ivy, ragweed, and hogweed. The chemicals may be industrial chemicals encountered at work, detergents, cosmetic ingredients, or chemical residues in rubber gloves and condoms. Metals in bracelets, watch straps, earrings, studs, sleepers, spectacles, and fasteners on clothing, can all cause contact dermatitis. Nickel is often the culprit though any metal can cause dermatitis; gold and gold plate is usually safe.

Contact dermatitis usually clears up quickly once the cause is removed. Never persevere with a cosmetic or a piece of jewellery, hoping you will get used to it. The condition may become much worse and require treatment with corticosteroids prescribed by your doctor.

Seborrheic Dermatitis

Seborrheic dermatitis is a red, scaly rash that appears on the scalp, nose, eyebrows, chest, and back. It often itches. On the scalp it is associated with dandruff but seldom responds to antidandruff shampoos, which can sometimes aggravate it. A variety of treatments are available but corticosteroid drugs applied with antimicrobial substances are usually effective. The condition should be treated early and all skin irritants, such as harsh detergents, should be avoided. Try avoiding conditioners and switching to a mild shampoo that contains sodium laureth sulfate or ammonium laureth sulfate instead of SLS (sodium lauryl sulfate) until the condition improves.

Cosmetic Ingredients that Can Cause Dermatitis

Over 300 cosmetic ingredients have been linked to dermatitis. Of these some of the most commonly used ingredients are shown below:

2-Bromo-2-nitropropane-1,3-diol
Alcohol (including Denat.)
Ammonium Glycolate
Benzyl Alcohol
BHA
BHT
Cetearyl Alcohol
Cetyl Alcohol
Chloroacetamide
Cocamide DEA, MEA and MIPA
Cocamidopropyl Betaine
Bi-t-Butylhydroquinone
Diammonium Dithiodiglycolate
DMDM Hydantoin
Glyceryl Thioglycolate
Glycolic Acid
Imidazolidinyl Urea

Lanolin and Lanolin derivatives
Methyldibromo Glutaronitrile
Oxybenzone (Benzophenone-3)
p-Phenylenediamine (including HCl and Sulfate)
Propylene Glycol
Ricinoleic Acid
Sorbitan Palmitate
Sorbitan Sesquioleate
Stearamidoethyl Diethylamine (and Phosphate)
Stearyl Alcohol
t-Butyl Hydroquinone
TEA-Cocoyl Hydrolyzed Collagen
TEA-Cocoyl Hydrolyzed Soy Protein
TEA-Stearate
Tocopherol (Vitamin E)

Photodermatitis

People who are photosensitive are abnormally sensitive to light, especially sunlight which, even on an overcast day, is many times brighter than any form of artificial lighting. These people can develop photodermatitis, which is a rash consisting of small spots or blisters that appears on any part of the body exposed to direct sunlight. Photosensitivity can be a symptom of a more serious disease, or it can be caused by some prescription drugs, cosmetic ingredients, or extracts from plants such as butter-cups, parsnips, or mustard. If you develop a rash on any part of your body exposed to the sun, and you are not taking drugs that can have this side effect, stop using your current personal care products and try another brand. If the condition does not clear up quickly or becomes severe, you should consult your doctor.

ECZEMA

Eczema is an inflammation of the skin resulting in itching, scaling of the skin, and sometimes blisters which occasionally become infected. There are many forms of eczema, including dermatitis, atopic eczema, nummular eczema, stasis eczema, and hand eczema. Of these, only hand eczema and dermatitis can be linked to cosmetics and toiletries, but the other forms of eczema may be irritated by personal care products, dishwashing liquids, rubber gloves, some fabrics, and detergent residues or fabric conditioners in clothing.

Atopic eczema runs in families where there is a history of allergies, such as hay fever or asthma. It is common in babies, first appearing between the ages of two months and eighteen months. For mild cases, simple, home remedies can be used and generally involve the application of a moisturizing (emollient) cream such as petroleum jelly. If the eczema patches are scratched, weeping may occur, the patches may enlarge and infections may set in, requiring treatment by a doctor. Antibiotic ointments may be prescribed to treat infections and the eczema itself may be treated with corticosteroids. Sometimes antihistamine drugs will reduce itching. Infant atopic eczema often clears up by itself when the child reaches puberty. Where the condition runs in families, it may last for several years. Exposure to the sun often reduces the size of the eczema patches.

The cause of nummular eczema is unknown and it is resistant to all and any form of treatment. It mainly occurs in adults. Stasis eczema occurs on the legs of older people who have varicose veins. Like nummular eczema, it is difficult to treat, but corticosteroid creams may give some temporary relief.

Hand eczema is usually caused by chemical contact on the skin. It often occurs on the hands as a reaction to dishwashing liquids and detergents. Cosmetics and toiletries can have a similar effect on other parts of the body. In these cases the condition is called contact eczema and usually clears up if the offending chemicals are kept away from the skin. These may be difficult to identify in cosmetics and toiletries since the eczema may be caused by a combination of ingredients that, individually, have no adverse effects on the skin. You should stop using any personal care product you suspect may be causing your skin problems. If you continue to use it, the eczema may become chronic and difficult to treat. These severe cases may require treatment with corticosteroid drugs prescribed by your doctor.

In all cases of eczema, the sufferer should avoid the use of potent cosmetics and toiletries, such as exfoliants and skin lighteners. They should discontinue using any product that causes soreness or irritation, no matter how slight. They may find keeping cool relieves their symptoms, and they should avoid skin contact with artificial fabrics and materials containing wool or silk. Cotton is generally the most comfortable material for eczema sufferers. If cotton causes irritation, there may be chemical residues from washing powders or fabric conditioners in the material.

Eczema in a Bottle

The following cosmetic ingredients have all been linked to eczema:

1,2-Dibromo-2,4-dicyanobutane	Methyl Alcohol
Alcohol	Methyldibromo Glutaronitrile
Alcohol denat.	Potassium Tallowate
Butadiene/Acrylonitrile Copolymer	Sodium Lauryl Sulfate (SLS)
Diammonium Dithiodiglycolate	Sodium Tallowate
Glycol	Styrene/Acrylates/Acrylonitrile Copolymer

PSORIASIS

Psoriasis and eczema are often confused because they may share a similar outward appearance of thickened patches of scaly skin. Psoriasis tends to cause red, inflamed patches covered by silvery scales, which seldom itch unless a large part of the body is affected. The cause of psoriasis is not known but it tends to run in families. Psoriasis most commonly appears as red, scaly patches on the elbows, knees, and scalp – where it may be mistaken for dandruff as the excessive growth of skin leads to the constant shedding of large clumps of dead skin cells. While the condition may be made worse by cosmetics, there is no evidence that is it caused by them or by any other chemical that comes in contact with the skin. It tends to appear and disappear and seems to be triggered by a number of factors including diet, emotional stress, physical illness, and skin damage. Psoriasis can be treated with corticosteroids and other drugs.

Cosmetic Ingredients that Can Cause Psoriasis

Only two cosmetic ingredients have been reported to be linked to psoriasis. These are:

Linalool (or Linalol)

Hydroxycitronellal

ACNE AND BLACKHEADS

Blackheads occur when hair follicles or sebaceous glands of the skin become blocked with an oily mixture of sebum (the skin's natural oil) and keratin (the tough, fibrous protein that makes up skin, hair, and nails). The mixture hardens and becomes a plug that blackens where it meets the air. If bacteria become trapped in this plug and are able to breed, the blackheads may become infected, in which case, red pimples (known as papules) appear. If the infection worsens, the follicle becomes inflamed and filled with puss and leads to whiteheads and acne.

The most common type of acne is adolescent acne (*acne vulgaris*), which is brought about by a change in hormones during puberty. A sudden change to a hot, humid climate can trigger tropical acne, which mainly affects young, white travelers. Chloracne is not common and is caused by skin contact with toxic chlorinated compounds which are not used in cosmetics.

Old Wives' Tales – Herbal Acne Cure

Thyme is said to cure spots, zits, and pimples. It may work, but it may also cause contact allergies and may make the condition worse.

Chemical acne is caused by comedogenic (acne promoting) substances. These are often oily or greasy substances that get into the skin pores and block them, causing sebum to build up in the follicles. Exposure to mineral oils and cooking oils can cause chemical acne or they can worsen the condition. A wide range of cosmetic ingredients are also comedogenic and should be avoided by acne sufferers. If you experience a sudden outbreak of blackheads or acne try a different cosmetic for a while.

Comedogenic (Acne Promoting) Ingredients

The following ingredients are either known or suspected comedogens and should be avoided if you suffer from blackheads or acne:

Butyl Stearate	Myristyl Propionate
Coal Tar	Octyl Stearate
Decyl Oleate	Olea Europaea (Olive oil)
Isocetyl Stearate	Oleic Acid
Isopropyl Isostearate	Potassium Tallowate
Isostearyl Neopentanoate	Propyleneglycol-2-myristyl Propionate
Lanolin	Sodium Tallowate
Lanolin Alcohol	Theobroma Cacao (Cocoa butter)
Lauryl Alcohol	Xanthene
Linum Usitatissimum (Linseed oil)	Zea Mays (Corn oil)
Methyl Oleate	

Several ingredients containing Myristate, Palmitate and Laneth- have also been linked to acne and blackheads.

Acne often clears up by itself in a few days. Squeezing pustules is discouraged as it can lead to small scars and can also spread the bacteria to other parts of the body. Ultraviolet light or direct sunlight helps acne to clear, but severe cases may need medical treatment. Benzoyl peroxide (now banned from cosmetics and toiletries in the EU), retinoic acid, and antibiotic creams and lotions may be prescribed for persistent acne. If these fail, long-term treatment with oral antibiotics or retinoid drugs may be prescribed, but these have unpleasant side effects and are used only as a last resort.

CANCER AND COSMETICS

The cause of many cancers is still unknown but there are many factors, known as carcinogens, which can increase the risk of our developing the disease. Cancer usually develops after a long term, low-level exposure to the carcinogen.

There are many different types of carcinogen. Chemical carcinogens are chemicals that cause cancer. A notorious example is cigarette smoke which contains tar rich in polycyclic aromatic hydrocarbons. Benzene vapor, present in unleaded petrol, is also a known carcinogen. Physical carcinogens include such things as asbestos dust, ultraviolet rays from sunlight, X-rays and other forms of radiation. Some viruses have been linked to cancer. These are rare and are called biological carcinogens.

Several chemicals are cancer suspects which means that animal experiments may have resulted in cancer but the evidence linking the cancer to that chemical is currently uncertain. In 1960, this uncertainty spawned the infamous Delaney Amendment to the FDA's Food, Drug and Cosmetic Act of 1938. In a nutshell, this amendment meant that any substance that was suspected of causing any type of cancer in any laboratory test, no matter how the test was carried out, would be banned from use in any food product, cosmetic, or oral drug, even if the risk was minute. Delaney's critics asked the question whether sugar would be banned if a laboratory rat developed a tumor after being force-fed a vast quantity of it day-in and day-out for its entire life? Presumably, this experiment has never been carried out.

No such rule exists in the EU. Each chemical is tested separately and ruled upon individually. If the risks are sufficiently high, the chemical is banned. Where the risk is uncertain, for example in the case of formaldehyde, a preservative used in cosmetics, the chemicals are still used but are subject to restrictions.

Ingredients that Can Cause Cancer

The following ingredients have all been implicated in a cancer scare, linked to cancer or are cancer suspects, or they may contain carcinogenic residues; however, we have not found any evidence that cosmetics containing these ingredients have directly caused cancer in individuals.

1,2-Phenylenediamine

2,4-Diaminoanisole

2,4-Diaminoanisole Sulfate

2,4-Toluenediamine

2,5-Diaminoanisole

2-Chloro-p-phenylenediamine

2-Chloro-p-phenylenediamine Sulfate

2-Methoxyaniline

2-Nitro-p-phenylenediamine

2-Nitropropane

4-Chloro-1,2-phenylenediamine

4-Methoxyaniline

BHT

CI 77266

CI 77268:1

Coumarin

DEA (ingredients containing
DEA may contain DEA residues)

Diamine

Dimethicone

Direct Black 38

Direct Blue 6

FD&C Red #3

Formaldehyde

Hydrogen Peroxide

Naphthalene

Nitrilotriacetic Acid

o-Nitro-p-Aminophenol

Phenacetin

Phthalic Acid

Ingredients containing Phthalate

Steramidopropyl Diamethylamine

Tocopherol

Trisodium NTA

MUTAGENS AND TERATOGENS

A mutagen is an agent that can cause mutations in living cells. A mutagen can be a virus, a chemical, or one of several types of radiation – naturally occurring radiation (from rocks or the sun), the result of nuclear fallout from atomic tests, radiation leaks, medical X-rays, or radiotherapy. The changes take place in the nucleus of the cell, potentially giving rise to cancer or an inherited disease. Mutagens that cause cancer are called carcinogens.

Teratogens (from the Greek "terat," meaning monster) are mutagens that cause changes in the cells of embryos or fetuses, resulting in malformed babies. The most notorious examples of teratogens are the rubella virus and thalidomide, a drug used to reduce nausea and morning sickness during pregnancy.

Mutagens and Teratogens

The following cosmetic ingredients and oxidation hair dyes have been linked with cell mutations; however, we have found no evidence that cosmetics containing these ingredients have directly caused harm to any individuals.

2,4-Diaminoanisole (and Sulfate)	Dimethicone
2,4-Toluenediamine	m-Phenylenediamine
2-Nitro-p-phenylenediamine	m-Phenylenediamine Sulfate
4-Nitro-o-phenylenediamine	p-Phenylenediamine (and HCl and Sulfate)
4-Nitro-o-phenylenediamine HCl	Phthalate (family)

Boric Acid and Borates have been linked to fetal malformation.

CONTACT LENS INFECTIONS

There have been a number of scare stories associated with the wearing of contact lenses. Eye infections caused by a microbe called acanthamoeba have been increasing rapidly with the growing number of contact-lens users. This microbe causes acanthamoeba keratitis, a painful and disabling eye disease. Acanthamoeba keratitis can be treated if it is diagnosed early, but some patients have required corneal transplants and a few patients have lost an eye. Poor contact-lens hygiene has been linked to 85 percent of the diagnosed cases of this infection in the UK. Some medical experts suggest, in fact, that the number of cases of acanthamoeba keratitis has not been increasing, but that doctors and opticians have simply become better at recognizing and diagnosing it.

Make sure your lens-cleaning solution can kill acanthamoeba. This microbe is the most common amoeba (single-celled protozoan), and occurs in soil, fresh and brackish water, airborne dust, hot tubs, air-conditioning units, and in the noses and throats of humans and animals. This is why you should never clean grit from your contact lenses or moisten them by licking or putting them in your mouth.

It's a Fact

Each year misdirected champagne corks and sporting accidents claim more eyes than acanthamoeba infections caused by poor contact-lens hygiene.

Always use a quality contact-lens cleaning solution and then rinse the lenses in sterile water or saline solution before putting them back in your eyes. A large number of contact-lens cleaning solutions contain hydrogen peroxide, which is extremely effective at killing the vast majority of microbes. It is also highly corrosive and damaging to eyes, and must be neutralized completely before the contact lenses are used after cleaning. This is usually achieved by adding an enzyme that slowly breaks down the hydrogen peroxide to water and bubbles of oxygen. Some brands of cleaning solution use a chemical catalyst instead of an enzyme to break down the hydrogen peroxide. In either case the neutralizer can be added as a tablet or it can be built into the contact-lens case. If you use the latter system, the case should be changed regularly in accordance with the manufacturer's instructions.

The hydrogen peroxide system can lead to two problems. If you are in a hurry and leave insufficient time for the hydrogen peroxide to break down, or if you use an old lens case where the built-in neutralizer has become less effective, you risk getting this corrosive chemical in your eyes. As long as there are bubbles around the lenses, hydrogen peroxide is present; wait until the bubbling has completely stopped before reusing the lenses. The other problem is that if the neutralizer breaks down the hydrogen peroxide too quickly, it may not have sufficient time to kill all of the microbes. This can happen if too much neutralizer has been added or if the solution becomes too warm, for example, if the lens case is kept on a hot, sunny windowsill. It may also happen if the hydrogen peroxide has become weak with age, so never use solutions that have passed their sell-by date.

As an alternative to hydrogen peroxide, cleaning solutions can be based on surfactants (detergents) and antimicrobials. These can leave residues on the lenses which may cause irritation if they are not thoroughly rinsed off. Whatever system you use, it should be perfectly safe providing you always follow the manufacturer's instructions.

EYE WHITENERS

The so-called eye whitener drops that are available over the counter reduce the red appearance of tired, bloodshot eyes by narrowing the tiny blood vessels that cover the surface of the eyes. When the medication wears off the blood vessels dilate again, but all too often they become larger and redder than they were before the treatment. The natural response is to use more of the whitening drops and before you know it you are locked into a cycle of using these products habitually. These products should be restricted to occasional use only, and should not used as a routine cosmetic.

Eyes commonly become red through tiredness, allergy, cold winds or dryness caused by environmental conditions, and (less frequently) as a result of injury or infection. The redness may be nature's way of warning us of a more serious condition that requires medical treatment. Eye-whitening drops will remove the redness but they will not treat the underlying cause of the problem. Delaying essential medical treatment by masking the symptoms may allow the condition to worsen.

Eye-whitening drops usually contain vasoconstrictors which narrow the blood vessels, and may also contain antihistamines to alleviate allergic reactions. Both of these ingredients may cause adverse effects such as irritation, allergies, or local toxicity. If your red-eye condition is painful, has a discharge, or impairs your vision, do not use eye whiteners but seek medical advice.

16 salons and surgeons

Just lie back and relax
While I do your bikini wax.
Perhaps a spot of liposuction,
Dermabrasion or breast reduction?

If you want to pamper yourself, then a day at a salon or health spa might be in order. This might make you feel good, and an expert makeover may improve your looks, hide your fine lines and reduce the appearance of your wrinkles but, unfortunately, it only lasts as long as the make-up does. If you really want to change your looks and actually get rid of those wrinkles, then you will have to spend some serious money on cosmetic surgery. This chapter looks at what the salon can do for you, and then briefly reviews some of the more common cosmetic surgery procedures. Some of the procedures carried out in salons such as waxing and eyelash tints (which are banned in the USA), have been dealt with in previous chapters (see *Chapter 5 – Skin Care* and *Chapter 9 – Hair Care*).

SALONS

Cosmetics and toiletries used by professional hairdressers and beauticians are different to those you can buy in the high street. Professional toiletries often contain higher concentrations of active ingredients such as hair-perming solutions and hair-removal formulations, and they have special labeling rules, usually involving additional health and safety information. This assumes the professionals are highly trained and know how to use these products correctly. Make sure you visit a qualified beautician and not someone who is inexperienced, otherwise you risk your skin being burnt or your hair damaged by strong solutions being used incorrectly. A good, qualified hairdresser will know if your hair is too brittle to be permed or the strength of the solution that can be applied safely. A good, qualified beautician will know or be able to establish whether your skin is too sensitive for a product, or be able to tell whether the marks on your fingernails are due to normal wear and tear or to a fungus which should be treated by a doctor.

Electrolysis

Electrolysis results in the permanent removal of unwanted hairs. There are two methods – the tried-and-tested needle epilator, or the recently introduced tweezer epilator.

A needle epilator consists of a fine needle, which is pushed into the skin, alongside the hair shaft, and into the hair follicle. A small electric current is then passed through the needle, to kill the hair root. The hair is then removed with a pair of tweezers and, if the treatment is successful, it will not grow again.

Treatment using professional epilators should only be carried out by a qualified beautician or electrologist. In the wrong hands, there is a risk of infection, electrical shock, or permanent disfigurement. Even in the right hands, electrolysis can be uncomfortable or painful. Electrolysis on the forearms or legs can prove expensive and time consuming, requiring many sessions to remove all the hairs. It is possible to buy needle epilators for home use and these are generally safe since they produce lower voltages than are used in salons, but the risk of infection remains. It is not recommended to have this type of electrolysis on the lower margins of the eyebrows where the skin is thin and easily damaged, nor on the armpits where there is an abundance of bacteria that increases the risk of infection.

Tweezer epilators are a more recent development and are less painful than needle epilators because they do not penetrate the skin. The hair is grasped in an insulated pair of tweezers, through which the electric current flows. The electricity travels down the hair shaft and into the root, destroying it. The hair, along with its dead root, is then pulled out with the tweezers.

Both needle and tweezer epilators can give a small, painful electric shock if the needle or tweezer accidentally touches the skin and both methods will require several treatments. Even if all the hairs are removed from an area of skin, there may be other hair follicles lying dormant, ready to appear in their next growth cycle. As a rough guide, to remove all the hairs from one forearm, you will require approximately eight hours of treatments over a period of two months, then once a month for the next eight to ten months to clear any new hairs that may appear.

Research into the use of lasers for permanent hair removal is currently under way. A black dye is applied to the skin and soaks into the hair follicle. The excess dye is then washed away and a laser beam scanned across the skin. The heat of the laser beam is absorbed by the dye in the hair follicle but not by the surrounding skin tissue. The laser overheats the hair roots and kills them. At the time of writing, the tests show this process permanently removes about 30 percent of the hairs in each treatment.

As an alternative to hair removal on large areas such as the forearms and legs, you can disguise the appearance of dark hairs, making them less obvious by lightening or bleaching them. This can be achieved by using a mixture of hydrogen peroxide and dilute ammonia.

Ear Piercing

The way that ear piercing used to be carried out was to puncture the ear lobe with a needle, then to push a gold stud through the hole to prevent it from healing. This procedure is no longer used by professionals, as it carries a risk of transmitting infections, although some brave people still use this method on themselves, or cajole friends into helping them.

The preferred professional method now is to use a piercing gun, which fires the stud through the ear lobe without first puncturing it. The stud comes in a sealed, sterile package and is not touched by the person operating the gun, nor does the gun come into direct contact with the ear. Once in place, the stud is covered with a sterile dressing for a few days. Then for the next four to six weeks the stud is rotated twice daily to stop the skin from attaching itself to it, and the ear lobe is cleaned with surgical spirit or hydrogen peroxide to prevent any infections.

Generally, piercing your ear lobes in this way carries little risk, but studs that contain nickel can cause dermatitis. If an infection occurs, it can be easily treated with antibiotics prescribed by your doctor. Recently it has become fashionable to wear an earring, or a number of earrings, through the top part of the ear. This part of the ear is composed of cartilage which has a poor blood supply. If an infection takes hold here, it may be difficult to treat and, in some cases, may require the surgical removal of a portion of the infected outer ear, causing permanent disfigurement.

A blow to the side of the head caused, for example, in a side-on car collision, or from a sporting accident, will always be potentially dangerous, but this danger is increased by wearing earrings or studs in the top of the ear. The impact may drive the stud or earring into the side of the skull causing a fracture, or possibly worse. Earrings worn on the ear lobe would merely be pushed into the fleshy recess above the jaw joint, causing little damage.

Aromatherapy

Aromatherapy is a branch of complementary (alternative) medicine used to treat a wide range of ailments by massaging essential oils onto the skin. Aromatherapists offer treatments for coughs, colds, burns, headaches, insomnia, viral, bacterial and fungal infections, fatigue, psoriasis, and eczema. Mental and emotional disorders are also treated but, as with all branches of alternative medicine, most of the claims are unscientific and little or no clinical evidence is available to support them. The medical profession does, however, agree that aromatherapy sessions are extremely relaxing and can successfully treat stress-related ailments and psychosomatic illnesses.

The treatment relies on the essential oils, or components dissolved in the oils, entering the body, either by absorption through the skin or by inhalation of the vapors. As with most chemicals, the skin is an effective barrier and few, if any, oils will penetrate deep enough to enter the bloodstream. The essential oils most often used are those from bergamot, geranium, lavender, rosemary, tea tree, and ylang ylang (*Cananga odorata* or poor man's jasmine).

Bergamot oil contains 5-methoxypsoralen, which is known to cause photosensitivity. Patients are advised to avoid direct sunlight for some time after treatment using this oil. 5-Methoxypsoralen is banned from cosmetics in the EU except for the normal content in natural essences used. Rosemary oil has also been reported to cause photosensitivity and it is an irritant that can cause allergic dermatitis.

Geranium oil is known to cause skin irritation and has been linked to contact dermatitis. Linalool (also spelled linalol and linalool) has been reported to cause facial psoriasis. It is a component of both lavender oil and bergamot oil.

Are aromatherapy products cosmetics or medical products? This is not easy to answer. Aromatherapy products sold over the counter in the UK fall within the scope of the General Product Safety Regulations 1994, unless they claim to have, or are intended to have, medical or cosmetic functions. They are classified as cosmetics if they are intended to be placed on the skin (or any other external parts of the body including the mouth and teeth) for the purpose of cleaning, changing the odor or appearance, or to protect it or keep it in good condition. If the product makes medical claims or if it is intended to be used for medical reasons, then it becomes a medicinal product and is regulated as such.

SURGEONS

It is not the aim of this book to advise on cosmetic surgery. However, the only realistic way to remove fine lines and wrinkles is through medical intervention, whether by the use of retinoid drugs or surgical procedures. Therefore, some of the more common cosmetic treatments available are discussed below.

Collagen Replacement Therapy (CRT) and Fat Transplants

CRT is the simplest and least invasive of the procedures available for the reduction of fine lines and wrinkles.

Collagen, a tough, fibrous, flexible protein, occurs naturally in the deeper layers of our skin and is responsible for its elasticity. As we age, the network of collagen fibers gradually weaken and become damaged through the constant stretching of the skin, exposure to ultraviolet radiation, cigarette smoke, and injury. Every time we smile, frown or squint, we put stress on the collagen in our facial skin and weaken it further. Over the years collagen is damaged and lost from our skin, making it less elastic. The creases that appear when we smile no longer vanish when we cease smiling, and when we stop squinting, the crow's feet in the corners of our eyes stay with us. Collagen replacement therapy (CRT) restores the levels of collagen and improves the appearance of fine lines and wrinkles. It can also be used to disguise pock marks, minor scars, and unwanted dimples.

A month before treatment the patient is given a patch test on the arm to make sure they are not allergic to the collagen; this is usually bovine collagen (from cattle), although collagen extracted from other animals is also used. The replacement therapy is painless and takes about 15 to 20 minutes. Anesthetic creams are applied to the skin and the collagen is injected directly into the dermis (deeper layer of skin) using a fine hypodermic needle. Minor defects can be treated in one session but deeper blemishes may require two or more treatments. There is usually some swelling and redness immediately after the treatment but this fades within a week and the skin then appears normal, although it looks fuller, smoother, and feels firmer and younger.

The injected collagen gradually breaks down and is absorbed by the body. To maintain an improved appearance, between two and four top-up treatments are needed each year.

Collagen implants involve exactly the same techniques but they are used to give more volume to eyebrows, chins, and lips, improving their proportions to match the rest of the face. As an alternative to rhinoplasty (surgery to alter the size or shape of the bridge of the nose – a nose job), collagen implants are often used to enhance the chin, making the nose appear smaller and more in proportion with the rest of the face. Again, regular top-up treatments are required. More permanent results can be achieved by implanting persistent materials such as silicone or PTFE (the same materials are used to make non-stick pans). Implants of this nature require more invasive surgery, often under general anesthetic.

A safer alternative to collagen implants is a fat transplant. Fat cells are taken from another part of the body, often the hips, and injected into the face. This has two advantages over CRT. First, there is no chance of an allergic reaction since the fat comes from your own body, and second, it lasts longer than CRT. About 80 percent of the transplanted fat cells die and are reabsorbed into the body, but those that are implanted near to blood vessels survive. This can give a permanent improvement to the contours of the face.

Face-lift

A face-lift is a surgical procedure to smooth out fine lines and wrinkles, and lift sagging skin under the chin and below the cheeks. The effect is to make an aging face look between five and ten years younger. The operation is often carried out under local anesthetic, as an out-patient procedure. It causes discomfort and bruising, and sometimes swelling, which lasts between a few days to two weeks after the operation. Stitches are removed after three to five days, and the scars are usually hidden under the hairline or in natural folds in the skin. Residual scars usually fade within a year. The cosmetic improvement may not be apparent until all of the bruising and swelling has subsided.

The operation involves the removal of a strip of skin starting at the top corner of the forehead, following the hairline down to the top of the ear where it meets the cheek, then down the front of the ear to the point where the ear lobe joins the cheek. The skin covering the cheeks is undercut all the way to the nose and corner of the mouth. This flap of skin is then pulled up and back, and sewn together again at the hairline. It is usual to do both sides of the face at the same time.

There are always a few risks associated with any surgical procedure but the outcome is usually very good, and only rarely do patients find the results are not what they expected. After the operation, the face will continue to age normally and fine lines and wrinkles will return after five to ten years, but at that time, the patient will still look five to ten years younger than their real age. Despite the expense, it is essential to find a cosmetic surgeon who has a good reputation.

Liposuction and Microsuction

Also called suction lipectomy or vacuum-assisted lipectomy, liposuction is a surgical procedure carried out by a cosmetic surgeon to physically remove excess body fat (lipids), thereby improving the contours of the body. It is usually carried out under general anesthetic and involves making a small incision in the skin where the scar can be hidden in the natural folds of the skin. A hollow, stainless steel tube is then inserted into the fatty, subcutaneous layer which lies just below the dermis, and suction is used to remove unwanted fat, in the same way that a vacuum cleaner picks up dust. It is normal practice to treat both sides of the body during the operation. After the procedure there is usually some swelling, bruising and soreness. The resulting reduction in weight will last until you start to over-eat again.

When you put on weight, you do not increase the number of fat cells in your body, but rather the size of the existing cells as they swell up with the excess fat. If you only seem to gain fat on your thighs it is because you have a lot of fat cells in that part of your body. If you reduce the number of fat cells in your thighs by liposuction, you will permanently reduce the amount of fat that can be stored there. This means that if you over-eat and gain weight, the fat will be more evenly distributed over your body, maintaining its improved contours.

Microsuction is a similar procedure to liposuction. It is used to remove excess fat cells from the delicate tissues of the face using very fine tubes.

Eyelift

Blepharoplasty, commonly referred to as an eyelift, is a cosmetic operation to remove bags, sagging skin, folds, and wrinkles from the eyelids. It can be carried out on both the upper and lower eyelids but is most commonly used to remove the pads of fat that collect under the eyes, forming unsightly bags.

For bag removal, an incision is made inside the lower eyelid, through which the fat is removed by suction. If it is also necessary to tighten and smooth the skin over the bag, the incision is made on the outside of the eye, just below the eyelashes.

To tighten the skin under the eyes, a thin, horizontal strip of skin is removed just below the eyelashes, allowing the scars to be disguised by the natural folds in the skin, and the remaining skin is stretched to close the incision, thereby removing its loose or wrinkled appearance. For the upper eyelids, a horizontal fold of skin is removed from the center of each lid, allowing the resulting scars to be hidden in the natural folds of the eyelids.

Eyelifts usually take about 90 minutes and are normally carried out under local anesthetic, the patient being allowed home the same day. Swelling and bruising usually subside in three to ten days and are assisted by the application of cold pads soaked in a mild astringent solution, such as witch hazel. A reputable cosmetic surgeon may advise people against this procedure if they have a tendency to scar easily or if their scars persist for a long time.

Deep Skin Peels

The appearance of fine lines and wrinkles can be reduced temporarily by peeling off the outer layer of skin from the face. This makes the face red, raw, and sore for a few days before new skin grows, but this new skin will appear to have fewer fine lines and wrinkles. Cosmetic surgeons use chemical skin peels such as strong acids, or physical skin peels such as dermabrasion or (more commonly now), laser planing.

Originally, phenol-based skin peelers were used to dissolve the outer layer of skin cells, but this is a highly corrosive and unreliable technique and has been superseded by the use of trichloroacetic acid (TCA). These chemicals are far more corrosive than any skin peel (exfoliant) you can buy over the counter or use in a salon, and they burn much deeper into the skin. Results are generally good, but there are some horror stories of permanent disfigurement and eye damage.

Dermabrasion involves a tiny, high speed, rotating abrasive pad which is used to skim off the outer layer of skin cells in the same way that a large sanding disk is used to smooth wooden floors. Technology moves very quickly and dermabrasion is rapidly being replaced by laser planing, in which a powerful laser beam burns off the outer layer of skin cells. Results are generally good and at the time of writing, there have been no headline horror stories of which the authors are aware.

Other Procedures

The ingenuity of cosmetic surgeons knows no bounds and they come up with some amazing solutions to improve our looks. For example, when we frown a tiny pair of muscles, called corrugators, contract causing vertical furrows to appear above the nose. As we get older, the furrows become more obvious and persistent. Cosmetic surgeons have come up with two solution to this. An operation called a corrugator resection simply cuts these muscles to stop them causing the furrow lines. Since these muscles do nothing else, all other facial expressions are unaffected.

If you do not like the sound of cutting the muscles, you can paralyze them instead using a drug called Botox. Each treatment lasts about six months and the results are immediate. The only risk is that the muscles on one side may recover before the other, giving the face an unbalanced frown. This drug can also be used to paralyze the muscles that cause horizontal furrows on our forehead. The only alternative currently available to removing these horizontal furrows is a forehead lift – a more invasive and extensive procedure.

Botox, is made from botulism toxin, a deadly poison, but it is, nevertheless, a safe drug.

17 animal products and animal testing

The use of animal products in cosmetics and toiletries, and animal testing, have been the subject of much controversy. This chapter examines the need for animal testing and looks at the alternatives. It alerts vegetarian readers to the ingredients in cosmetics and toiletries that may be derived from animals, and it reveals what manufacturers really mean when they claim their products have not been tested on animals.

ANIMAL TESTING

In a perfect world there would be no animal testing. However, we all use modern medicines, cleaning chemicals, cosmetics, and toiletries, and we benefit from the cheap food produced using modern agricultural chemicals. At the same time we demand that these substances are proved to be perfectly safe before they are used in the products we buy and consume. It is essential, therefore, to find realistic and reliable safety tests that provide alternatives to animal testing.

The big players in the cosmetics game are the USA and the EU in the West, with Japan dominating the Eastern market. These countries/unions have been working together to find reliable *in vitro* methods (non-animal, literally meaning "in glass" such as test-tubes or petri dishes), using tissue cultures for testing the safety of cosmetic ingredients. The search to find an acceptable alternative to animal testing has been fraught with difficulties and, despite the advances that have been made in using these techniques, there are many critics who believe they are unreliable or limited in some way, and that a certain amount of animal testing will always be necessary.

In 1993 the EU produced a directive that all animal testing of cosmetic ingredients or their combinations would be banned after January 1, 1998. This ruling was in conflict with the requirement that any cosmetics sold in the EU must not cause damage to human health when used under normal or reasonably foreseeable conditions. To this end the deadline for the animal-testing ban was postponed until June 30, 2000. On June 19, 2000 the deadline was further postponed until June 30, 2002. It would be reasonable to assume that this new deadline is likely to be extended until non-animal testing techniques have been proved completely reliable. Until that time, animal testing will continue.

The animals used are mainly albino rabbits, for testing cosmetics and toiletries, and mice and rats for most other substances. Cats, dogs, primates, and farm animals account for less than one percent of all animal tests, and some cosmetics are tested for skin irritation on human volunteers. The most common test for cosmetics is the Draize test, where the chemicals are placed directly into the eye or onto the skin of an albino rabbit to test for irritation and damage.

Tissue cultures used in non-animal tests often consist of a mass of living cells taken from a mouse and then grown on a culture medium in a glass dish. Many hundreds of dishes of cells can be grown from just a few cells taken from just one living animal. Cosmetics or individual cosmetic ingredients are added to the cells in the dish, and any changes in the cell's biochemistry may indicate an adverse reaction to a chemical. However it is difficult to say exactly how that change will translate to irritation or harm in humans.

Cosmetic labels may carry phrases like "Cruelty Free," or "Not Tested On Animals," but this may be misleading. If these phrases are used in the EU, regulations require the label to state if the testing was carried out on the finished cosmetic or on individual ingredients or combinations of ingredients. No such regulations exist in the USA. The product may say that there has been no animal testing, but the manufacturer may have arranged for the supplier of the ingredients to do the tests for them. Alternatively they may simply check the scientific literature to see if the tests have been carried out in the past and only use those ingredients that have already been tested. Many ingredients have been around for years. You can be certain that someone, somewhere, has thoroughly tested them on animals on more than one occasion.

Even if all the ingredients in a cosmetic have previously been tested and found to be harmless, combinations of these ingredients may have a combined irritant effect, or they may react together in an unpredictable way, forming harmful products. It is for this reason that tests on the finished product are important. In the EU's guidelines for testing cosmetic safety, it is noted that, currently, there is no *in vitro* test that has been successfully validated for use on finished cosmetics. In the interests of animal welfare the finished cosmetic may be sold without further animal tests, providing that:

1 the toxicity of all the ingredients is known,
2 the combined ingredients are unlikely to react together in an adverse way, and
3 the ingredients do not include something that is likely to cause other ingredients to penetrate the skin to a greater extent than they penetrated when they were originally tested.

Tests for toxicity, phototoxicity, cell mutation, gene mutation, and a range of other potentially damaging effects are generally carried out reliably on tissue cultures. A microscope will show up any cells that are dying or growing in an abnormal way. Despite these tests, however, some of the ingredients that cause these effects still find their way into cosmetics.

ANIMAL PRODUCTS

As the name suggests, animal products come from animals, often from parts of the animals that are not suitable for human consumption. The use in cosmetics of products derived from human tissues, endangered, or protected species is banned. The main animal products used are proteins (and the amino acids obtained from them), and fats and oils used for making soaps and detergents – although some of these can also be obtained from plant sources or synthesized from petroleum products. Relatively few fragrances are obtained from animals, although musk is a valued scent secreted from the scent glands of the male Tibetan musk deer, musk ox, civet cat, otter, and several other species, and ambergris from the sperm whale and castoreum from the beaver have also been used in expensive fragrances.

Soap

Soap is made when natural fats and oils are boiled with sodium hydroxide, a strong, corrosive alkali. Sodium stearate is the most common ingredient in bars of soaps and other soap-based cleansing products. Sodium and potassium tallowate are also common ingredients of soap. They are produced from beef, or sometimes lamb fat. There is currently no vegetable source of tallowates, but it is possible to obtain stearates from non-animal sources.

Since the BSE crisis (bovine spongiform encephalopathy, or "mad cow disease"), EU regulations required beef tallow to be processed at extreme conditions. Saponification (soap making) must be carried out using 12M sodium hydroxide – an enormously concentrated solution of caustic soda. During batch processing, temperatures of at least 95°C must be used for at least three hours, to ensure all microbes or proteins contaminating the tallow are completely destroyed. For continuous processes, a temperature of 140°C and a pressure of at least 2 bars (that is twice normal atmospheric pressure) must be used for at least eight minutes. Additionally, cosmetics and toiletries must not contain any part of the skull, brain, eyes, tonsils, or spinal cord of cows, sheep, or goats aged 12 months or more, or the spleens of year-old sheep or goats. This age limit for sheep and goats is reduced if the animal's permanent incisor teeth have erupted through their gums.

Mink Oils

Mink are bred for their superior fur. The oils that keep the mink's fur in perfect condition are secreted by glands in the subcutaneous layers of their skin. These oils are extracted from the fatty tissues under the skin when the mink are killed. It is assumed that they will impart the same qualities to human hair and skin as they did for the ill-fated animal. Several semisynthetic derivatives of mink oil are also used in cosmetics. These can be easily recognized since part of the INCI name will include the word "mink."

Proteins and Amino Acids

Elastin, keratin, and collagen are all animal proteins that find their way into cosmetics and toiletries. Elastin is an elastic protein which is extracted from the artery walls of mammals, and sometimes from their skin tissues. Collagen is the tough, fibrous protein that forms tendons, ligaments, and connective tissues. It is claimed that elastin and collagen penetrate the skin and rejuvenate its elasticity lost during the normal aging process. Another myth is that keratin, the tough, fibrous protein that makes up skin, hair, and nails can, when added to shampoos and conditioners, enter the hair and repair any damage. This notion is as ludicrous as the idea that rubbing sawdust into a storm-damaged tree can mend the broken branches.

Placenta

The placenta (afterbirth) is the organ that allows nutrients, oxygen, and waste materials to be exchanged between a female mammal's blood and her unborn infant. It is rich in proteins, hormones, and vitamins. Placental extract, both from human and bovine placentas, is valued for its supposed ability to rejuvenate the skin, and is widely used in cosmetics. Placental proteins are used as antistatic agents and humectants, and placental lipids (fats) are used as emollients.

Some manufacturers remove the hormones and other biologically active substances from the placentas before using them as placental extract in their cosmetics. In this case, the FDA recommends that manufacturers should not state that the product contains placental extracts. Currently, cells, tissues, or other products of human origin are banned from use in cosmetics in the EU. Any placental extract in products purchased in the EU will, therefore, be of bovine origin.

Animal Products

The following ingredients have been taken from animals. Look out for these names on their own or as part of the ingredient name. If you want to avoid animal products, make sure the cosmetic or toiletry states that it is free from animal products on the label.

Products obtained from animals that have been killed:
- Adeps Bovis (obtained from tallow)
- Animal Tissue Extract

- Aorta Extract
- CI 77267 (bone charcoal)
- CI 77268: 1 (black bone charcoal)
- Collagen
- Elastin
- Fish Glycerides
- Fish Oil
- Gelatin
- Hyaluronic Acid (from the synovial fluid that surrounds the joints in animal skeletons)
- Keratin
- Mink Oil and Mink Oil derivatives
- Musk (Muscone)
- Placenta
- Serum Albumin (from blood serum)
- Squali Iecur, Squalene and Pentahydrosqualene (from shark liver oil)
- Tallow and many ingredients containing the name "Tallow" or "Tallowate"
- Unipertan

Egg products including chicken and fish eggs obtained from fish roe:
- Albumen
- Ovum
- Phosphatidylcholine
- Roe Extract
- Salmo

Ingredients that can be obtained from both animal and vegetable sources:
- Lecithin
- Phospholipids
- Tyrosine
- Fatty acids and their derivatives that contain the names "Stearate," "Laurate," "Myristate," "Palmitate," "Oleate," "Linoleate," and "Linolenate." The corresponding fatty acids have names such as "Stearic Acid," "Lauric Acid," and so on. Some are converted to "-eth" ingredients, such as "Steareth," "Laureth," etc.
- Glycerin and many ingredients containing the names "Glyceryl" and "Glycereth"

Other products:
Ceresin is a petroleum product, but it is sometimes purified using animal charcoal.

18 labels and legal matters

"If the law supposes that," said Mr Bumble ... "the law is a ass – a idiot."

(*Oliver Twist*, Charles Dickens)

Although this chapter comes at the end of this section, it is perhaps the most important. It's all very well knowing about the adverse effects of individual cosmetic ingredients and how they work, but this is of little use if you do not know how to interpret the label and read between the lines. This chapter explains the law relating to the labeling of cosmetics and toiletries, including the names that must be used for ingredients and how they must be listed. It also points out some legal loopholes that a number of manufacturers eagerly exploit. The regulations relating to cosmetic labeling are remarkably similar on both sides of the Atlantic and, therefore, what follows applies equally to products sold in any EU country or in the USA.

LISTING THE INGREDIENTS

The law requires all cosmetics and toiletries to be clearly and correctly labeled. If it is not obvious, the label should state the purpose of the product and give simple instructions for its safe use. For example, if it is shampoo it should say so – in case you mistake it for mouthwash. The label must clearly show any restrictions, such as "Must not be used on children under the age of three," and it must highlight any harmful, corrosive, or active ingredients. For example, if a sunscreen contains oxybenzone the label must state, "Contains Oxybenzone." The label should also carry a list showing all of the ingredients in descending order of weight, and the INCI (International Nomenclature of Cosmetic Ingredients) name should be used wherever possible (see p.195).

Ingredients need not be listed on products supplied to professional salons in the USA, providing they are used exclusively in the salon and not sold to customers. "Best before" dates are required in the EU if the product is expected to deteriorate within 30 months of manufacture but they are not required in the USA, although many manufacturers do use them. The EU also requires product codes and the manufacturer's batch numbers to be included.

In practice things are not as simple as this. The product may be too small to carry a list of ingredients, or the manufacturer may want to keep the ingredients secret for valid commercial reasons. In both the USA and the EU the regulating authorities recognize that manufacturers may wish to keep certain ingredients secret and in this event, they may apply to the regulating authorities for an exemption to the labeling regulations. Before it is granted, however, the manufacturer must supply extensive proof that their product is safe and that they have a genuine reason for requiring trade secrecy.

A list of ingredients must be made available to the customer. If the container is too small to carry this list, as in the case of lipsticks, the ingredients may be written on the box (if there is one), or on a leaflet included in the box or a tag attached to the product. Failing this, the ingredients must be displayed on a notice where it can be easily seen, near to where the product is sold. In practice the notice is usually hidden away under the counter and you have to ask for it. As a last resort the manufacturer must send you a list of ingredients if you request one. The authors put this to the test and received by post, product information on six items, within two weeks of e-mailing one particular manufacturer.

The list of ingredients does not have to show substances that were used during the production of the cosmetic but are no longer present. For example, an acid may have been used to neutralize an alkali present in the cosmetic during manufacture, but is no longer present in the finished product. Impurities in the raw materials, such as pesticide residues in plant extracts, or chemical by-products formed accidentally during manufacture, do not have to be listed. Similarly, small amounts of solvents used as a carrier for fragrance chemicals will not be shown separately on the list of ingredients. Ingredients do not have to be listed on sample products that come with a monthly magazine or in junk mail, nor on small courtesy bottles or sachets provided in hotels.

The ingredients should be listed in descending order of weight so you can judge how much of each chemical is present. Water (Aqua) is often the main ingredient in liquid cosmetics and toiletries (80–90 percent in some products such as mild shampoos). Minor ingredients that each make up less than one percent of the finished product may be listed in any order after those ingredients that make up one percent or more. Active ingredients – that is, those that may have a therapeutic or medicinal effect (such as in a medicated shampoo or mouthwash) – should be listed under the heading "Active Ingredients," before the main list of other ingredients.

In the case of decorative cosmetics that come in a range of colors or shades, such as lipstick, eye shadow, mascara, foundation, and hair color, manufacturers may economize on their label-printing costs by producing one label for all of the shades – providing they show all of the colorants used in the entire range. In the EU these are listed at the end of the ingredients in square brackets, like this: [+ /- CI 77491, CI 77492, CI 77499]. In the USA they are listed after the words "May Contain: ... " This means the particular shade of make-up you are looking at *may contain* at least one of the colors listed, but probably not all of them and, in fact, may contain no color at all. This does not help the individual who knows they are allergic to CI 77491 but not to the other two in the above example. Does this product contain it or not?

READING BETWEEN THE LINES

The label can be very revealing if you read between the lines. If you are worried about buying anything with a harmful ingredient look for the word, "Contains ... " The EU Commission have identified a number of ingredients that are not entirely safe and require them to be clearly labeled separately from the main list of ingredients; for example, "Contains Alkali," "Contains Hydrogen peroxide," "Contains Thioglycollate," and so on. You can also look out for warnings. If the label says, "Not for use on children under the age of 3," you may decide that you don't wish to use it on yourself.

Another way to gain more information is to look at the order in which the ingredients are listed and locate the ingredient you are interested in. For example, if you want to buy a product that contains mainly natural ingredients, you can find out how much of the natural ingredient it contains by reading between the lines. First you need to know that plant extracts are always listed using their Latin names, to avoid confusion caused by regional variations of common plant names. On the sample label shown below for Dewberry Shampoo, you can see the fruit extract's name given in Latin. Next, you must know that the ingredients are listed in decreasing order by weight if there is one percent or more of the ingredient, followed by those ingredients that each make up less than one percent of the finished product, in any order.

TYPICAL INGREDIENTS – NATURAL COLLECTION DEWBERRY SHAMPOO

Ingredients:

Aqua, Sodium lauryl sulfate (SLS), Sodium chloride, Cocamide DEA, PEG-6 cocamide, PEG-55 propylene glycol oleate, Polyquaternium-7, Citric acid, Parfum, 2-Bromo-2-nitropropane-1,3-diol, Rubus fruticosus, Magnesium nitrate, Methylparaben, Sodium benzoate, Denatonium benzoate, Benzoic acid, Magnesium chloride, Propylparaben, Methylchloroisothiazolinone, Methylisothiazolinone, CI 17200, CI 42090

Aqua	Water – the main ingredient.
Sodium lauryl sulfate (SLS)*	Anionic surfactant.
Sodium chloride	Common salt – astringent.
Cocamide DEA*	Emulsifier and high-foaming surfactant. Helps to produce a lather. Between 1 and 5 percent is typically added.
PEG-6 cocamide*	Emulsifier and surfactant.
PEG-55 propylene glycol oleate*	Thickening agent to give the shampoo body.
Polyquaternium-7	Antistatic agent. Also forms an oily film on the hair, i.e., it is a hair conditioner.
Citric acid	Used to adjust the pH of the shampoo.
Parfum	A mixture of fragrance chemicals, often more than 50 in number many of which are artificial.

2-Bromo-2-nitropropane-1,3-diol*	Preservative limited to 0.1 percent.[+]
Rubus fruticosus	Blackberry extract – a close relative of the dewberry (Rubus caesius).
Magnesium nitrate	Improves the action of Methylchloroisothiazolinone and Methylisothiazolinone (see below).
Methylparaben*	Water-soluble preservative, limited to 0.4 percent.[+]
Sodium benzoate*	Water-soluble preservative, limited to 0.5 percent.[+]
Denatonium benzoate	Denaturant – imparts an unpleasant taste to discourage consumption.
Benzoic acid*	Water-soluble preservative limited to 0.5 percent.[+]
Magnesium chloride	Improves the action of Methylchloroisothiazolinone and Methylisothiazolinone (see below).
Propylparaben*	Oil-soluble preservative, limited to 0.4 percent.[+]
Methylchloroisothiazolinone* and Methylisothiazolinone*	Preservative mixture, limited to 0.0015 percent.
CI 17200*	Red dye (synthetic azo dye).
CI 42090*	Blue dye (synthetic coal tar dye).

* These ingredients are subject to restrictions or have been linked to harmful or adverse effects.

+ Indicates that this ingredient may be used in larger quantities if it is used for another specified purpose other than as a preservative.

The product in this example is part of the manufacture's "Natural Collection" of toiletries and the consumer is lead to believe that this is, somehow, better for you, or at least less synthetic, than products that are not "natural." Careful reading of the ingredients shows that this is far from true. The natural ingredient is listed after 2-Bromo-2-nitropropane-1,3-diol. This is used mainly as a preservative and is known to have some harmful effects. For this reason, EU regulations restrict the amount that may be used to 0.1 percent of the finished product, although the manufacturer is allowed to use more than this if the chemical is used for another purpose other than a preservative. For example, it may be used as an antimicrobial to control the growth of bacteria on the scalp. Even so, the manufacturer is unlikely to use more than one or two percent of this chemical, as such a high concentration would probably be harmful. If the manufacturer has used a larger amount of this harmful substance, the word "natural" becomes meaningless. And even if there is as much as two percent of it present, the dewberry extract is lower on the list, meaning there must be less than two percent of the "natural" extract present in the shampoo – not enough even to give it a color! If, however, the 2-Bromo- 2-nitropropane-1,3-diol is used for its usual function, as a preservative, then there is less than one percent of dewberry extract in this product – again making the word "natural" completely meaningless. In fairness, the main ingredient here is water, and one would have to admit that this is a natural ingredient.

It is worth pointing out that the manufacturer has used the more common *Rubus fruticosus* (blackberry or bramble) extract, rather than the closely related but less common *Rubus caesius* (dewberry) in this product. Perhaps the name "Dewberry Shampoo" was used as it sounds more appealing than "Bramble" or "Blackberry Shampoo."

Natural, Hypoallergenic, Dermatologically Tested, and Alcohol Free

As explained in *Chapter 2 – Marketing: Myths and Magic*, there are no legal definition of the terms "Natural," "Hypoallergenic," or "dermatologically tested" in the USA and this appears also to be the case in the UK. These terms, and others like "allergy tested," and "non-irritating," carry no guarantee that the products will not cause skin irritation or allergic reactions.

Two other phrases used on labels are often a cause of confusion. "Alcohol Free" literally means that the product contains no Ethyl alcohol (INCI name – Alcohol or Alcohol denat.). Some consumers prefer to avoid alcohol because it can cause a stinging sensation in products like deodorants and aftershave lotions, and many people believe it dries out the skin. It can also cause systemic eczematous contact dermatitis. A product labelled "Alcohol Free" may, however, contain traces of alcohol used as a carrier for fragrance chemicals, and it may also contain other alcohols such as Cetyl alcohol, Lanolin alcohol, or Benzyl alcohol. These alcohols do not have the same effect on the skin as Ethyl alcohol and their inclusion in a list of ingredients should not be taken to mean that Ethyl alcohol is present.

Brands which claim to be "Unscented" or "Fragrance Free" do often contain small quantities of fragrance chemicals, added by the manufacturer to cover up the unpleasant, natural odors of other ingredients. If this is the case the list of ingredients will include "Fragrance," "Flavor," "Parfum," or "Aroma." If you want to avoid fragrance chemicals altogether, check the list of ingredients on the back of the product rather than the banner on the front.

NAMING THE INGREDIENTS

The International Nomenclature Committee (INC) is based in Washington, DC and has members from both American and European companies. Their function is to provide simple, systematic names for all existing cosmetic ingredients, and for new ingredients as they are developed. Cosmetic manufacturers that introduce new ingredients must apply to the INC for an INCI name (International Nomenclature of Cosmetic Ingredients). These INCI names have replaced the older CTFA (Cosmetic, Toiletry and Fragrance Association) names. Chemicals used for fragrance or flavor do not have INCI names and do not have to be listed individually in the ingredients. In the EU, fragrances are listed simply as "parfum," flavors are listed as "aroma."

EU ingredient labels should list colors at the end of the list using their CI (colour index) numbers or HD (hair dye) numbers. In the USA the FD&C (food, drug, and cosmetic) numbers are still used. Where colors are banned from food products but allowed in drugs and cosmetics, the numbers become D&C numbers.

Apart from colors, there are other differences between the USA and the EU in the use of INCI labeling conventions. For example, in the USA, English names are always used instead of Latin for plant extracts and the so-called "trivial ingredients" such as water (the EU prefers to use Latin names to avoid the problem of regional variations in the common names of plants). Using both names on the labels – for example, Water (Aqua) or Cocoa butter (Theobroma cacao) or CI 14700 (FD&C Red #4) – easily overcomes these differences.

The American spelling of sulfur, instead of the English, sulphur, has been adopted as the INCI standard and passed on to derivatives of sulfur such as sulfuric acid, sulfate, sulfide, and sulfite, instead of sulphuric acid, sulphate, sulphide, and sulphite.

The EU Commission maintains a list of these INCI names which it updates from time to time, but this must not be mistaken for a list of authorized ingredients.

BANNED INGREDIENTS

Manufacturers are free to use almost any ingredient they like providing suitable safety tests have been carried out and it does not appear on a list of banned ingredients. This is where the FDA and the EU Commission differ. In the USA, the FDA has banned or restricted nine chemicals or families of chemicals from cosmetics and toiletries. These are biothionol, hexachlorophene (except where a manufacturer can demonstrate that it is more effective than a safer alternative), mercury compounds (except when used as preservatives in eye cosmetics), CFC (chlorofluorocarbon) propellants, vinyl chloride and zirconium salts in aerosol products, halogenated salicylanilides, chloroform, and methylene chloride. In the EU there are over 400 prohibited chemicals or families of chemicals, although it must be said that this list is way over the top and includes unlikely substances such as radioactive materials and deadly poisons like thallium compounds, cyanide, and strychnine. Interestingly, the EU allows cosmetics to contain up to 35 percent by weight of methylene chloride, the active ingredient in most solvent paint strippers, while the FDA has prohibited it altogether.

LOOPHOLES IN THE LAW

Currently, a loophole in the EU Commission's regulations could allow a manufacturer to sell a potentially dangerous cosmetic simply by having it classified as a drug. For example, the EU Cosmetics Directive restricts the amount of hydrogen peroxide (and substances that liberate hydrogen peroxide) to 0.1 percent in oral care products – implying that these ingredients are considered to be harmful in larger quantities. The EU Medical Devices Directive, however, allows larger amounts of these chemicals to be used in oral care preparations – suggesting that hydrogen peroxide is safe if it is sold by the pharmacist but dangerous if sold over the cosmetics counter.

In a recent case, the UK Secretary of State for Trade and Industry banned the sale of a tooth-whitening product in the UK on the grounds that it was a cosmetic, and as a cosmetic, did not meet the requirements of the Cosmetics Directive. The product was classified as a drug in Germany and was sold freely over pharmacy counters there. The manufacturer asked the courts to rule that the UK authorities should respect the German decision that their product was, in fact, a drug and allow it to be sold in the UK, but in July 1999, the Court of Appeal upheld the decision that it was a cosmetic. The UK consumer's safety has not been jeopardized in this case, but one wonders whether other cosmetic products that do not comply with the EU's cosmetic safety standards have found their way onto pharmacy counters instead.

In the USA the issue is more clear cut. Cosmetics and drugs are clearly defined by the FDA and a product may be classified as a cosmetic, a drug, or a cosmetic which is also a drug. A cosmetic is essentially something that is applied to the body to temporarily change its appearance or odor. Cosmetics that make a medical claim, such as shampoos that treat dandruff, toothpastes that reduce cavities, sunscreens that prevent sunburn, or preparations that reduce wrinkles, are classified as cosmetics that are also drugs. Providing the product is proved to be safe and complies with the regulations for cosmetics, or drugs, or both, it may be freely sold either as a cosmetic or as an over-the-counter drug.

ABRASIVE

Abrasives are scratchy substances that are added to cosmetics and toiletries to remove materials from the skin by mechanical rubbing, or to gently scrape deposits from the teeth. They often act as polishes and improve the gloss of nails and teeth. Soft abrasives, such as bran or oatmeal, are added to bars of soap to gently massage and temporarily improve the blood supply to the skin.

ABSORBENT

Absorbents are added to cosmetic preparations to remove unwanted substances such as droplets of water or oily liquids that might spoil the appearance of the product. They may also be used in body and face powders to absorb excess moisture or oil from the skin. Absorbent ingredients are added to decorative cosmetics such as lipstick, foundation, and eye shadow to absorb sebum, the skin's natural oil, preventing it from darkening or discoloring the make-up.

ACNE

Acne occurs when bacteria infects hair follicles or sebaceous glands of the skin that have become blocked with an oily mixture of sebum (the skin's natural oil) and keratin (a tough, fibrous protein that makes up skin, hair, and nail). Some cosmetic ingredients are comedogenic, i.e., acne promoting. See *Chapter 15 – Medical Matters*. See also *Comedogen*.

ADDITIVE

Substances that are added to cosmetics in small amounts to improve the product are called additives. They may impart a desirable sheen or enhance the effect of other ingredients, or they may suppress the undesirable effects of other ingredients. They may even be added purely for marketing reasons and add nothing to the quality of the product whatsoever.

AGING

The gradual deterioration of living things caused by the inability of cells to regenerate correctly. The first signs of aging are fine lines and wrinkles caused by loss of elasticity of the skin. Skin discoloration is also common. See *Chapter 5 – Skin Care*.

AHA

See *Alpha-Hydroxy Acid*.

ALLERGIC REACTION

An allergic reaction is an immune-system response to a substance that does not normally cause symptoms in the majority of the population. See the main entry in *Chapter 15 – Medical Matters*.

ALPHA-HYDROXY ACID (AHA)

Alpha- (and beta-) hydroxy acids are cosmetic ingredients that soften and remove the outer layer of skin. They can temporarily improve the appearance of discolored or flaking skin and may even disguise fine lines. See *Chapter 5 – Skin Care*. See also *Exfoliant*.

AMINO ACIDS

Amino acids are the building blocks of proteins. If amino acids were represented by colored beads, a protein would be a long, colorful necklace. In all there are 20 amino acids found in human proteins. Twelve of these, the non-essential amino acids, can be manufactured in our bodies, but the remaining eight, essential amino acids come from proteins in our diet. The digestion process breaks down plant and animal proteins in our food, into individual amino acids. We join these together again in our cells to manufacture fibrous human proteins to grow hair, skin, nail, muscle, and soft tissue, and globular proteins such as enzymes. The amino acids present in cosmetics and toiletries cannot be incorporated into our proteins by applying them externally to the skin or hair. Drinking shampoo would allow you to metabolize the amino acids in it, but this is not recommended.

Amino acids and protein fragments are used in cosmetics for a number of reasons, not least of which is to mislead the consumer into believing the product will somehow improve the proteins in their skin and hair. They are used as antistatic agents in shampoos and conditioners and they can be chemically modified, forming emulsifiers and surfactants. Tyrosine is added to sunscreens to boost the tanning process. (See *Tanning Agent* and *Suntan*.)

A mixture of amino acids and protein fragments is obtained when the long protein molecules are broken down (hydrolyzed) by boiling protein-rich materials with strong acids or alkalis, or by the action of digestive enzymes on proteins. The proteins come from a variety of sources, for example, silk, wheat, hair, hoof, horn, and milk.

ANIMAL PRODUCTS AND ANIMAL TESTING

See *Chapter 17 – Animal Products and Animal Testing.*

ANION

(Pronounced *an-eye-on*.) A negatively charged ion. See *Ion*.

ANIONIC DETERGENT

These are by far the most common type of surfactant, or cleaning chemical, and are widely used in any product that is designed to clean dirt and grease from any surface, including skin and hair. They are synthetic or semisynthetic in origin. See *Anionic Surfactant, Surfactant, Detergent* and *How Soaps and Detergents Work* in *Chapter 6 – Soaps, Shower Gels, and Cleansing Lotions.*

ANIONIC SURFACTANT

A surfactant (cleaning chemical, i.e., soap or detergent) that carries a negative electrical charge on the water-soluble part of the surfactant molecule. It is usually associated with a positively charged ion such as sodium, potassium, or ammonium, which plays no significant part in the cleaning process. These are by far the most common surfactants and include sulfated detergents such as sodium lauryl sulfate (SLS) and ammonium laureth sulfate, which are used widely in shampoos, shower gels, bubble baths, liquid soaps, and cleansing lotions. Soaps such as sodium stearate, potassium tallowate, and sodium palm kernelate (used in bars of toilet soap, moisturizing soap, and dermatological soap) are similar in structure to anionic detergents. See *Surfactant* and *How Soaps and Detergents Work* in *Chapter 6 – Soaps, Shower Gels, and Cleansing Lotions.*

ANTICORROSIVE

These chemicals are added to cosmetics to prevent corrosion of the packaging or the machinery used to produce the cosmetic. Corrosion is generally a problem suffered by metals. Since most cosmetics and toiletries are packaged in plastic, or occasionally glass, the packaging corrosion problem does not exist. If anticorrosion agents are present in the list of ingredients on glass or plastic containers, you can be sure they have been added for the convenience and profits of the manufacturer. Aerosols, however, are packaged in steel or aluminum containers and may require the addition of anticorrosion agents.

Corrosion occurs when acids, alkalis, or a combination of water and oxygen (present in air) attack the metal. The acid and alkali problem can be solved by regulating the level of acidity or alkalinity. The water/oxygen problem is solved by adding chemicals that react with the oxygen and remove it. Rust inhibitors in central heating systems work in much the same way. The problem is that these chemicals are not desirable in cosmetics, and are strictly regulated in the EU. Look out for sodium nitrite and nitromethane, two commonly used but hazardous anticorrosion additives.

ANTIDANDRUFF AGENT

Antidandruff agents are added to shampoos, conditioners, and other hair-care products to control dandruff. See *Dandruff* and *Chapter 9 – Hair Care* for more details.

ANTIFOAMING AGENT

Many toiletries contain surfactants (soaps and detergents) that tend to form a foam or lather when agitated with water. This may be desirable in some products but not in others. It is certainly not desirable during the production process and antifoaming agents are often added for the convenience of the manufacturer. Antifoaming agents reduce the amount of foam formed or prevent it altogether. It is rather like the effect mayonnaise has on the suds in the washing-up bowl.

Antifoaming agents are generally oily or water-repellent chemicals such as silicone oils, which are strongly attracted to the surfactant and tend to gather up the surfactant molecules. Other antifoaming agents are surfactants themselves, which act by reducing the surface tension of the water, preventing the formation of the thin films from which bubbles are made. Look out for names containing "cone", such as methicone and dimethicone, although these are also used as film formers, moisturizers, and antistatic agents.

ANTIMICROBIAL

Antimicrobials are chemicals that control the growth of microbes on the body. They are used in shampoos, toothpaste, mouthwash, antiseptic lotions, and deodorants, and are added to other cosmetics and toiletries where they may act as preservatives. See *Chapter 4 – Preservatives*. See also *Preservative*.

ANTIOXIDANT

Antioxidants block the reaction of fats and oils with oxygen and prevent the breakdown of cosmetic ingredients which may lead to rancid odors. Some antioxidants are also used as food additives to preserve the fats and oils present in pre-cooked foods. Both citric acid and lactic acid can improve the efficiency of antioxidants, allowing smaller quantities of these to be used in the product. See *Chapter 4 – Preservatives*.

ANTIPERSPIRANT

Antiperspirants reduce the skin's ability to perspire. They are commonly used to reduce body odor. Antiperspirants are frequently aluminum compounds, sometimes mixed with zirconium salts. These reduce sweat production by the sweat glands and block the ducts that carry the sweat to the skin. See *Chapter 7 – Deodorants and Antiperspirants*. See also *Deodorant* and *Astringent*.

ANTISTATIC AGENT

Static electricity causes hair to cling to your hairbrush and clothes, and stand out, becoming uncontrollable. Moistening your hair will remove the static charge but it will return as soon as the hair dries again. Antistatic agents are added to hair conditioners and some shampoos to prevent the build up of static electricity in your hair. They are often cationic surfactants – molecules that cling to surfaces and carry a positive electrical charge, which effectively neutralize or carry away the unwanted static electricity. See also *Conditioner*.

AROMA

The European word used in a list of ingredients to indicate that flavorings have been added to an oral care product. See *Flavor*.

AROMATHERAPY

Aromatherapy is a branch of complementary (alternative) medicine used to treat a wide range of ailments by massaging essential oils onto the skin. See *Chapter 16 – Salons and Surgeons*. See also *Essential Oils*.

ASTRINGENT

Astringents close the pores of the skin, improving its tone and texture, making it feel firmer. They work by reducing the water content of skin cells and can aid the healing of broken or inflamed skin. They can also be used to reduce tear production by inflamed or infected eyes. See *Chapter 5 – Skin Care*.

AZO DYES

Azo dyes are artificial colorants made from a coal tar extract or chemicals derived from crude oil. Artificial colors and fragrance chemicals have been implicated in a large number of adverse reactions to cosmetics and toiletries. See *Chapter 3 – Colorants and Fragrances*. See also *Coal Tar Dyes*.

BENZOATES

Benzoic acid, sodium benzoate, and a host of related compounds such as the parabens, are widely used in foods and cosmetics. They are antimicrobial preservatives – chemicals that kill cells or prevent them from reproducing and infecting the food, toiletry, or cosmetic. They have been linked to a large number of health problems such as asthma and eczema. See *Chapter 4 – Preservatives*. See also *Preservative*.

BETA-HYDROXY ACID

These are exfoliating chemicals similar to alpha-hydroxy acids. See *Alpha-Hydroxy Acid* for more details.

BINDER

Binding agents are often very large molecules (polymers) which are added to solid or very thick cosmetics to help hold the mixture together, to give it solidity and to help the cosmetic spread on the skin and stay there.

BIODEGRADABLE

Most cosmetics end up in the drains after being washed off. The chemicals in the cosmetics are often quite resilient and survive the journey through the sewers and into the rivers, lakes, and eventually the sea. Microbes may try to break these down and use them for food. If they succeed the chemical is said to be biodegradable and, therefore, environmentally friendly. If they cannot be broken down, the chemicals are said to be non-biodegradable and they add to the global pollution problem. Most modern surfactants are biodegradable, but early petroleum-derived detergents made from branched-chain alkylbenzene sulfonates, were not. When they were first sold in the 1950s, they immediately became popular because they did not leave white deposits of scum on clothing, in the same way as soap powders did. They also produced little lather and were ideal for front-loading washing machines and dishwashers. Unfortunately they were not biodegradable because bacteria could not digest the branched-chain hydrocarbons. In the sewers they mixed with protein fragments which acted as foam boosters, producing vast amounts of lather which covered the rivers and streams and, in urban areas, was blown through the streets by the wind. These surfactants were quickly replaced by biodegradable straight-chain alkylbenzene sulfonates, derived from petroleum.

Another notorious example of a pollutant which has its origins in household chemicals, is nonylphenol. This is a common ingredient in cleaning agents, detergents, and some cosmetics. It is an EDC (endocrine disrupting chemical, or "gender bender") which mimics estrogens (the female sex hormones). Nonylphenol, along with other EDC pollutants, have recently been found to be responsible for a fall in the sperm count in males of every species of animal, including humans. They are also responsible for the feminization of males and the malformation of male genitalia in all animal species. See *Chapter 13 – Common Sense and Cosmetic Safety* for a full account of gender benders.

BIOLOGICAL ADDITIVE

These are cosmetic ingredients that are derived from animals or plants and are used for a variety of reasons, including marketing. Currently human products are banned from cosmetics in the EU, and it is illegal to use products from endangered species or plants that are known to produce controlled poisons such as belladonna (atropine – a nerve poison), or foxgloves (digitalis – a heart stimulant).

Vitamins, pro-vitamins, amino acids, and partly digested proteins are commonly added to cosmetics, and advertisers would have us believe they do remarkable things for us. In fact they have little or no effect on the skin or hair. They do, however, make the cosmetic highly nutritious and susceptible to microbial infection, so a cocktail of preservatives is added to prevent this. It has been suggested that the main effect of adding biological additives to cosmetics is to expose us to unnecessary levels of harmful preservatives.

Some plant extracts do have beneficial effects, for example, aloe vera extract and aloe vera gel are known to have a soothing effect on the skin and are commonly used in shampoos, conditioners, skin-care lotions, and after-sun lotions to relieve burning. (Aloe vera is a member of the lily family.) In most cosmetics, however, the amount added is insufficient to have any therapeutic value and it is an irritant for some individuals.

Amongst the animal products used are mink oil products, derived from the fatty subcutaneous tissue of mink; elastin, an elastic protein extracted from artery walls of mammals and sometimes from skin tissues; keratin, the tough, fibrous protein that makes up skin, hair, and nail; and collagen, another tough, fibrous protein that forms tendons, ligaments, and connective tissue. See *Chapter 17 – Animal Products and Animal Testing* for more details.

BLACKHEADS

Blackheads are black specks that appear on the face, shoulders, upper arms and chest, and occasionally elsewhere on the body. They occur when hair follicles or sebaceous glands of the skin become blocked with the skin's natural, oily secretions or with some oily chemicals or cosmetic ingredients. The mixture trapped inside the follicle hardens and becomes a plug that blackens on the surface where it meets the air. The incidence of blackheads can be reduced by regular washing and by avoiding comedogenic (acne promoting) chemicals.

There is rarely a bacterial infection in blackheads but, if they do become infected, red pimples (papules) appear. Whiteheads and acne occur when the infection has developed. See *Chapter 15 – Medical Matters* for more details.

BLEACHING AGENT

Bleaching agents are used to lighten the color of hair or skin. They are often potent chemicals and must be used with caution. Dental bleach, under the influence of ultraviolet light, may be used by a dentist to whiten discolored teeth. Denture cleaners sometimes contain sodium hypochlorite, sodium perborate, or sodium percarbonate, which both whiten the dentures and kill bacteria.

Hair is commonly bleached using a mixture of hydrogen peroxide and a mild alkali such as ammonia. This mixture can also be used to bleach stains on fingernails but fresh lemon juice can also remove many unsightly marks from the nails, especially those caused by processing some types of fruit or vegetables.

Hydroquinone is used to lighten dark patches on the skin caused by hyperpigmentation, which is the over production of melanin, the skin's natural pigment. Hydroquinone reduces the ability of the melanocytes in the skin to produce melanin. It takes three to four weeks for the darker skin to shed and lighter skin to show through. During this time exposure to sun should be avoided as sunlight promotes melanin production by the melanocytes and defeats the use of skin lighteners. The use of Hydroquinone in skin-lightening products is now banned in the EU. See also *Oxidizing Agent* and *Skin*.

BOTANICAL ADDITIVE

These are plant extracts that are added to cosmetics for a variety of reasons. Some are alternatives to synthetic ingredients, for example, oils pressed from seeds can replace mineral oils obtained from petroleum. Others have a therapeutic function, for example, tea-tree oil has a deodorant and antimicrobial effect. Farnesol is another plant extract with deodorant qualities. Plants also provide natural fragrances and can contribute to the color and appearance of a product.

The marketing people would have us believe these plant extracts somehow make the cosmetic wholesome and natural. We see the perfect, virginal blonde drifting sylph-like through the soft-focus autumn woodland, gracefully gathering nature's bounty, fresh and glistening with morning dew. In fact it couldn't be further from the truth. The plants are grown in extensive fields using all of the techniques of modern, intensive agriculture to maximize the profits. This investment is zealously protected by using a cocktail of herbicides and pesticides, and the residues of these chemicals can potentially contaminate the cosmetic.

The INCI name for botanical ingredients is usually the botanical, Latin name for the plant, but the common name is often prominent on the label.

BSE

BSE is an abbreviation for bovine spongiform encephalopathy or "mad cow disease." Fears that this disease can be passed on to humans via cosmetic products derived from cattle, sheep, and goats caused the EU Commission to regulate the use of certain parts of these animals in March 1998. See *Chapter 17 – Animal Products and Animal Testing* for further details.

BUFFER

A buffer is a mixture of chemicals, usually two, that can resist changes in levels of acidity or alkalinity and, therefore, control the pH (acidity level) in a personal care product. Some ingredients in cosmetics and toiletries are fairly acidic or alkaline. Both acids and alkalis are eye and skin irritants. Addition of a buffer to a product will counteract the unwanted acidity or alkalinity caused by the other ingredients, producing a neutral pH.

Skin secretes a cocktail of chemicals which tend to increase its acidity during the day. Since many colorants and dyes change color in the presence of acids or alkalis, make-up tends to change its shade as the day wears on. To combat this, many decorative cosmetics, such as foundation, lipstick, mascara, eye shadow, and eye liner contain buffers to resist changes in the acidity levels and thereby maintain their colors. See also *pH Control*.

CARCINOGEN

A carcinogen is something that causes cancer. Chemical carcinogens are chemicals that cause cancer. Physical carcinogens include such things as asbestos dust, ultraviolet rays from sunlight, X-rays, and other forms of radiation. Some viruses have been linked to cancer. These are rare and are known as biological carcinogens. See *Chapter 15 – Medical Matters*. See also *Mutagen* and *Phototoxin*.

CATEGORY (1 OR 2)

Category-1 personal care products are those that are for use on children under the age of three, for use on or near the eyes or for use on or near mucous membranes. All other cosmetics and toiletries are Category-2 products. The level of microbial contamination for each category has been defined by the EU Commission and the level set for Category-1 products is 50 times lower (i.e., 50 times fewer microbes) than Category-2 products. Products must meet these standards when they are supplied and must contain sufficient quantities of preservatives to maintain these levels during normal use. See *Chapter 4 – Preservatives*. See also *Microbe*.

CATION

(Pronounced *cat-eye-on*.) A positively charged ion. See *Ion*.

CATIONIC SURFACTANT

A synthetic surfactant (cleaning chemical) that carries a positive electrical charge on the surface-active part of the surfactant molecule. Cationic surfactants are commonly used in hair and fabric conditioners. See *Surfactant, Conditioner* and *How Soaps and Detergents Work* in *Chapter 6 – Soaps, Shower Gels, and Cleansing Lotions*.

CHELATING AGENT

Chelating agents are chemicals that wrap themselves around metal ions rather like an octopus might envelop its prey. In doing so they effectively remove the metal ion from the cosmetic and prevent it from affecting its appearance, shelf life, or effectiveness. They also wrap themselves around calcium and magnesium ions present in hard water and prevent them from forming a powdery scum with some soaps. They are, in effect, softening the hard water. (These hard-water ions reduce the cleaning action of soaps and detergents.) Chelating agents also prevent metal ions that form part of the cosmetic from being removed by alkaline ingredients or ingredients that might bond to them and form an insoluble compound.

The most common chelating agents are salts of EDTA (also called edetates), which can be found in almost all soaps, cleansing lotions, shampoos, conditioners, and many other products. They also serve a similar function in foods, where they have been linked to adverse effects such as diarrhea, vomiting, and abdominal cramps.

COAL TAR DYE

These are artificial dyes made from coal tar. Artificial colors and fragrance chemicals have been implicated in a large number of adverse reactions to cosmetics and toiletries. See *Chapter 3 – Colorants and Fragrances*. See also *Azo Dyes*.

COLLAGEN

Collagen is a tough, fibrous but flexible protein that occurs in tendons, ligaments, bones, and connective tissues. It is also found in deeper layers of the skin (the dermis) and gives skin its elasticity. As we grow older, the number of collagen fibers in the dermis is reduced and our skin becomes less flexible. Collagen replacement therapy (CRT) is used to reduce the appearance of fine lines and wrinkles in aging skin. Collagen implants are used to improve the contours of the face and lips. See *Collagen Replacement Therapy*.

Some cosmetics and toiletries contain hydrolyzed collagen (collagen from the bones, ligaments, and tendons of animals (mainly cattle), that has been partially broken down by the action of acids, alkalis, or enzymes), or derivatives of hydrolyzed collagen. Contrary to what the manufacturers would like us to believe, these ingredients will not be absorbed by our skin to reverse the natural loss of collagen. See also *Chapter 17 – Animal Products and Animal Testing*.

COLLAGEN REPLACEMENT THERAPY (CRT)

Collagen replacement therapy (CRT) is a cosmetic procedure which temporarily restores the levels of collagen and improves the appearance of fine lines and wrinkles. It can also be used to disguise pock marks, minor scars, and unwanted dimples. Collagen of animal origin is injected directly into the dermis (the deeper layers of skin) using a fine hypodermic needle. See *Chapter 16 – Salons and Surgeons*. See also *Collagen*.

COLORANT

A colorant is a pigment or colored chemical. Colorants are used on their own or mixed with other colorants to impart a certain color or shade to cosmetics and toiletries. Some are used to color the product to improve its appearance or to temporarily impart that color or hue to the skin. Other colorants, for example hair dyes, are designed to produce a longer-lasting color change.

The range of colors available to cosmetic manufactures is vast. The EU inventory of cosmetic ingredients includes over 470 hair dyes, colorants, and other ingredients designed to alter the appearance of cosmetics. In the EU colorants are named using the colour index numbers, e.g., CI 10316, or by simple names such as Titanium dioxide and Mica. In the USA they are named using their FD&C or D&C designations, e.g., D&C Red #33.

See *Chapter 3 – Colorants and Fragrances*. See also *Azo Dyes* and *Coal Tar Dyes*.

COMBINATION SKIN

People with combination skin usually have a triangle of greasy skin which encompasses the forehead, nose, parts of the cheeks either side of the nose, and the chin but the sides of the face have dry skin. See *Chapter 5 – Skin Care*.

COMEDOGEN

(Pronounced *comm-ed-O-jen*.) A comedogenic chemical promotes acne and blackheads. Comedogens are often oily or greasy substances, found in a wide range of cosmetics and toiletries, that block hair follicles which subsequently become filled with a mixture of sebum and keratin where bacteria can breed and cause a localized inflammation or infection. See *Chapter 15 – Medical Matters*.

CONDITIONER

Conditioners are applied to the hair after shampooing to improve its sheen, feel, and controllability. They are usually rinse-off preparations but recently many more non-rinse-off conditioners have come onto the market. The main ingredients are generally water emulsified with an oily substance, non-ionic and cationic surfactants, and anti-static agents. See *Chapter 9 – Hair Care*. See also *Hair* and *Shampoo*.

CONTACT ALLERGY

A contact allergic reaction is an immune-system response to a chemical or other substance that comes into contact with the skin. See *Chapter 15 – Medical Matters*.

CONTACT DERMATITIS

This is an inflammation of the skin caused by a chemical or other substance that comes into contact with the skin. For full details see *Chapter 15 – Medical Matters*.

CONTACT ECZEMA

This is an inflammation of the skin resulting in blistering, scaling, or flaking and is triggered by chemicals or other substances coming into contact with the skin. See *Chapter 15 – Medical Matters* for full details.

CONTACT URTICARIA

This is urticaria (nettle rash or hives) caused by a chemical or other substance that comes into contact with the skin. See *Urticaria* and *Chapter 15 – Medical Matters* for more details.

COSMECEUTICAL

This is an invented word that is supposed to suggest that a cosmetic ingredient can have a physiological effect on the body tissues, rather like a powerful drug causing actual changes in the cells, thus producing a real rejuvenation of the skin. In the real world few such chemicals exist, and those that do have effects like this, such as retinoic acid, are banned from cosmetics and are controlled by the medical authorities.

COSMETICS

The word cosmetics is generally taken to include all toiletries and personal care products such as sunscreens, insect repellents, contact-lens cleaning products, hair dyes, make-up and make-up removers, and implements such as nail boards, tweezers and exfoliating pads, and everything else you use to take care of your appearance and personal hygiene. Globally, cosmetics is a multi-billion dollar industry, with decorative make-ups accounting for about 30 percent of the total. Much of the research into the safety of cosmetic ingredients is funded by the industry. In the EU the industry is regulated by the EU Commission; in the USA the Cosmetic Ingredient Review Panel (CRIP) is the cosmetic industry's self-regulatory body for addressing the safety of cosmetic ingredients. The FDA, however, has powers to intervene and seize any product that proves to be harmful or does not conform to the FDA's regulations.

CUTICLE

The outer layer of cells on the hair shaft (see *Hair*) or a thin flap of skin that joins the lunula (half-moon shaped, lighter colored part of the nail) to the nail fold (fold of skin that surrounds the nail). During a manicure at home or in a salon, the cuticle is sometimes softened with cuticle softener and pushed back towards the nail fold, to expose more of the lunula and to lengthen the nail. This can push bacteria and dirt under the nail fold, resulting in an infection. Fragments of previously used nail builders, such as nail hardeners and enamels, can also be pushed under the nail fold – resulting in irritation, soreness, and allergic reactions. See *Chapter 9 – Hair Care* and *Chapter 12 – Nail Care*.

CUTICLE SOFTENER

Before the cuticle (See *Cuticle*) is pushed back during a manicure, a cuticle softener is applied to both loosen and soften the cuticle. A cuticle softener usually contains water to soften the skin and surfactants to speed up the wetting and softening process. Exfoliants such as alpha or beta-hydroxy acids may be added to dissolve the proteins in skin and soften the cuticle more effectively. See *Chapter 12 – Nail Care*. See also *Alpha-Hydroxy Acid* for adverse effects of exfoliants, and *Cuticle Solvent*.

CUTICLE SOLVENT

A solution containing a strong alkali such as sodium, or potassium hydroxide, which dissolves the cuticle (the flap of skin joining the nail to the nail fold). These are highly corrosive toiletries and should be used with caution. See *Chapter 12 – Nail Care*. See also *Cuticle* and *Cuticle Softener*.

D&C

D&C colorants have been certified by the FDA for use in any drugs or cosmetics sold in the USA, but not for use in food. See *Chapter 3 – Colorants and Fragrances*. See also *Colorant, Coal Tar Dye* and *Azo Dye*.

DANDRUFF

Dandruff is a common, harmless condition where there is excessive shedding of specks or flakes of dead skin cells from the scalp. It is most common in adolescents and young adults, and diminishes in middle years, although older people can suffer from it, especially stroke victims. Men are more likely to have dandruff than women and people with greasy skin and hair suffer more from it than people with dry skin.

Dandruff is one of the top ten problems for which people seek over-the-counter medical treatments, usually in the form of medicated or antidandruff shampoos. The condition generally returns if the treatment is stopped. If the treatment is not effective the shedding may be caused by a more serious condition, such as eczema, psoriasis, or seborrheic dermatitis. See *Chapter 9 – Hair Care*.

DEA

Diethanolamine (DEA) is not itself commonly used in cosmetics and toiletries but chemicals that contain DEA are widespread. They include ingredients such as Cocamide DEA, a high foaming surfactant used in a large variety of shampoos, foaming bath oils, shaving foams, liquid soaps, shower gels, and specialist bars of soap. Oleamide DEA and Lauramide DEA are also common cosmetic ingredients acting as emulsifiers and foam boosters.

In 1998 the FDA issued a fact sheet outlining a study that linked DEA and DEA-related ingredients to cancer in laboratory animals when the chemicals were applied to their skin. The results suggest that the carcinogen is DEA itself, which is present in residual levels in the DEA-related ingredients. The FDA are currently assessing the risks, if any, to consumers of cosmetics containing DEA-related ingredients.

DEEP SKIN PEEL

A surgical procedure that removes a substantial layer of skin in order to eradicate fine lines and wrinkles. Chemical skin peels require the use of strong exfoliants such as trichloroacetic acid (TCA), which are not available in home skin peels or other cosmetics. Physical skin peels include dermabrasion carried out using a rotating abrasive pad, or laser planing using a powerful laser beam. See *Chapter 16 – Salons and Surgeons*.

DEMULCENT

Demulcents have a soothing effect on irritated, inflamed, or injured skin.

DENATURANT

Products that contain a substantial amount of ethanol (alcohol) have denaturants, such as benzyl alcohol or methanol, added to them to make the ethanol unpalatable. This discourages people from drinking the product. In countries where alcoholic drinks carry a large tax or excise duty, rendering the alcohol undrinkable reduces this tax burden and lowers the price of the product. The amount of denaturant that is added depends on national laws and levels of taxation. Generally speaking, in countries where taxation is high, greater quantities of denaturant are added.

DENTAL BLEACH

Seriously discolored or stained teeth can be whitened by a dentist. A bleaching agent is painted onto the teeth and then activated by shining an ultraviolet light onto the chemicals.

DENTIFRICE

Still available but rather old fashioned, dentifrice is similar to toothpaste but is sold in a block or cake. The abrasive is usually chalk, which is softer and less damaging than modern abrasives such as hydrated silica. See *Chapter 8 – Teeth and Oral Care Products*. See also *Toothpaste*.

DEODORANT

Deodorants reduce or mask unpleasant body odors. They generally work by preventing bacterial growth in warm, damp areas of the body and, at the same time, provide a masking fragrance. They are often used in association with antiperspirants and come in a variety of forms, including aerosols, deodorant sticks and gels, and roll-on deodorant lotions. See *Chapter 7 – Deodorants and Antiperspirants*. See also *Antimicrobial* and *Antiperspirant*.

DEPILATORY AGENT

Depilatory chemicals remove unwanted body hair by dissolving the protein structure of the hair, thus weakening it and allowing it to be detached at skin level. Metal sulfides and thioglycolates are the most common depilatories. They are often alkaline and the chemicals are quite toxic. Depilatories work at the surface of the skin and do not affect the hair root, so the hair will reappear in two to three weeks. See *Chapter 5 – Skin Care*. See also *Electrolysis* and *Hair Removal*.

DERMABRASION

This is a physical skin peel carried out by a cosmetic surgeon to eradicate fine lines and wrinkles. The procedure involves the use of a rotating abrasive pad which removes the outer layer of skin. See *Chapter 16 – Salons and Surgeons*.

DERMATITIS

Dermatitis is an inflammation of the skin that is related to eczema. It may be caused by an allergy or a reaction to something that comes into contact with the skin, or there may be no easily identifiable cause. For full details see *Chapter 15 – Medical Matters*. See also *Eczema* and *Photosensitivity*.

DERMIS

The dermis is the layer of living skin cells just below the outermost layer of dead cells. It contains fibers of collagen, which give skin its elasticity, small blood vessels called capillaries, nerve endings, hair follicles, hair erector muscles, sweat glands, and sebaceous glands. See *Chapter 5 – Skin Care* for full details.

DESQUAMATE

This is the correct term for shedding the outermost layer of skin cells – a completely normal process that never stops. See *Chapter 5 – Skin Care*. See also *Dandruff*.

DETERGENCY, THEORY OF

The theory of detergency is an explanation of how soaps and detergents are able to remove grease and other water-insoluble dirt. For full details see *Chapter 6 – Soaps, Shower Gels, and Cleansing Lotions*.

DETERGENT

A detergent is a surfactant (cleaning compound) used as an alternative to soap. The most common detergents are anionic detergents. These are made by the reaction of concentrated sulfuric acid with hydrocarbons (oily compounds) derived from petroleum, or by the action of sulfur trioxide on fatty acid alcohols, which are obtained from either natural fats and oils or from petroleum. In contrast to soaps, which are made by the action of strong alkalis on animal or vegetable fats and oils, detergents do not make scum – a white or grey, powdery deposit formed when soap chemically reacts with the calcium or magnesium present in hard water. See *Chapter 6 – Soaps, Shower Gels, and Cleansing Lotions*.

DIETHANOLAMINE

See *DEA*.

DIOXANE (1,4-DIOXANE)

1,4-Dioxane is accidentally formed as an undesirable by-product in the manufacture of some cosmetic ingredients when two molecules of ethylene oxide combine together in an unwanted chemical reaction. It must be carefully removed by vacuum stripping before the ingredient is used. 1,4-Dioxane is a carcinogen (cancer-causing agent) which is known to cause systemic cancer in rodents when painted on their skin, and liver and nasal cancer when fed to test animals. It is known that this compound is readily absorbed through human skin, although much of it is thought to evaporate before it is absorbed. See *Chapter 13 – Common Sense and Cosmetic Safety*.

DRY SKIN

A type of skin which is characterized by a lack of sebum secretions. See *Chapter 5 – Skin Care* for full details.

DYE

A dye is a colorant that is soluble in water. Dyes can be either natural extracts or synthetic coal tar or azo dyes. Because they dissolve in water, dyes disperse evenly through cosmetics and toiletries producing clear, colored liquids. They can also be absorbed into hair and fibers of textiles. Some dyes fade when exposed to bright lights. They can also fade from hair or fabrics if they are leeched out during washing, or subjected to bleaching agents such as chlorine in swimming pools. See *Chapter 3 – Colorants and Fragrances*. See also *Lake, Colorant, Coal Tar Dye* and *Azo Dye*.

EAR PIERCING

The latest and most hygienic method for ear piercing is to use a piercing gun, which fires a stud through the ear lobe without first piercing it. The stud comes in a sealed, sterile package and is not touched by the person operating the gun. Similarly, the gun does not come into contact with the ear. Once in place, the stud is covered with a sterile dressing for a few days, then for the next four to six weeks it is rotated twice daily and the ear lobe is cleaned with surgical spirit or hydrogen peroxide to prevent any infections. For further details see *Chapter 16 – Salons and Surgeons*.

ECZEMA

Eczema is an inflammation of the skin resulting in itching, scaling of the skin, and sometimes blisters, which occasionally become infected. There are many forms of eczema but of these, only hand eczema and dermatitis can be linked to cosmetics and toiletries. See *Chapter 15 – Medical Matters* for full details. See also *Dermatitis*.

ELASTIN

Elastin is a flexible, elastic protein found in the walls of arteries and veins. It is an animal product used as a source of proteins and amino acids for cosmetic ingredients. There is no mechanism by which it can penetrate the skin, thereby rejuvenating its elasticity.

ELECTROLYSIS

Electrolysis results in the permanent removal of unwanted body hair using a needle epilator, or the recently introduced tweezer epilator. In both cases a small electric current is passed through the apparatus to kill the hair root. The hair is then removed with a pair of tweezers and, if the treatment is successful, it will not grow again. See *Chapter 16 – Salons and Surgeons*. See also *Hair Removal*.

EMOLLIENT

Emollients are applied to the skin or mucous membranes to increase the moisture content of the skin. They work by forming a thin layer of oil or grease on your skin, trapping water beneath it and acting as a barrier to water vapor, preventing loss of water by evaporation. The extra moisture soaks into the outer layer of skin cells, making them swell. This has the effect of making the skin feel softer and smoother, and it makes dry or cracked skin more flexible, alleviating any pain or soreness. See *Chapter 5 – Skin Care*. See also *Moisturizing Cream, Humectant, Emulsion* and *Emulsifier*.

EMULSIFIER

Oil and water do not mix. Since many personal care products contain both oils and water, chemicals that help them to mix must be added. When they mix, a creamy substance called an emulsion, is formed. Milk, cream, mayonnaise, and most cosmetic creams and lotions are emulsions.

A simple oil and vinegar dressing for your salad must be shaken vigorously before you use it. Soon after you set it down, the oil floats to the top. If you now add a teaspoonful of mustard and shake it, a thicker, creamy emulsion forms which remains mixed for several minutes, or longer. The mustard acts as an emulsifier or emulsifying agent. In cosmetics, the emulsifiers are often surfactants. Emulsion stabilizers are also added to cosmetic emulsions, to prevent the oil and water from separating, thereby increasing their shelf life. See *Emulsion* and *Emulsion Stabilizer*.

EMULSION

Personal care products are often emulsions, an intimate mixture of oils and water that contain emulsifiers and emulsion stabilizers to prevent them from separating. A mixture that contains more oil than water is called a water-in-oil (W/O) emulsion. These are thick creams or fairly solid, waxy substances. Butter, moisturizing cream, and lipstick are water-in-oil emulsions, containing between 20 and 30 percent water dispersed through wax or oil.

Emulsions that are mainly water and contain only 20 to 30 percent oil, are called oil-in-water (O/W) emulsions. These tend to be thin lotions. Single cream, moisturizing milk, and many shampoos and conditioners are oil-in-water emulsions.

See *Emulsifier* and *Emulsion Stabilizer*.

EMULSION STABILIZER

Emulsion stabilizers are added to emulsions to prevent them from separating into their component parts, thus improving their shelf life. See *Emulsion* and *Emulsifier*.

EPIDERMIS

The epidermis is the outermost layer of skin, consisting mainly of dead skin cells arranged in layers, which resemble paving slabs when viewed under a microscope. It is an effective barrier to water, most chemicals, some UV rays, and microbes. It varies in thickness, being thinnest on the eyelids and thickest on the soles of the feet and palms of the hand. It is thicker in men than women and thinner in both infants and the elderly.

The extreme outermost layer of the epidermis is called the stratum corneum (or horny layer or keratinized layer). Below the stratum corneum are four more layers of cells that make up the epidermis. The deepest layer is called the basal layer, which is composed of living cells and melanocytes which produce melanin, the skin's natural pigment. When these cells die, they gradually migrate to the surface of the skin.

After leaving the basal layer the cells enter the prickle-cell layer (stratum spinosum, also called the stratum malpighii or stratum aculeatum), named after the fine threads that link the cells together. They then move up to the granular layer (stratum granulosum) where the process of changing to keratin first starts. The cell nuclei start to shrink and are gone by the time the cells reach the fourth layer, the stratum lucidum, where the cells start to flatten and come to resemble thick, uneven paving slabs. The fifth and final layer is the stratum corneum where the cells are flat like paving stones, almost completely dehydrated and composed almost entirely of keratin. See *Chapter 5 – Skin Care* for further details.

ESSENTIAL OILS

The term "essential oils" has two quite different meanings. Oils which have strong essences are used as fragrances in cosmetics and flavorings in food. They are also used in aromatherapy, a branch of alternative medicine. (See *Aromatherapy*.)

The second meaning refers to fats and oils which are necessary (essential) to maintain our health. Our body can make some of them naturally but those we cannot make must be included in our diet. These are known by dieticians as essential (necessary) oils.

ETHYLENE OXIDE

Ethylene oxide (oxirane) is a chemical derived from petroleum and is used to produce ethoxylated ingredients such as PEG and PEG derivatives, and any ingredient that ends with the letters "eth." There are worries that residues of a chemical suspected of causing cancer – 1,4-Dioxane – produced accidentally from ethylene oxide, may contaminate cosmetics. See *Dioxane*.

EXFOLIANT

Exfoliants are chemicals that soften or dissolve the outer layers of the epidermis (outer layer of dead skin cells, also called the horny layer, keratinized layer or stratum corneum), allowing this layer to be removed. The widely held belief is that fine lines and wrinkles are removed along with the outer layer of skin cells. In fact, exfoliants can slightly improve the appearance of fine lines, help to remove discolored or flaking skin, and reduce the incidence of blackheads.

Ingredients such as salicylic acid, alpha- and beta-hydroxy acids, phenols, trichloroacetic acid (TCA), and glycolic acid are exfoliants. Abrasive pads and bars of soap containing bran or oatmeal are also used to exfoliate skin. See *Alpha-Hydroxy Acids* in *Chapter 5 – Skin Care* for full details of exfoliants.

EXT. D&C

Ext. D&C colorants are harmful if swallowed. They are certified by the FDA for use in externally applied drugs and cosmetics only. See *Chapter 3 – Colorants and Fragrances*. See also *Colorant, Coal Tar Dye* and *Azo Dye*.

EYELIFT

Blepharoplasty, commonly referred to as an eyelift, is a cosmetic operation to remove bags, sagging skin, folds, and wrinkles from the eyelids. It can be carried out on both the upper and lower eyelids but is most commonly used to remove the pads of fat that collect under the eyes, forming unsightly "bags." See *Chapter 16 – Salons and Surgeons*. See also *Liposuction*.

EYE LINER

Eye liners are decorative cosmetics used to highlight or accentuate the eyes. They are used to draw a thin line on the upper eyelid, following just above the line of the eyelashes. They may also be drawn on the lower eyelid, below the lower eyelashes. They are either colored, water-based paints applied with a fine brush, cakes of pressed talc and magnesium stearate consolidated with oily ingredients, or thick, waxy creams that are supplied in the form of a pencil. See *Chapter 11 – Make-up*.

EYE SHADOW

Eye shadow is a decorative cosmetic used to enhance the appearance of the eyes. It is commonly available in the form of creams, powders, cakes, and gels. See *Chapter 11 – Make-up*

FACE-LIFT

A face-lift is a surgical procedure which can make an older face look between five and ten years younger. Fine lines and wrinkles are smoothed out, and sagging skin under the chin and below the cheeks is lifted and tightened. The operation is often carried out under local anesthetic, as an out-patient procedure. See *Chapter 16 – Salons and Surgeons.*

FACTOR

Also called the sun-protection factor (SPF), this is an indication of the level of protection afforded by a sunscreen. The larger the number, the greater the protection. For example, if your skin is not used to the sun and is likely to burn in 20 minutes, a factor 6 sunscreen will allow you to stay in the sun for six times longer, i.e., 6 times

20 minutes, or 120 minutes, i.e., two hours before you risk burning. See *Chapter 14 – Sun and Skin*.

FD&C

FD&C colorants have been certified by the FDA for use in any food product, drug, or cosmetic sold in the USA. See *Chapter 3 – Colorants and Fragrances*. See also *Colorant, Coal Tar Dye* and *Azo Dye*.

FILM FORMER

Film formers are cosmetic ingredients that stick to skin, hair, or nails, forming a thin, unbroken layer or film. They are also used to aid the spreading of cosmetics. There are almost 300 film formers available to manufacturers and many of these have dual roles, doubling up as antistatic agents, thickeners, binding agents, moisturizers, and emulsion stabilizers.

Generally speaking, film formers fall into three groups: water-soluble film formers; waxes and oils; and polymer- (plastic-) based film formers.

Water-based film formers include surfactants, protein derivatives, and amino acids. They occur widely in products such as conditioners, moisturizing creams, and hair mousse. Oils are also important film formers in these products. They are usually applied as emulsions in water-based formulations, the film remaining on the hair or skin after the water has dried. Proteins and amino acids will prevent complete drying of the water and aid the moisturizing properties of these products.

Waxes are commonly found in products such as lipstick, foundation, mascara, eye shadow, and eye liners. They can be of a natural origin, such as beeswax or waxes extracted from plants, petroleum-based waxes, or even synthetic silicone waxes similar to furniture polish. Formulations containing waxes also contain ingredients such as alcohols or oils to soften the waxes, helping them to spread evenly.

Nail polish and hair sprays often contain polymer-based film formers. These are generally applied as a solution that contains a solvent, and the film is left behind when the solvent evaporates. Hair sprays, and some mousses, contain resin-based polymers, vinyl acetate polymers, or silicone polymers. As the solvent evaporates, a thin film of the polymer hardens and sticks the hair shafts together, thus holding the hair firmly in place. Of these, the vinyl acetate films are favored, as they are easily washed out using water. Inhaling film-forming chemicals, in the form of aerosol sprays, can cause lung damage, breathing difficulties, sensitization, and allergic reactions.

Nail builders, such as nail polish and nail varnish, often contain acrylic polymers that are dissolved in alcohol-based solvents. These are painted onto the nails and the film of polymer is left behind when the solvent evaporates. These solvents are usually flammable and should be kept away from sources of ignition until the nails are completely dry. The films are usually insoluble in water and can remain in place for several days. They are removed using a nail-polish solvent. These often contain acetone, ethyl acetate, butyl acetate, or amyl acetate, all flammable liquids, mixed with oils to prevent the nails from drying out. Oil-in-water emulsions are also used as nail-polish removers.

FINE LINES

Fine lines are the first sign of aging skin, usually appearing around the eyes, then the corners of the mouth. As you age they become larger and are called wrinkles. See *Wrinkles*. See also *Chapter 5 – Skin Care*.

FLAVOR

Ingredients added to impart a flavor to oral care products do not have to be listed separately. Instead, the word "Flavor" (in the USA), or "Aroma" (in the EU) is used in the list of ingredients to indicate that flavoring chemicals have been added. These may be natural flavors or artificial flavors, made by mixing a number of synthetic chemicals.

FLUORIDE

Fluoride-containing compounds are added to toothpastes, mouthwashes, and other oral care products to prevent cavities and dental caries (tooth decay). It is thought to be absorbed into the minerals that make up the tooth enamel, making it more resistant to acid attack. See *Chapter 8 – Teeth and Oral Care Products* for full details.

FOAMING AGENT

Foaming agents are chemicals that form a foam, or lather, when shaken with water. Since lather has a strong psychological link with cleaning, even though it plays little part in the cleaning process, foaming agents (foam boosters) are often added to toiletries that contain low-lather detergents, to compensate for the lack of foam produced by them. They are also important in foaming products such as shaving foam and some hair mousse. The foam helps to maintain a high concentration of the product in the place where it is required.

FOAM BOOSTER

Another name for a foaming agent. See *Foaming Agent*.

FOUNDATION

Foundation forms a base over which other make-up is applied. It comes in a variety of forms such as powders, cakes, or creams, having a subtle color designed to tone in with the skin and to give an even hue to the whole of the face. It can also cover up minor skin blemishes such as spots or zits and freckles, or skin that had been darkened or reddened by the sun. See *Chapter 11 – Make-up*.

FRAGRANCE

Fragrances are added to cosmetics to impart a specific smell to the product. They are indicated on the list of ingredients by the word "Fragrance" in the USA, or "Parfum" in the EU. The fragrance may be a natural plant extract or a cocktail of several artificial fragrance chemicals. There are 932 fragrance chemicals listed by the EU Commission, and none of these has to be named separately on the list of ingredients. Fragrances and colorants are often the cause of adverse reactions to cosmetics. Hypoallergenic products often do not contain fragrance chemicals or colorants. See *Chapter 3 – Colorants and Fragrances* for further details. See also *Musk*.

FREE RADICAL

A free radical is an atom or molecule that possesses an unpaired electron, which makes the free radical extremely reactive, usually in a destructive way. Strong sunlight causes premature aging of skin. The sun's ultraviolet rays generate free radicals in the skin and it is thought that these cause the breakdown of the collagen, which gives skin its elasticity. Free radicals also play a vital role in the formation of a suntan. They convert tyrosine, an amino acid, to melanin, the skin's natural brown pigment. See *Chapter 14 – Sun and Skin* for further details.

GENDER BENDER

This is a popular name for endocrine disrupter chemicals (EDCs) or hormone disrupter compounds (HDCs). These are chemicals that can act like hormone molecules, causing changes in growth or body chemistry. They can even disrupt the correct gender development of males. See *Chapter 13 – Common Sense and Cosmetic Safety* for full details.

GREASY SKIN

A skin type characterized by the over-production of sebum. See *Chapter 5 – Skin Care* for details.

HAIR

Hairs of varying length, thickness, and color grow from almost every part of your body. Each hair grows from a pit called a follicle and is composed of dead cells that contain a tough, fibrous protein called keratin, and pigments called melanin. Whether hair is straight or curly depends on the cross-section of the hair. Round hairs tend to be straight while oval shapes are usually curly. See *Chapter 9 – Hair Care* for full details. See also *Conditioner, Hair Dye, Hair Perm, Electrolysis, Hair Removal, Depilatory Agent, Dandruff* and *Shampoo*.

HAIR DYE

Hair dyes are used to color hair, either temporarily or permanently. They come in four varieties: progressive hair colors, temporary hair colors, semi-permanent hair colors, and permanent (oxidation) hair colors. For full details see *Chapter 9 – Hair Care.*

HAIR PERM

Hair perms are chemical treatments that permanently change the shape of the hair shaft. They are used to make straight hair curly, or to straighten curly or frizzy hair, in which case they are called hair straighteners. See *Chapter 9 – Hair Care* for full details.

HAIR REMOVAL

There are several ways to remove unwanted body hair. Physical methods include shaving or pulling out the hairs. Chemical methods involve the application of strongly alkaline creams called depilatories, which dissolve the unwanted hair at the surface of the skin. These methods are temporary solutions and the hair soon reappears at its normal rate of growth. Electrolysis, using needle or tweezer epilators, can permanently remove unwanted body hair. See *Chapter 5 – Skin Care* and *Chapter 16 – Salons and Surgeons* for full details.

HAIR STRAIGHTENER

Hair straighteners are chemical treatments similar to hair perms that are used to straighten curly, wavy, or frizzy hair. They can be applied by a hairdresser or they are available as kits for home use. See *Chapter 9 – Hair Care* for details of how they work.

HARD WATER

Hard water contains small amounts of calcium or magnesium that is leeched from rocks such as chalk, limestone, or gypsum as rain water drains into rivers and reservoirs. In areas where there is no chalk, limestone, or gypsum the water is said to be soft. Hard water is an important source of calcium in our diet and some water companies add calcium, in the form of lime, to the water supply. EU health regulations require a minimum calcium content in drinking water. Many people believe that the presence of these minerals improves the taste of water, while others claim that tea tastes better if brewed with soft water.

Some individuals claim that hard water leaves their skin and hair feeling dry after washing. After shampooing in hard water, some of the minerals remain on your hair and can affect its texture but conditioners usually compensate for this. The feeling of dry skin may be caused by the mild astringent properties of calcium or magnesium ions. Astringents cause the skin to retain less water.

The feeling of dry skin could also be caused by scum. In its simplest terms, soap is a sodium salt of a fatty acid. As a general rule, all sodium compounds are soluble in water. When soap is dissolved in hard water, some of the sodium swaps places with the calcium (or magnesium), and a new compound is made, which is a calcium salt of a fatty acid. This is not soluble in water and forms a solid, white or grey deposit called scum or soap scum, some of which remains on your skin making it feel powdery, and much of which forms the familiar ring in the bath tub or dulls the shine on the basin. Shampoos contain detergents rather than soap. These do not react with hard water and so no scum deposits are left in your hair.

After washing, soap seems to rinse off more quickly in hard-water areas than in soft-water areas. Any soap that clings to your skin chemically reacts with hard water and no longer behaves like soap. It no longer feels soapy and you are satisfied that the soap has been rinsed away. But in fact your skin is not completely free of chemical residues. A thin, powdery film of scum is left on your skin, some of it being removed by the towel when you dry yourself. In soft-water areas, your skin can still feel slightly soapy, even after thorough rinsing, because soft water is less effective at removing the soap. The presence of a residual film of soap on your skin may act as a lubricant and give the impression that the soft-water has not dried out your skin, while making you think that hard water does.

The scum problem means that soap cannot be used in shampoos and conditioners. Soap powders for washing clothes often contain water-softening chemicals such as washing soda (sodium carbonate), or zeolites that remove the calcium from hard water before it has a chance to react with the soap and produce scum. Detergents avoid the scum problem altogether and are a better choice for shampoos and conditioners. Most brands of toilet soap contain tetrasodium EDTA, which combines with the calcium or magnesium ions and prevents the formation of scum. This is only effective in small amounts of water, for example, in the lather you work up in your hands. In a large volume of water the tetrasodium EDTA is overwhelmed by the calcium and magnesium ions, the result being scum in the wash basin or bathtub.

HIGHLIGHTS

Highlights are decorative streaks of colored or bleached hair. The color can be a temporary or permanent hair dye. Permanently dyed and bleached highlights will eventually grow out. It is also possible to remove them by coloring all of the hair. Some people have natural highlights, usually in the form of a patch of light or white hair that contains less pigment or no pigment at all. See *Hair Dye*.

HORMONES

Hormones are chemicals that stimulate changes in our bodies. Some of these, notably the sex hormones, are known to have an instantly noticeable effect on our skin. We all remember the appearance of adolescent pimples and greasy skin during puberty, and changes in skin condition often accompany menstruation, pregnancy, menopause, and sometimes, HRT (hormone replacement therapy) or the contraceptive pill. For this reason, some manufacturers have added estrogens (female sex hormones) to cosmetics, especially to skincare creams and lotions that claim to rejuvenate skin and reduce wrinkles, lotions that claim to restore hair or prevent hair loss, and some products used to treat skin conditions such as seborrhea.

Most estrogens have been banned from cosmetics in the EU, and the FDA has strictly limited the amounts of these hormones that may be present in the finished product. The FDA's *Cosmetics Handbook* states that these products are ineffective and that there is insufficient data to establish the safety of hormones in cosmetics.

HUMECTANT

Humectants prevent personal care products from drying out. They are also used in food products. Most water-based cosmetics and toiletries contain humectants. There are many to choose from but the most commonly used is glycerin, although sorbitol is rapidly establishing itself as the humectant of choice. Both of these are natural substances.

Sorbitol occurs naturally in fruit, but it can be manufactured on a large scale from glucose. It is used in the food industry as a thickening agent for jellies or jams, and is particularly useful in the preparation of food products for diabetics.

Glycerin is a by-product of the soap-manufacturing industry. It is found in all fats and oils and is released when these are broken down by alkalis. It is used in fondant icing to retain moisture and prevent it from becoming rock-hard.

Humectants actually absorb moisture from the air and become damp. If you mark the level of the liquid in a bottle of glycerin, then leave it on a shelf for a week or two with the lid off, when you come back to it the level will have gone up. This happens because the glycerin literally sucks the moisture out of the air and dilutes itself. This is how glycerin or sorbitol keeps toothpaste moist when you leave the cap off.

HYDRATION

When a substance is thoroughly wetted and water molecules are clinging to the molecules of that substance, we say that substance is hydrated. The water molecules form weak chemical bonds – hydrogen bonds – to the other molecules. A hair shaft takes between three and six minutes to become completely hydrated and softened, depending on residual surface films of conditioner, mousse, hair spray, or your own natural oils. In this case, the water molecules soak into the hair shaft and attach themselves to the strands of protein from which the hair cells are composed. Surfactants assist this process by lowering the surface tension of the water, allowing it to form a film over the entire surface of the substance being hydrated.

HYPERSENSITIVITY

Hypersensitivity is a severe over-reaction of the body's immune system to a causative substance called an allergen. It is a form of extreme allergic reaction that can be life-threatening, although the number of cases of hypersensitivity caused by personal care products is extremely small – less than one in a million. See *Allergy* in *Chapter 15 – Medical Matters* for full details of Types I, II, III, and IV hypersensitivity.

HYPOALLERGENIC

A hypoallergenic cosmetic or toiletry should cause fewer allergies than personal care products that do not claim to be hypoallergenic. Colorants and fragrances are often not added to hypoallergenic products, as they are frequently implicated in adverse reactions to cosmetics. For further details, see *Chapter 2 – Marketing: Myths and Magic*.

INCI

An abbreviation for International Nomenclature of Cosmetic Ingredients. For more details, see *Chapter 18 – Labels and Legal Matters*.

ION

An ion (pronounced *eye-on*) is an atom or molecule that carries an electrical charge. Atoms bond together to make new chemicals. One method of bonding involves a metal atom passing an electron (a minute, negatively charged particle) to another, usually non-metal atom. The metal atom is left with a positive electrical charge and is called a cation (*cat-eye-on*). The non-metal atom gains the negative electrical charge of the electron, and is called an anion (*an-eye-on*). Now that the cation and anion have opposite electrical charges, they attract each other and bond together.

Ionic bonding is important in many cosmetic ingredients. Soap is a compound made when a positive sodium ion bonds to a negative ion derived from a natural fat or oil. Since the main part of soap is a negative ion (anion), we call soap an anionic surfactant. The most common synthetic detergents are anionic detergents. They also carry a negative charge on the surface-active (cleaning) part of the detergent, and are associated with positively charged sodium, potassium, or ammonium ions.

Ions are important in cosmetics and toiletries because they have a natural liking for water and often dissolve or easily mix with water. Oils do not mix with water because they contain no ions. Their atoms bond together using non-ionic methods.

The positive charge on cationic surfactants is important in hair and fabric conditioners. Since they carry their own positive electrical charge, they can neutralize, or discharge, any static electricity that builds up in dry hair, making it more controllable.

IRRADIATION

Irradiation is a method for sterilizing personal care products using ionizing radiation – usually gamma rays emitted from a highly radioactive material such as cobalt-60. After the product is sealed in its container, any microbes that are contaminating it are killed by an intense beam of gamma rays, which can penetrate all materials used for packaging. The radioactive source is kept some distance from the items being irradiated, and never comes into direct contact with them. Intense ultraviolet rays from a powerful UV lamp can also be used to kill microbes, but these rays have a poor penetrating power and cannot pass through most plastic, glass, or metal containers.

Some products that have been sterilized by irradiation do not mention this on the label. This is because many consumers do not understand the nature of gamma rays and are worried about using products that have been irradiated. However, after irradiation there is no residual radiation left in the product. Gamma rays are rays of extremely high-energy, electromagnetic radiation. Light is much the same except its rays have a vastly lower energy. When a spotlight is turned off at the theatre, the stage becomes completely dark. No residual light is left in the auditorium, nor in the performers. It is the same with gamma rays. They vanish completely when the radioactive source is removed.

Some fresh foods and most medical equipment are sterilized using gamma rays. When a gamma ray strikes a molecule of water, the molecule absorbs the energy of the ray and is split into two smaller, highly energetic particles called free radicals. Many of these join together again and the water molecule is reformed as though nothing had happened. However, the additional energy from the ray cannot remain in the newly formed water molecule and is released in the form of heat and an eerie, but harmless blue glow. Free radicals, however, are extremely reactive and can cause chemical changes in other substances instead of changing back into water molecules. If the free radicals are formed inside the cell of a microbe, they damage essential chemicals in the cell and kill the microbe. Insects and insect eggs are destroyed in the same way, but some mold spores do not contain water and can survive irradiation.

Too much irradiation can cause a product to deteriorate. Strawberries that have been irradiated have a much longer shelf-life than non-irradiated strawberries, but over-irradiation can give them a metallic flavor. Products with a high oil or wax content do not take well to irradiation. The free radicals attack the waxes and oils, breaking them down to smaller molecules that have an unpleasant, sometimes rancid, odor. See also *Microbe* and *Preservative*.

KERATIN

Keratin is a tough, fibrous protein used by the body to make hair, skin, and nail. It is resistant to damage from wind and weather, and some chemicals in the environment. It is extracted from animal skins, hair, hooves, and horns, and is added to some cosmetics and toiletries, usually in the form of hydrolyzed keratin or keratin amino acids, broken down or partly broken down using acids, alkalis, or enzymes. Proteins and amino acids play a number of roles in personal care products such as antistatic agents, emulsifiers, pH-controlling additives, and surfactants, but they are not absorbed by the skin, hair, or nail and they do not become incorporated into our body tissues to repair or improve them. See also *Amino Acid*.

LAKE

Lakes are colorants made by combining dyes with metals, usually chromium, aluminum, zirconium, or manganese. They are usually more durable than dyes because they are insoluble in water and are not leeched-out during washing. They are often used in make-up because they do not run and stain clothing. See also *Dye, Colorant, Coal Tar Dye* and *Azo Dye*.

LIPID

Lipids are natural fats, oils, or waxes that occur in plant and animal tissues. They are insoluble in water and contain a variety of substances including tocopherol (vitamin E), cholesterol, and lanolin. The most common lipids are combinations of fatty acids and glycerin, and are a valuable source of cosmetic ingredients.

Tallow (animal fat) contains many different lipids but glyceryl tristearate is one of the most abundant. It consists of three molecules of stearic acid (a fatty acid) combined with one molecule of glycerin. These four molecules can be separated from each other by saponification – a chemical reaction carried out by boiling the tallow with sodium hydroxide (caustic soda, a very strong, highly corrosive alkali). The sodium hydroxide releases the glycerin and combines with the stearic acid to form sodium stearate, which is used as soap.

Glycerin is used elsewhere in the cosmetic and food industries as a humectant, and the fatty acids are used as surfactants, emulsifiers, and emulsion stabilizers. Fatty acids can be further modified by chemical processes, producing a vast range of cosmetic ingredients. They can, for example, be reduced to fatty alcohols which are used as film formers, surfactants, and emulsifiers, and these can be modified by ethoxylation with ethylene oxide, forming a range of non-ionic surfactants. These surfactants can in turn be treated with sulfur trioxide to make a range of anionic surfactants, such as the extremely common sodium laureth sulfate.

Waxes and oils, which are extracted from petroleum (crude oil), are not referred to as lipids. They are more accurately called hydrocarbons but, like lipids, they are useful cosmetic ingredients. Examples of these petroleum-based hydrocarbons include ozokerite, a hard wax used in lipstick, and paraffinum liquidum (liquid paraffin), widely used in moisturizing creams and lotions. Hydrocarbons can be chemically modified to make fatty acid alcohols, which are identical in every respect to the fatty acid alcohols obtained from lipids. These can then be ethoxylated, then sulfated, forming the same range of surfactants as can be made from natural fats and oils.

Beeswax, spermaceti, and carnauba wax are solid lipids used as thickeners and film formers in a wide range of decorative cosmetics such as lipstick, mascara, foundation, eye shadow, and eyeliner. Mixed with resins, they form the base for depilatory waxes used for hair removal.

LIP GLOSS

Lip gloss is a lightly colored or neutral, non-greasy gel that gives a shine to the lips. It is often an oil-in-water emulsion or a mineral oil made into a gel by mixing it with bentonite clay. It is sometimes used on top of a lipstick to enhance its gloss. See *Chapter 11 – Make-up*. See also *Lipstick*.

LIPOSOME

A liposome is a microscopic bubble of fat filled with another substance. Liposomes were first produced in 1965 and are used as a delivery system for drugs. For example, the fat bubbles can be filled with an anticancer drug and, after injecting it into the patient, the liposomes find their way to the cancer tumor and release the drug, preventing it from having a toxic effect on healthy tissues in other parts of the body. They also allow drugs that only dissolve in water to be delivered to fatty tissues. As well as anticancer drugs, liposomes have been used to deliver antibiotics and antiviral drugs, including AZT, the anti-AIDS drug.

Liposomes vary in size and composition. The fatty membrane is composed of various lipids but natural, non-toxic phospholipids (a fatty substance containing phosphate), mixed with cholesterol are commonly used. Some companies have tweaked their design and patented them under various names, such as lipospheres, nanosomes and Nanosomin. Nanospheres are similar to liposomes, but are microscopic spheres made of a variety of plastics.

Cosmetics manufacturers eagerly embraced this technology as a vehicle to deliver cosmetic ingredients to deeper layers of the skin. They are essentially natural and harmless, and the word, "liposome", rolls off the tongue easily and adds scientific credibility to the manufacturers' claims. Many of these claims, however, are exaggerated. Research has demonstrated that liposomes can penetrate into the stratum corneum layer of the skin. This sounds impressive, until you realize that this is the extreme outer layer of the epidermis (the outer layer of dead skin cells), and that there are three more layers of dead cells to go through before you reach the living, basal cell layer which sits on top of the dermis, the main living tissue of the skin.

Some manufacturers will tell you that cell membranes, the tissue that surrounds living cells, are made of protein strands and phospholipids, the same material that liposomes are made of. For this reason, they claim that liposomes can get inside cells to deliver the cosmetic ingredients, and sometimes they can even collect cholesterol and carry it out of the cell. Cell membranes carefully control what goes into and out of the cell. Any unwanted chemicals inside the cell are likely to damage it, and perhaps you are better off storing your cholesterol inside your cells rather than releasing it into your circulatory system, where it can settle and block your arteries.

Cosmetic liposomes commonly deliver vitamins A, C, and E to the skin where, it is claimed, they act as antioxidants and free radical scavengers. This is claimed to reverse or reduce the aging effect that excessive exposure to the sun has on the skin. (See *Vitamins*.)

If you buy a product that contains liposomes, make sure it is a water-based gel rather than an oily or creamy emulsion that contains waxes and oils, as these may interact with the fat bubble of the liposome and cause it to deteriorate. Some liposomes can become oxidized during manufacture, often by overheating them at a crucial stage. It has been suggested that oxidized phospholipids can damage any cells they enter. Therefore, accidentally overheated liposomes containing phospholipids may present a danger to health.

LIPOSUCTION

The common name for suction lipectomy or vacuum-assisted lipectomy, liposuction is a surgical procedure carried out by a cosmetic surgeon to physically remove excess body fat (lipids), thereby improving the contours of the body. See *Chapter 16 – Salons and Surgeons*. See also *Eyelift*.

LIPSTICK

Lipsticks can be purchased in the form of waxy sticks, pencils, creams, liquid paints, and gels. They are used cosmetically to highlight the lips or can be applied as a medical treatment for damaged, infected, or inflamed lips. Since lipstick is used near the mucous membrane of the mouth, it is a Category-1 cosmetic and subject to strict regulations concerning levels of microbial contamination. See *Chapter 11 – Make-up*. See also *Microbe*.

MASCARA

Mascara is applied to the eyelashes to both thicken and darken them. This frames the eyes, making them appear larger and more alluring. As you age, your eyelashes become thinner and lighter in color and mascara has the effect of making the eyes appear more youthful. It is available in both liquid and cake form. Since mascara is intended for use near the eyes it is a Category-1 cosmetic and subject to strict microbe contamination standards. See *Chapter 11 – Make-up*. See also *Microbe*.

MELANIN

Melanin is the skin's natural pigment produced by melanocytes in the basal cells of the epidermis (outer layer of skin). It is also the pigment that gives hair its color. See *Chapter 5 – Skin Care* for full details.

MICROBE

Microbe is a common word for micro-organism. It is a general term used to describe any microscopic, single-celled, living organism. It is often extended to include some multi-celled, complex organisms such as mold and fungi, and viruses which do not have cells. Cosmetics can become infected with molds, fungi, yeasts, bacteria, and protozoa. Microbes enter personal care products during manufacture, when the containers are being filled, and while you are using them at home. There is a danger that microbes in cosmetics and toiletries may be transferred to your body and start an infection.

If a cosmetic or toiletry becomes infected, the rapidly reproducing microbes often produce a bad smell and may cause some clear products to become cloudy. Sometimes visible patches of mold appear on the surface. The microbes can chemically alter cosmetic ingredients, causing colors and odors to change. The altered substances may be poisonous or harmful.

For the purpose of setting acceptable levels of microbial contamination, the EU Commission has divided cosmetics and toiletries into two categories. Category-1 products are those for use on infants under the age of three, for use on or near the eyes, or for use on or near mucous membranes. All other personal care products are Category-2 products. See *Chapter 4 – Preservatives* and *Chapter 13 – Common Sense and Cosmetic Safety*. See also *Irradiation, Preservative* and *Antimicrobial*.

MOISTURIZING CREAM

Moisturizing creams contain emollients, which are substances used to moisturize the skin by preventing loss of water from the skin through evaporation. The emollient forms a thin, oily or slightly greasy layer which keeps water in the skin. The simplest moisturizing substance is petroleum jelly, a purified grease made from crude oil, or a simple vegetable oil such as coconut oil or olive oil. Humectants such as glycerin or sorbitol may also be added to retain moisture and hold it in the skin. Water is included in the mixture to accelerate the hydration (moistening) of the dry, outer layer of skin cells. As water enters the cells they plump up, giving a smoother appearance and feel to the skin, and reducing the appearance of fine lines. The effect lasts for six to twelve hours before the cells dry out and shrink again. See *Chapter 5 – Skin Care*. See also *Emollient, Emulsion, Emulsifier* and *Emulsion Stabilizer*.

MUCOUS MEMBRANE

Mucous membranes line the mouth, the digestive tract, the respiratory tract of the nose, wind pipe and lungs, the genital and urinary passages, and the eyelids. They appear as soft, moist, pink surfaces that secrete a lubricating, mucus-containing fluid from special cells called goblet cells. They help to keep our body cavities moist, lubricated, and clean.

Many cosmetic ingredients can penetrate mucous membranes more easily than they can penetrate skin. If they come into contact with mucous membranes they usually cause irritation, inflammation, and sometimes pain. Some ingredients are considered too harmful to come into contact with mucous membranes and are banned from cosmetics and toiletries designed for use on or near those parts of the body.

Since mucous membranes are more easily infected by microbes, all personal care products designed for use on or near them, for example, lipstick, eye make-up, toothpaste, mouthwash, eye drops, and contact-lens rinsing solutions, are classified as Category-1 products for the purpose of microbial contamination. They will therefore contain sufficient amounts of preservatives to prevent microbial contamination from rising above the prescribed levels. Some brands of contact-lens rinsing solutions do not contain preservatives. Instead, they are sterilized by heating the solution to a high temperature or by irradiation using gamma rays. The sterilized solution may be sealed in a pressurized dispenser, making it difficult for microbes to enter and contaminate the product. Non-pressurized products are susceptible to infection and are often packaged in sealed, single-dose units. Larger containers carry instructions that they should be disposed of after a certain period of use, in case they have become contaminated.

Personal care products that are not specifically intended for use on or near the mucous membranes should not be used in those areas. They may contain microbes above the recommended levels, or they may contain ingredients that can be absorbed through the mucous membrane causing irritation, sensitization or allergic reactions, or they may have a toxic effect when they enter the bloodstream.

MUSK

Musk is a scent secreted from the scent glands of the male Tibetan musk deer, musk ox, civet cat, otter, and several other species. It is used as a pheromone to attract and impress females of the same species. The odor of musk is not particularly pleasant to humans but, despite this, many females are attracted to it. It has the effect of heightening and increasing the persistence of scents from flowers. Musk is, therefore, a valued fragrance chemical and is used in many perfumes and deodorants.

Nitro-musks are simple molecules that are easily and cheaply made. They are chemically unrelated to muscone or civetone but they have odors that are remarkably similar. Some of these compounds have been found to be harmful and are banned from cosmetics in the EU. See *Chapter 3 – Colorants and Fragrances*.

MUTAGEN

A mutagen is an agent that can cause mutations in living cells. The changes take place in the nucleus of the cell, potentially giving rise to cancer or an inherited disease. Mutagens that cause cancer are called carcinogens. Teratogens (from the Greek *terat*, meaning monster) are mutagens that cause changes in the cells of embryos or fetuses, resulting in malformed babies.

Some cosmetic ingredients are known to be mutagenic, teratogenic, or carcinogenic. These include several of the "diamino" hair dyes such as 2,4-diaminoanisole, antimicrobials and preservatives such as formaldehyde and boric acid, and additives such as tocopherol (vitamin E). See *Chapter 15 – Medical Matters* for lists of mutagenic and carcinogenic cosmetic ingredients.

NAILS

Like hair and skin, nails (properly called onyx) are composed of the tough, fibrous protein, keratin. The main part of the nail is called the nail plate. It is attached to the underlying skin which is called the nail bed. Around the edges of the nail, the skin forms a nail fold that wraps around and overlaps the edges of the nail. The cuticle is a thin flap of skin that covers the nail fold and is attached to the nail plate. Its job is to prevent dirt and microbes going under the nail fold where they may start an infection. See *Chapter 12 – Nail Care* for full details of nail structure, growth and nail cosmetics. See also *Cuticle* and *Cuticle Solvent*.

NATURAL

Natural substances used in cosmetics include plant or animal extracts, and minerals obtained from the earth. Many people regard natural substances as being more wholesome or more healthy than artificial chemicals. See *Chapter 2 – Marketing: Myths and Magic* for full details of the use of the word "natural." See also *Botanical Additives* and *Chapter 17 – Animal Products and Animal Testing*.

NEEDLE EPILATOR

A needle epilator is the device used to permanently remove unwanted body hair by a process called electrolysis. See *Chapter 16 – Salons and Surgeons* for full details.

NITROSAMINES

Nitrosamines (pronounced *night-row-za-means* or sometimes *night-russ-A-means*) are potent carcinogens (cancer-causing chemicals), which can be accidentally formed during the manufacture of cosmetic ingredients or by the interaction of two, otherwise harmless, ingredients in the finished product. It has even been reported that chemicals secreted by our skin can react with some cosmetic ingredients to form nitrosamines. Despite rigorous testing for these contaminants, nitrosamines have been detected in many cosmetics. See *Chapter 13 – Common Sense and Cosmetic Safety* for full details.

NON-IONIC SURFACTANT

A non-ionic surfactant is a surfactant (cleaning chemical) that consists of a single molecule and carries no electrical charge. Fatty acid alcohols such as cetearyl alcohol or stearyl alcohol are the simplest non-ionic surfactants. These can be bonded to ethylene oxide, forming polyethylene glycol (PEG) derivatives and "eth" surfactants, such as the laneth, steareth or ceteareth family. Many of these produce little, if any, lather and are particularly useful where lather is undesirable, for example in hair conditioners and detergents for front-loading washing machines and dishwashers. See *Surfactant* and *How Soaps and Detergents Work* in *Chapter 6 – Soaps, Shower Gels, and Cleansing Lotions*.

NON-RINSE OFF

Any personal care product that remains on your skin for a lengthy period of time is called a non-rinse off (or non-rinse out) product. These include moisturizing creams, deodorants, lipsticks, eye shadows, mascaras, eye liners, foundations, mousse, and hair dyes to mention but a few. Since they are in contact with your skin for a long time, some cosmetic ingredients are banned from non-rinse-off products. These include the preservatives sodium iodate, 5-bromo-5-nitro-1,3-dioxane, and phenoxy-isopropanol; the antidandruff agent zinc pyrithione; the anticorrosion agent sodium nitrite; and depilatory agents containing thioglycolates. These substances are considered to be too harmful to remain on your skin for more than a few minutes and are, therefore, restricted to rinse-off (rinse out) products such as shampoos, cleansing lotions, and hair-removal creams, which are washed off soon after they are used. For a list of colorants that are banned from non-rinse-off products, see *Chapter 10 – Baby Products*.

OPACIFIER

Opacifiers reduce the amount of light that can pass through a liquid. They are used in conjunction with thickeners to make clear or slightly cloudy (translucent) liquids appear rich and creamy. Since water is the main ingredient in products such as shampoos, conditioners, shower gels, and cleansing lotions thickeners, and sometimes opacifiers and colorants, are added to make them seem less watery and to improve their pouring properties.

Some opacifiers give the product a sheen or a pearlized appearance, making it look more attractive to the consumer. There is a strong psychological link between the appearance and the perceived quality or effectiveness of medicines and toiletries, and therefore it is extremely important for manufacturers to make their products visually appealing to their customers.

Manufacturers have a vast range of opacifiers to choose from. The list includes insoluble minerals like chalk and silica, metal salts of fatty acids such as calcium stearate or aluminum behenate, and both natural and synthetic polymers. Many opacifiers have a dual role. Chalk can reduce unwanted acidity in a product, and polymer-based opacifiers can also act as film formers and thickeners.

ORAL CARE AGENT

Oral care agents are added to oral care products to clean and protect the oral cavity. Antimicrobials and surfactants are added to mouthwash to clean and sterilize the mouth. Abrasives and surfactants in toothpaste and dentifrice help to clean and polish teeth, while fluoride strengthens tooth enamel and strontium salts reduce the sensitivity of teeth to sudden temperature changes.

Since the mouth is lined with mucous membrane, several ingredients, including some preservatives and colorants, are not permitted in oral care products. See *Chapter 8 – Teeth and Oral Care Products*.

OXIDIZING AGENT

Oxidizing agents are chemicals that cause other chemicals to become oxidized. Oxidizing agents remove electrons from other chemicals. When this happens, oxygen atoms are added to, or hydrogen atoms are removed from the chemical that is being oxidized. In cosmetics this often produces desirable effects. Oxidizing agents, often hydrogen peroxide, are added to oxidation hair dyes to develop the color and fix it into the hair shaft. (See *Hair Dye*.) When hair is permed or straightened, the protein strands in hair are weakened and separated using a reducing agent (a chemical which acts in the opposite manner to an oxidizing agent); the hair is then reshaped under tension and finally the protein strands are rejoined using an oxidizing agent.

Oxidizing agents often have a whitening or bleaching effect and they are also disinfectants. Hydrogen peroxide can be used to bleach hair and to sterilize contact lenses, and it is used as an antiseptic mouthwash. Sodium hypochlorite is found in domestic bleach, but it is also used in conjunction with water softeners and detergents to clean and sterilize dentures and oral braces. It is also used in sterilizing solutions for baby feeders. Since oxidizing agents kill bacterial cells, they also damage skin and eyes, so great care should be taken when using any product that contains oxidizing agents.

OXIRANE

Another name for ethylene oxide. See *Dioxane*.

PERSPIRATION

Perspiration is water secreted by sweat glands onto the surface of your skin where it evaporates and keeps your body cool. Most of your body, and especially your palms, soles of your feet, and forehead, are covered with eccrine sweat glands that empty directly onto the surface of your skin. At puberty, a second type of sweat gland develops under your arms and around your genitals. These apocrine sweat glands empty into the hair follicles of your pubic hair and underarm hair, where the sweat picks up sebum and protein fragments before flowing out of the follicle and onto the skin. The breakdown of these substances by bacteria produces the well-known underarm odor. See *Chapter 7 – Deodorants and Antiperspirants*.

pH CONTROL

pH is a measurement of the strength of an acid or alkali. Alkalis are the chemical opposites of acids but, like acids, they can be highly corrosive to a wide range of materials, especially the skin, hair, and eyes.

The pH scale is a series of numbers from zero to 14. All acids and alkalis can be assigned a number on this scale according to their strength. The strongest acids are placed at zero or 1 on the scale. The numbers gradually increase as the acids become weaker. The weakest acids have a pH of about 6. Neutral substances such as water, which are neither acidic nor alkaline have a pH of 7. As numbers increase above 7, we enter the realm of alkalis. The weakest alkalis have a pH of 8 or 9. As the numbers increase, the alkalis become stronger until the strongest of all are placed at pH 14.

Any acids stronger than pH 3 (i.e., pH zero, 1, or 2) are likely to cause severe skin burns. Likewise, any alkali stronger than pH 11 (i.e., pH 12, 13, or 14) will quickly damage skin. You are unlikely to encounter such strong solutions in cosmetics designed for home use. Cosmetic surgeons may use trichloroacetic acid, which has a pH of about 1, as an exfoliant (skin peeler), and skin peelers used by professionals in beauty salons may have a pH of 3, but the strongest exfoliant you are likely to encounter for home use will probably have a pH of 3.5 or 4. Even so, prolonged skin contact can result in severe burns.

Nail-cuticle solvent contains caustic alkalis such as sodium hydroxide. These are usually supplied in formulations that contain a maximum of 5 percent of the alkali and the pH will not exceed 12.7. This is more than strong enough to cause severe eye damage and painful skin burns. Other alkaline products, such as hair-removal creams and perming solutions, may also have pH values of 11 to 12.

The pH of body fluids is 7.4 and skin has a pH of between 5 and 5.6, men's skin being slightly more acidic than women's. Skin pH varies from person to person and becomes slightly more acidic throughout the day as the body secretes a cocktail of chemicals from sweat glands and sebaceous glands, but it seldom goes below pH 5. This acidity on the skin helps to control the growth of unwanted bacteria.

Eyes and skin are sensitive to acids stronger than pH 4 and alkalis stronger than pH 10. For this reason, manufacturers must remove unwanted acidity or alkalinity in cosmetics and toiletries. Excess acidity is reduced by adding an alkali, usually sodium hydroxide, while unwanted alkalis are neutralized with weak acids such as citric acid, lactic acid, or fatty acids. Chemicals added to remove unwanted acidity or alkalinity do not have to be listed with the other ingredients, although several manufacturers volunteer this information.

Once the desired pH has been achieved, buffers are added to maintain it. A buffer is usually a combination of two simple chemicals that work together to resist changes in pH during use or storage.

So what do the letters "pH" stand for? Nothing. They do not stand for anything. All acids contain hydrogen ions. H is the chemical symbol for hydrogen. Stronger acids have a greater concentration of hydrogen ions than weaker acids. The amount of hydrogen present in an acid can be measured and expressed as a number, but this number is often unwieldy. Therefore, the "p" in pH, represents a simple mathematical operation that is applied to this unwieldy number in order to convert it into a simple number between zero and 14 – 14 being directly related to the number of hydrogen ions found in pure water.

See also *Buffer*.

PHOTODERMATITIS

Photodermatitis is a form of dermatitis caused by an abnormal sensitivity to sunlight. It appears as a series of blemishes or blisters on those parts of the body that are exposed to sunlight. See *Photosensitivity, Dermatitis* and *Phototoxin*.

PHOTOSENSITIVITY

A photosensitive person has an abnormal sensitivity to sunlight, the consequence usually being a rash on those parts of the body that have been exposed to the sun. It may also be the result of a more serious disease of the internal organs, such as porphyria or systemic lupus erythematosus: these conditions are often worsened by exposure to sunlight. More commonly, the photosensitivity is caused by a drug which is being taken or by chemicals, including cosmetics and plant extracts, that are present on the skin. Juices from buttercups, mustard, strawberries, parsley, and parsnips are well known to cause photosensitivity and are called photosensitizers.

Drugs that are known to cause photosensitivity include:

- Antibiotics containing tetracyclines, oxytetracyclines, naladixic, and some sulfonamides.
- Diuretics containing cyclopenthiazide (Navidrex and Navidrex K), benzofluazide (Neo-naclex), and hydrochlorothiazide (Moduretic).
- Some antidepressants, sedatives, and tranquillizers such as lithium, amitriptyline (Lentizol or Limbitrol), trifluoperazone (Stelazine), fluphenazine (Modecate, Moditen, Motipress, and Motival), and prochloroperazine (Stemetil and Vetigon).
- Insulin.
- Some antimalarial drugs such as quinine, quinine derivatives, Daraprim, and Nivaquine.
- Some contraceptive pills.
- Some hormone replacement therapies.

If you are taking any of these drugs you should not use sunbeds and you should avoid the noonday sun. At all other times you should use a sunscreen with a high sun-protection factor.

If you are not taking any of these drugs and you develop a rash when you are exposed to the sun, change the cosmetics you are using and apply a good quality sunscreen. If the rash persists, avoid the sun, especially when it is strongest between 11:00 a.m. and 3:00 p.m., and consult your doctor. See also *Dermatitis* and *Phototoxin*.

PHOTOTOXIN

Phototoxins are chemicals that undergo changes when they absorb the energy of sunlight, and are converted into poisonous substances that are absorbed through the skin and into the bloodstream. These photochemical reactions may also produce photoirritants (new chemicals that are skin irritants), or photomutagens (new chemicals that cause cell mutations by damaging genes, which could result in fetal malformations, inherited diseases, or cancer).

Many compounds absorb light. Whenever you take a photograph, the chemicals in your film are altered by the light. Light can also cause colors to fade, such as those in curtains, wall coverings, and furnishings. Sunscreens contain UV absorbers that absorb the energy of ultraviolet radiation and disperse it harmlessly before it reaches the deeper layers of you skin. During the design and testing stage of sunscreens, stringent safety tests must be applied to ensure they do not form phototoxins, photoirritants or photomutagens. Generally speaking, the sunscreen is subjected to artificial sunlight consisting of all frequencies of light, including UV-A and UV-B. During the test there should be no significant changes in the chemicals. If changes do occur, the toxicity of the new substances must be tested on living cells, from both bacterial and mammalian origin. If there are no significant chemical changes after 10 hours of simulated irradiation, the cell tests for photomutagens are not required. In order to ensure the tests are working correctly, they must be carried out in duplicate: once using the new sunscreen and once using 8-methoxypsoralen, a known phototoxin which is now banned from use in cosmetics in the EU.

PIGMENT

Pigment is another word for colorant. See *Chapter 3 – Colorants and Fragrances*. See also *Colorant*, *Dye*, *Lake*, *Azo Dye* and *Coal Tar Dye*.

PLACENTA

Also called the afterbirth, placental extract, both from human and bovine (cattle) placentas, is a valued cosmetic ingredient that is widely believed to rejuvenate the skin. Currently, cells, tissues, or other products of human origin are banned from use in cosmetics in the EU. Any placental extract in products purchased in the EU will therefore be of bovine origin. See *Chapter 17 – Animal Products and Animal Testing.*

POLYMER

Polymers are giant molecules that are made by joining many thousands of smaller molecules together, rather like joining beads to make a long necklace. They are widely used in plastics, fabrics, and paints, and in cosmetics as thickeners, film formers, antistatic agents, opacifiers, and emulsion stabilizers.

Natural polymers used in cosmetics include proteins, cellulose derivatives, and starch derivatives (modified starch). Artificial polymers that commonly appear in lists of ingredients are acrylates, carbomers, methicones (silicone polymers), PEG derivatives, and PVP (polyvinylpyrrolidone). PVP is commonly used in decorative cosmetics such as lipsticks and mascara, and has been linked to cancer.

Minute strands of nylon and other fibers are used to reinforce some brands of mascara to prevent them from cracking and flaking off. Microscopic nylon spheres (called nanospheres) have also been used as fillers in cosmetics, i.e., to fill in fine lines and wrinkles giving a smoother appearance to wrinkled skin.

POWDERS

Loose powders and pressed powders (cakes) are used to reduce the gloss of oily skin or foundation and form the base of blushers (rouge), highlighters, and shaders. They are often colored mixtures of minerals – mainly talc and kaolin with magnesium, calcium, or zinc stearate to aid adhesion. Care should be taken when using powders as inhaling mineral dust is harmful and can cause breathing difficulties, allergies, or more serious lung diseases. See *Chapter 11 – Make-up.*

PPM

Parts per million or particles per million. This is a unit to measure very small concentrations of chemicals, usually impurities or contaminants. 1 ppm means there is one particle of a contaminant in every million particles of the product. 1 ppm translates to 0.0001 percent. Modern chemical techniques, used for chemical analysis or forensic science, can detect chemicals in the order of 1 ppb (one particle per billion).

PRESERVATIVE

Preservatives are chemicals that are added to personal care products to prevent or control the growth of microbes in the product. Since they are designed to kill cells or prevent them from multiplying, preservatives are potentially harmful cosmetic ingredients and the vast majority of preservatives have restrictions on their use. Since there are also strict rules concerning levels of microbial infection in personal care products, virtually all products you buy will contain at least one preservative, making it almost impossible to avoid using potentially harmful chemicals on your body. See *Chapter 4 – Preservatives* for full details. See also *Benzoates, Microbe, Antimicrobial* and *Deodorant*.

PROBIOTICS

As the name suggests, probiotics are the opposites of antibiotics. Probiotics encourage the growth of bacteria. After an infection that has been treated with a course of antibiotics, bowel disorders may occur because the antibiotic has changed the normal, healthy bacterial flora of the gut. Foods like natural, live yoghurt can encourage a rapid restoration of the gut flora.

The word "probiotic" sounds healthy, wholesome, and scientific – an ideal word for cosmetic marketing. But there can be no excuse whatsoever for adding ingredients that encourage bacterial growth in cosmetic products.

PROPELLANT

Propellants are gases that are compressed into pressurized containers and used to expel the product when the pressure is released. They are used in aerosol sprays, pressurized dispensers for sterile contact-lens cleaning solutions, and some brands of shaving foam and hair mousse. The propellant is usually a gas that turns to a liquid under pressure. It must be non-toxic by inhalation, although the products dispensed may be harmful and, as a general rule, should not be inhaled.

Traditionally, CFCs (chlorofluorocarbons) were used but, despite being non-toxic, non-corroding, non-flammable, and cheap to produce, they have been superseded by hydrocarbons because of the damage CFCs have wreaked on the ozone layer. Nowadays a mixture of butane, isobutane, and propane is the most commonly used propellant. This is highly flammable and inhaled by solvent abusers, which can result in intoxication, hallucinations, nausea, vomiting, coma, and (occasionally) death.

PROTEIN

Proteins are large molecules formed when many hundreds or thousands of amino acid molecules join together. They fall into two groups: fibrous proteins like collagen and keratin, that make up muscle, skin, hair, nail, cartilage, ligaments, and tendons; and globular proteins, found in the body fluids and used as hormones, enzymes, antibodies, and hemoglobin in red blood cells. Glycoproteins are proteins that are attached to sugar molecules, and lipoproteins are proteins attached to lipid (fatty) molecules.

Proteins are added to some personal care products for a variety of reasons. They can act as emulsifiers, antistatic agents, film formers, thickeners, and humectants, but they have no biological significance. Contrary to advertisers' claims, they cannot be absorbed by hair, skin, or nail, and they cannot repair or improve our body tissues. See also *Amino Acid*.

PRO-VITAMIN

Pro-vitamins are substances in our diet that are absorbed by the body and converted into vitamins. Panthenol – pro-vitamin B_5 – and beta-carotene – pro-vitamin A – are the most common pro-vitamins used in cosmetics. Beta-carotene is a natural colorant found in many roots, including carrots. See *Chapter 2 – Marketing: Myths and Magic*. See also *Vitamins*.

REDUCING AGENT

A reducing agent is the chemical opposite of an oxidizing agent, and causes chemical changes in other substances. The first stage in perming or straightening hair is to weaken the protein strands using a reducing agent, consisting of an alkaline solution of a thioglycolate. Hydroquinone is also a reducing agent used in oxidation hair dyes and localized skin lighteners.

Technically speaking, reducing agents give electrons to other chemicals. In the process of doing this they often add hydrogen atoms to, or remove oxygen atoms from the chemical that is being reduced. They are often fairly potent chemicals and, when used in personal care products, they usually work in alkaline conditions, making them potentially harmful substances. See also *Hair Perm* and *Oxidizing Agent*.

RETIN-A

Retin-A is a brand name for tretinoin, a drug related to retinoic acid and used for the treatment of acne and other skin conditions. See *Tretinoin* and *Retinoic Acid*.

RETINOIC ACID

Retinoic acid is a retinoid drug related to vitamin A and used to treat acne when all other treatments, such as antibiotics, antimicrobials, and benzoyl peroxide have failed. It has the effect of reducing oil production in the skin and is useful in treating any skin condition that causes excessive oil production, or scaling or thickening of the skin. It is also being evaluated as a treatment to reduce wrinkles caused by the aging process or by excessive exposure to ultraviolet light.

When used to treat acne, the condition often worsens for a while, but does improve after about 10 weeks. It can cause serious side effects, such as irritation, skin peeling, discoloration of the skin (both darkening and lightening), and liver damage. For this reason it is available only on prescription and is banned from cosmetics in both the EU and the USA. See also *Tretinoin*.

RINSE OFF

Rinse-off products, also called rinse-out products, are those that are in contact with the body for only a short time before being rinsed off with water. Because of the short exposure time, these products are allowed to contain potent ingredients that could damage skin or hair if left on the body for any length of time. Rinse-off products include shampoo, shower gel, hair removers, cuticle solvents, and hair-perming formulations.

SEBUM

Sebum is the skin's natural oil and is produced in the sebaceous glands located next to hair follicles, into which the sebum is released. See *Chapter 5 – Skin Care*. See also *Hair, Blackheads* and *Acne*.

SEMISYNTHETIC

A semisynthetic substance is a natural substance that has been significantly modified by chemical reactions. The foam booster Cocamide DEA is one example of a semi-synthetic compound. You may read statements such as "derived from coconut oil" but you will be unable to find a single molecule of Cocamide DEA in any natural source. The bottom line is, semisynthetic compounds are not natural.

SENSITIZATION

Sensitization is an unwarranted action of the immune system that initiates an allergy. Normally, your immune system recognizes invading microbes and develops antibodies to kill them. Once the infection has been removed the antibodies are retained by the immune system so your body can "remember" these particular microbes and deal with them quickly if they ever re-infect you. This is why you can only catch some illnesses once.

Occasionally, for no reason, your immune system develops antibodies to harm-less substances such as pollen or cosmetic ingredients. You become sensitized when the antibodies are first produced, and the pollen or cosmetic ingredient is now called an allergen. You will have no symptoms, however, until you next meet the allergen, when you will experience an allergic reaction, which may be mild or severe. See *Chapter 15 – Medical Matters* for full details.

SENSITIVITY

If your skin has an adverse reaction to a cosmetic or toiletry, whether it is a mild irri-tation or a severe rash, you are sensitive to at least one of the ingredients in that product. Sensitivity is the degree to which you are sensitive. It varies from person to person and on different parts of your body. Greasy skin is more resistant to water-soluble irritants, and the thick skin on your palms is less sensitive than the thin skin on your eyelids and lips. Everybody is sensitive to corrosive chemicals such as strong acids or alkalis.

If you find you are sensitive to a personal care product, try a different brand. If you are sensitive to several products, read their lists of ingredients to see if there is one ingredient that is common to all of them; avoid it in future. If there is no common ingredient causing your sensitivity, it is probably a colorant or fragrance chemical causing the problem, and in this case you should try to avoid highly colored products and use unscented or fragrance-free products. It must be pointed out, however, that products labeled as unscented or fragrance free may contain some fragrance chemicals, to hide the unpleasant smells of other ingredients.

SHAMPOO

Shampoo is a mixture of detergent and water used to remove dirt and grease from hair. Sodium lauryl sulfate (SLS) is the most widely used detergent in shampoos and can be found in about 90 percent of them, usually in combination with other detergents such as sodium laureth sulfate. The detergent concentration varies between 5 and 20 percent of the shampoo, depending on whether it is for dry or greasy hair. For full details of the various types of shampoo, see *Chapter 9 – Hair Care*.

SHAVING FORMULATIONS (SOAP, GEL, FOAM, AND CREAM)

Wet shaving involves sliding a blade across the skin, which cuts off unwanted hairs at skin level. The process is made more comfortable and efficient if the blade is sharp, hair shafts are softened with water, and a lubricant is applied to the skin to prevent the blade from snagging and cutting the skin. This moisture and lubrication is supplied by the shaving soap, gel, foam, or cream. See the section on hair removal in *Chapter 5 – Skin Care*.

SHOWER GEL

Also called body shampoo or body gel, shower gel has essentially the same formulation as shampoo, but it is usually presented as a clear, colored gel rather than as an opaque, creamy liquid. See *Chapter 6 – Soaps, Shower Gels, and Cleansing Lotions*.

SKIN, SKIN COLOR AND SKIN TYPES

For a full description of the structure and color of skin, and the characteristics of normal, dry, greasy, and combination skin, see *Chapter 5 – Skin Care*.

SOAP

Soap is a basic surfactant (cleaning chemical) composed of sodium or potassium salts of fatty acids. The salts are made by boiling animal or vegetable fats or oils with a strong alkali such as sodium hydroxide (caustic soda) or, less commonly, potassium hydroxide (caustic potash). The excess alkali must be removed before the product can be used as a toiletry or cosmetic ingredient. See *Chapter 6 – Soaps, Shower Gels, and Cleansing Lotions* for full details of soap. See also *Hard Water* and *Detergent*.

SOAPLESS DETERGENT

This is another name for a detergent, an alternative to soap that is made from oils derived from petroleum and sulfuric acid, or from fatty alcohols and sulfur trioxide. See *Detergent*.

SOLVENT

A solvent is a liquid that can dissolve another substance. Water is the solvent used to dissolve and mix together the ingredients in most toiletries such as shampoo, conditioner, cleansing lotion, and make-up remover. Nail polish and nail-polish remover contain solvents such as ethyl acetate and amyl acetate. Occasionally oils are used to dissolve or soften waxes for lipstick and thick, water-in-oil emulsions like moisturizing cream for dry skin. Alcohol is frequently used as a carrier solvent for fragrance chemicals.

SPF

See *Sun-Protection Factor*.

STRATUM CORNEUM

The stratum corneum is the outermost layer of skin cells that are composed almost entirely of keratin, a tough, fibrous protein. It is the outermost part of the epidermis, which is composed of five layers, or strata, each containing skin cells at a different stage of development. It is also commonly called the horny layer or keratinized layer. See *Chapter 5 – Skin Care*.

SUNBLOCK

Another name for a sunscreen. See *Sunscreen*.

SUN-PROTECTION FACTOR (SPF)

Sometimes called SPF or reduced to just "Factor" on some brands of sunscreen, it indicates the level of protection given by the sunscreen. See *Chapter 14 – Sun and Skin*.

SUNSCREEN

The most common sunscreens, also called sunblocks or suntan lotions, are preparations that are rubbed onto the skin to prevent harmful ultraviolet rays from reaching the skin, or to reduce the intensity of the ultraviolet rays before they reach the skin. They fall into two groups: chemical sunscreens and physical sunscreens. Chemical sunscreens contain UV absorbers that absorb the ultraviolet rays and reduce their energy. Physical sunscreens contain reflective materials that reflect the ultraviolet rays away from the skin. Oral sunscreens, taken in the form of tablets, were once popular but they have now been banned by the FDA and are not licensed as a drug in the UK – hence they are not sold by pharmacists. For full details see *Chapter 14 – Sun and Skin*. See also *Ultraviolet Rays, Tanning Agent* and details of the structure of skin in *Chapter 5 – Skin Care*.

SUNTAN

Exposure to ultraviolet rays stimulates melanocytes in the basal layer of the epidermis (the outer layer of skin cells) to produce larger amounts of melanin, a brown pigment, to act as a natural barrier to the harmful effects of UV rays. See *Chapter 14 – Sun and Skin*.

SURFACTANT

A surfactant lowers the surface tension of a cosmetic or toiletry, allowing it to act as a cleaning agent or enabling it to spread easily and evenly. Many surfactants are anionic detergents found in shampoos, shower gels, and cleansing lotions. Soap is a surfactant that is similar in structure and action to anionic detergents. See *Detergent, Soap,* and *How Soaps and Detergents Work* in *Chapter 6 – Soaps, Shower Gels, and Cleansing Lotions.*

SYNERGIC EFFECT

A synergist is a substance that is capable of enhancing the effectiveness of another substance. This may have the advantage of reducing the amount of that substance used in a cosmetic or toiletry. Some antioxidants work better in the presence of small amounts of citric acid, lactic acid, or the sodium, potassium, or calcium salts of these acids – allowing smaller quantities of the antioxidant to be added. This reduces both the manufacturer's costs and the levels of chemical additives in the product. The preservative combination methylchloroisothiazolinone and methylisothiazolinone is more effective in the presence of small amounts of magnesium nitrate and magnesium chloride. In medicine, two antibiotics administered together may be far more effective at fighting an infection than either antibiotic taken on its own.

Of course the synergic effect can work against you. A cosmetic ingredient that normally has no adverse effects may be activated by another, equally harmless ingredient and cause an unexpected irritation or allergic reaction. Manufacturers avoid combinations of ingredients that are known to have adverse synergic effects, but these combinations are rare and often unpredictable. By using two different products at the same time you may unwittingly produce an undesirable combination of ingredients. There are no EU regulations relating to adverse synergic effects.

SYNTHETIC

Synthetic ingredients are made entirely by artificial means and are not found in nature unless they are exact copies of natural compounds. They are usually made from chemicals derived from crude oil, coal tar, or minerals obtained from the earth. Many people have an instinctive mistrust of synthetic ingredients but this is irrational and each substance must be judged on its own track record. Nylon is a completely synthetic material but few people have come to grief as a result of meeting this material. Indeed, millions of people world-wide have internal nylon sutures (stitches) that will remain harmlessly inside them for the remainder of their lives.

SWEAT

Another name for perspiration. See *Perspiration*.

TAN

Another word for suntan. See *Suntan*. See also *Chapter 14 – Sun and Skin*.

TANNING AGENT

Tanning agents encourage the formation of a suntan. For full details of bronzers, extenders, accelerators (boosters), and tanning pills, see *Chapter 14 – Sun and Skin*.

TINT

Another word for hair color. See *Hair Dye* and *Chapter 9 – Hair Care*.

TOOTH, STRUCTURE OF

For full details of the structure of teeth and oral care products, see *Chapter 8 – Teeth and Oral Care Products*.

TOOTHPASTE

Toothpaste is a mixture of cleaning agents, antimicrobials, preservatives, and other additives that remove bacteria, plaque, food particles, and minor stains from the teeth, gums, and oral cavity. See *Chapter 8 – Teeth and Oral Care Products*. See also *Fluoride*.

TOOTH POLISH

Tooth polish is similar to toothpaste but it is formulated to have a thinner, more fluid consistency and a shiny appearance. The abrasive is often finely ground, hydrated silica. See *Chapter 8 – Teeth and Oral Care Products*. See also *Fluoride*.

TRETINOIN

A generic drug related to retinoic acid and used for the treatment of acne and other skin conditions. It is also credited with the ability to reduce fine lines and wrinkles, but is banned from cosmetics in both the EU and the USA. Despite its unpleasant side effects, however, some cosmetic surgeons all to easily prescribe tretinoin and encourage its daily use as part of their skin-care regime. Retin-A is a brand name for tretinoin. See *Retinoic Acid*.

TWEEZER EPILATOR

This is a device that is used to permanently remove unwanted body hair by electrolysis. The hair is gripped by metal tweezers and a small electric current is passed through the hair to kill the hair root, before the dead hair is plucked out. See *Electrolysis* in *Chapter 16 – Salons and Surgeons*.

ULTRAVIOLET RAYS

Ultraviolet rays are high-energy electromagnetic rays similar to light rays, but they carry much more energy and are invisible to our eyes. They cause skin to tan, burn, and age prematurely, and they are known to cause some forms of skin cancer. For full details of Ultraviolet-A, B, and C (UV-A, B, and C) see *Chapter 14 – Sun and Skin*. See also *Suntan* and *Sunscreen*.

URTICARIA

Also known as nettle rash or hives, urticaria is a temporary skin condition in which a fluid appears in the dermis, causing raised yellowish patches or wheals surrounded by reddened skin. It usually itches but responds to antihistamine drugs, suggesting it is a form of allergic reaction. It can be caused by any number of things including foods, drugs, some plants and plant extracts, and contact with some chemicals, including cosmetic ingredients. When it is caused by skin contact it is called contact urticaria. It usually appears quite suddenly and disappears just as quickly after a few hours. See *Chapter 15 – Medical Matters*.

UV

An abbreviation for ultraviolet. See *Ultraviolet Rays*.

UV ABSORBER

UV absorbers are chemicals that absorb and dissipate the energy of ultraviolet radiation, preventing it from causing damage to the skin. They are common ingredients in sunscreens and can also be found in some daily skincare lotions. They may also be used to prevent ultraviolet radiation from fading the color of products, such as shampoo and foaming bath oil that are packaged in clear containers. In the EU, only permitted and provisionally permitted UV absorbers may be used in sunscreens. If the absorbers are used to protect a cosmetic or toiletry from the detrimental effects of ultraviolet rays, manufacturers are free to use a wider range of UV absorbers, including ingredients that are not on the permitted or provisionally permitted lists. See *Sunscreen*.

VISCOSITY ADJUSTER

Viscosity adjusters are added to cosmetics and toiletries to make them thinner or thicker. Shampoo contains mostly water so thickeners are added to improve its pouring properties. Nobody wants a shampoo or shower gel that gushes out of the bottle and then flows away through their fingers before they can use it. Similarly, no one wants a lipstick or eyeliner that is so hard that it cannot be easily spread. These products often contain light oils or fatty alcohols that soften the wax.

VITAMINS

Vitamins are important nutrients in our diet and are essential to maintain our health. They are also commonly used as cosmetic ingredients. Vitamins A, C, and E are the most commonly used vitamins, with vitamin B added occasionally in the form of cereals such as oat bran or hydrolyzed wheat proteins. Vitamin D_2 (ergocalciferol), and vitamin D_3 (cholecalciferol), are banned from cosmetics in the EU.

Vitamins A, C, and E have antioxidant properties. Vitamin C reacts with oxygen and is often used as an antioxidant in food products. In a similar way it can prevent the oxidation of cosmetics. Vitamins A and E are oil-soluble vitamins that can react with free radicals and destroy them. Apart from the banned D vitamins, little, if any of these vitamins are absorbed through the skin. See *Chapter 2 – Marketing: Myths and Magic*.

WAXING

Waxing is a method of hair removal that is suitable for large areas of skin such as the legs, bikini line, and forearms. Melted wax or cold wax tapes are placed over the skin and the hairs become embedded in the wax as it hardens. When the hardened wax is removed the hairs are pulled out. The hair roots are not usually killed and the hairs reappear in one to two weeks. Some people who regularly wax their legs claim that, eventually, the hairs no longer regrow. See *Hair Removal* in *Chapter 5 – Skin Care* for further details.

WRINKLES

Wrinkles are a sign of aging skin that has lost its elasticity. See *Chapter 5 – Skin Care* for details of aging skin, and *Chapter 16 – Salons and Surgeons* for wrinkle-reduction treatments.

index of cosmetic ingredients

HOW TO USE THIS INDEX

The ingredients that follow are listed alphabetically by their INCI (International Nomenclature of Cosmetic Ingredients) names, or other commonly used names. If you cannot find an ingredient, try looking in the list of alternative names that follows this section. If you still cannot find it, it is probably not listed in this book because it has no restrictions or harmful, adverse effects. With over 6000 cosmetic ingredients available to the manufacturers it is beyond the scope and scale of this book to list them all. For this reason, we have only included the most commonly used substances and those with restrictions or known harmful effects. Even so, over 2000 substances are covered in this index.

INCI Name

Treat this index like a phone book rather than a dictionary. INCI names often have two or more words. Look up whole words first. For example, "Ethyl urocanate" will come before "Ethylparaben" in the same way that "Williams Tom" will come before "Williamson Adam" in the phone book. Part of the reason for this is that the "space" character in "Ethyl urocanate" comes before the "p" in "Ethylparaben" in the computer's alpha-number-bet. The same is true of numbers and punctuation. These come before letters in the alpha-number-bet so "2,5-Diaminoanisole" comes before "2-Bromo-2-nitropropane-1,3-diol", and "o-Phenylphenol" comes before "Oak moss" because the "-" in "o-Phenylphenol" comes before the "a" in "Oak moss". Put simply, you must persevere; if you can't find an ingredient, look further up and down the list. Where there is a large family of related ingredients, for example the PEG family, these are covered under one entry.

Function

The most common functions of the ingredient are listed, but the manufacturer may use it for another purpose. For example, a substance normally used as a preservative in shampoo may be added to a deodorant to control bacteria on your body.

Origin

Many ingredients can be obtained from a number of raw materials and the most common sources are indicated. The term "Synthetic" means that the ingredient has been made by chemists and it has no natural origin. Sometimes a natural substance, which can be extracted from plants or animals, can also be made synthetically – for example vitamin E and some of the pro-vitamins. In a similar way, fatty acids and fatty alcohols can be obtained from animal and vegetable fats and oils, but they can also be made artificially by the catalytic cracking of petroleum (crude oil products). The term "Semisynthetic" indicates that a natural extract has been substantially chemically modified. For example, Laneth ingredients are made from Lanolin, a natural extract from the wool of sheep, which is then combined with varying amounts of ethylene oxide, a man-made chemical. Simply, you will not find a single molecule of a semisynthetic compound in any natural source.

Restrictions and Adverse Effects

Restrictions mainly refer to those imposed by the EU Commission. This is because there are fewer restrictions in the USA, but where FDA regulations apply these are mentioned. You should assume that restrictions have been applied because the ingredient would present a health risk to the consumer if it was added to cosmetics in amounts which are greater than specified, or used in products from which the ingredients are specifically prohibited. Presumably, if an ingredient is a potential danger to Europeans and subject to EU restrictions, it is probably harmful to Americans, and everyone else as well. If the ingredient has known or suspected adverse effects that have been reported in medical or scientific journals, or in texts or periodicals relevant to the cosmetics or chemical industries, these effects are listed. However, in many cases, only a very small number of individuals are likely to experience these adverse effects. Remember – the track record shows that the vast majority of cosmetics are perfectly safe if used properly. The term "No known adverse effects" means that the authors have not found any evidence that the ingredient can cause harm if the product is used correctly.

Usage

The term "EU/USA" indicates that the ingredients are used freely on both sides of the Atlantic. Where there are differences between EU and FDA regulations, these are indicated. The expression, "Not currently on the EU inventory of cosmetic ingredients" means exactly that. The EU inventory is not a list of approved ingredients. If a substance is not included in the inventory it does not mean that it is a restricted, harmful or banned substance. It simply means it has not yet been added to the list, which is constantly being updated, adding new ingredients (other than banned ones) as they come onto the market.

1,2-Dibromo-2,4-dicyanobutane

Function: Additive.

Origin: Synthetic compound.

Restrictions and Adverse Effects: Can cause contact eczema.

Usage: USA/Not currently on the EU inventory of cosmetic ingredients.

1,2-Phenylenediamine

(o-Phenylenediamine)

Function: Hair dye.

Origin: Synthetic compound.

Restrictions and Adverse Effects: Cancer suspect. Hair dyes sold in the EU that contain related phenylenediamines are subject to strict regulations; for example, see m-Phenylenediamine.

Usage: USA/Not currently on the EU inventory of cosmetic ingredients.

1-Naphthol

(Naphthol)

Function: Hair dye.

Origin: Synthetic compound.

Restrictions and Adverse Effects: Severe skin and eye irritant. Maximum amount allowed in the finished product is 0.5 percent. The name of this chemical must be clearly stated on the label separately from the list of ingredients.

Usage: EU/USA

2,4-Diaminoanisole

(4-MMPD)

Function: Hair dye.

Origin: Synthetic compound.

Restrictions and Adverse Effects: Mutagen. Cancer suspect. FDA rules require the following warning to appear on the label: "Warning – Contains an ingredient that can penetrate your skin and has been determined to cause cancer in laboratory animals."

Usage: USA/Not currently on the EU inventory of cosmetic ingredients.

2,4-Diaminoanisole sulfate

(4-MMPD sulfate)

Function: Hair dye.

Origin: Synthetic compound.

Restrictions and Adverse Effects: Mutagen. Cancer suspect. FDA rules require the following warning to appear on the label: "Warning – Contains an ingredient that can penetrate your skin and has been determined to cause cancer in laboratory animals."

Usage: USA/Not currently on the EU inventory of cosmetic ingredients.

2,4-Diaminophenol

Function: Hair dye.

Origin: Synthetic compound.

Restrictions and Adverse Effects: Irritant for some individuals. It is limited to 10 percent of the finished product. The label must clearly show the name of this chemical separately from the list of ingredients and it must carry the following warnings: "Can cause an allergic reaction. Do not use to dye eyelashes or eyebrows." Products supplied for professional use must carry the additional warning, "Wear suitable gloves."

Usage: EU/USA

2,4-Diaminophenol HCl

Function: Hair dye.

Origin: Synthetic compound.

Restrictions and Adverse Effects: Irritant for some individuals. It is limited to 10 percent of the finished product. The label must clearly show the name of this chemical separately from the list of ingredients and it must carry the following warnings: "Can cause an allergic reaction. Do not use to dye eyelashes or eyebrows." Products supplied for professional use must carry the additional warning, "Wear suitable gloves."

Usage: EU/USA

2,4-Toluenediamine

(m-TD, m-Toluenediamine, Toluene-2,4-diamine)

Function: Additive.

Origin: Synthetic compound.

Restrictions and Adverse Effects: Cancer suspect. Shown to be a mutagen on both the X-chromosome and RNA genes of human males. (RNA is a nucleic acid that works with DNA.) FDA rules require the following warning to be used: "Warning – Contains an ingredient that can penetrate your skin and has been determined to cause cancer in laboratory animals."

Usage: USA/Not currently on the EU inventory of cosmetic ingredients.

2,5-Diaminoanisole

Function: Hair dye.

Origin: Synthetic compound.

Restrictions and Adverse Effects: Cancer suspect.

Usage: USA/Not currently on the EU inventory of cosmetic ingredients.

2-Bromo-2-nitropropane-1,3-diol

(Bronopol)

Function: Preservative.

Origin: Synthetic compound.

Restrictions and Adverse Effects: Toxic. Irritant for some individuals. Can cause contact allergies and contact dermatitis. It is limited to 0.1 percent of the finished product if used as a preservative, but it may be added in larger quantities for other stated purposes. This compound is capable of interacting with amine-ingredients, forming carcinogens. See *A–Z of Cosmetic Terms – Nitrosamines*.

Usage: EU/USA

2-Chloro-p-phenylenediamine

Function: Hair dye.

Origin: Synthetic compound.

Restrictions and Adverse Effects: Cancer suspect.

Usage: EU/USA

2-Chloro-p-phenylenediamine sulfate

Function: Hair dye.

Origin: Synthetic compound.

Restrictions and Adverse Effects: Cancer suspect.

Usage: EU/USA

2-Ethylhexyl salicylate

Function: Additive.

Origin: Synthetic compound.

Restrictions and Adverse Effects: No currently known adverse effects.

Usage: USA/Not currently on the EU inventory of cosmetic ingredients.

2-Hydroxy-4-methoxybenzophenone-5-sulfonic acid

Function: UV absorber.

Origin: Synthetic compound.

Restrictions and Adverse Effects: This chemical causes little or no irritation to skin or mucous membranes in low concentrations, but it is restricted to a maximum amount of 5 percent of the finished product.

Usage: EU/USA

2-Methoxyaniline

Function: Hair dye.

Origin: Synthetic compound.

Restrictions and Adverse Effects: Cancer suspect.

Usage: USA/Not currently on the EU inventory of cosmetic ingredients.

2-Methyl-4-isothiazolin-3-one

Function: Preservative.

Origin: Synthetic compound.

Restrictions and Adverse Effects: Can cause contact dermatitis.

Usage: USA/Not currently on the EU inventory of cosmetic ingredients.

2-Nitro-p-phenylenediamine

Function: Hair dye.

Origin: Synthetic compound.

Restrictions and Adverse Effects: Cancer and mutagen suspect.

Usage: EU/USA

2-Nitropropane

Function: Additive / Solvent.
Origin: Synthetic compound.
Restrictions and Adverse Effects: Cancer suspect.
Usage: USA/Not currently on the EU inventory of cosmetic ingredients.

3-Benzylidene camphor

Function: UV absorber.
Origin: Synthetic compound.
Restrictions and Adverse Effects: The safety of this substance was uncertain and its use in cosmetics was only provisionally permitted in the EU, until June 30, 1998. On September 3, 1998, following further scientific tests, the provisional status was removed and this ingredient was permitted for use in cosmetics. It is limited to a maximum of 2 percent of the finished product. It may be used to protect the ingredients of other cosmetics and toiletries from the detrimental effects of sunlight.
Usage: EU/USA

3-Carbethoxypsoralen

Function: Tanning agent.
Origin: Synthetic compound.
Restrictions and Adverse Effects: Phototoxin.
Usage: USA/Not currently on the EU inventory of cosmetic ingredients.

3-Methylisothiazolin

Function: Preservative.
Origin: Synthetic compound.
Restrictions and Adverse Effects: Can cause contact allergies.
Usage: USA/Not currently on the EU inventory of cosmetic ingredients.

4,5,8-Trimethylpsoralen

Function: Tanning agent.
Origin: Synthetic compound.
Restrictions and Adverse Effects: Phototoxin.
Usage: USA/Not currently on the EU inventory of cosmetic ingredients.

4-Chloro-1,2-phenylenediamine

Function: Hair dye.
Origin: Synthetic compound.
Restrictions and Adverse Effects: Cancer suspect.
Usage: USA/Not currently on the EU inventory of cosmetic ingredients.

4-Hydroxybenzoic Acid

Function: Preservative.
Origin: Synthetic compound.
Restrictions and Adverse Effects: Benzoic acid, benzoates and parabens have been implicated in a large number of health issues. (See *A–Z of Cosmetic Terms – Benzoates*.) It is limited to 0.4 percent of the finished product if used on its own as a preservative, or 0.8 percent in total if used in combination with other parabens. Parabens may be added in larger quantities if used for other stated purposes.
Usage: EU/USA

4-Isopropyldibenzoylmethane

Function: Additive.
Origin: Synthetic compound.
Restrictions and Adverse Effects: Can cause contact dermatitis.
Usage: USA/Not currently on the EU inventory of cosmetic ingredients.

4-Methoxyaniline

Function: Hair dye.
Origin: Synthetic compound.
Restrictions and Adverse Effects: Cancer suspect.
Usage: USA/Not currently on the EU inventory of cosmetic ingredients.

4-Methylbenzylidene camphor

Function: UV absorber.
Origin: Synthetic compound.
Restrictions and Adverse Effects: The safety of this substance was uncertain and its use in cosmetics was only provisionally permitted in the EU, until June 30, 1998. On September 3, 1998, following further scientific tests, the provisional status was removed and this ingredient was permitted for use in cosmetics. It is limited to a maximum of 2 percent of

the finished product. It may be used to protect the ingredients of other cosmetics and toiletries from the detrimental effects of sunlight.

Usage: EU/USA

4-Nitro-o-phenylenediamine

(4-NOPD)

Function: Hair dye.

Origin: Synthetic compound.

Restrictions and Adverse Effects: Found to be a mutagen.

Usage: EU/USA

4-Nitro-o-phenylenediamine HCl

(4-NOPD Hydrochloride)

Function: Hair dye.

Origin: Synthetic compound.

Restrictions and Adverse Effects: Found to be a mutagen.

Usage: EU/USA

5,7-Dihydroxy-4-methylcoumarin

Function: Additive.

Origin: Semisynthetic or synthetic compound.

Restrictions and Adverse Effects: Skin sensitizer.

Usage: USA/Not currently on the EU inventory of cosmetic ingredients.

5,7-Dihydroxycoumarin

Function: Additive.

Origin: Synthetic compound.

Restrictions and Adverse Effects: Skin sensitizer.

Usage: USA/Not currently on the EU inventory of cosmetic ingredients.

5-Bromo-5-nitro-1,3-dioxane

Function: Preservative.

Origin: Synthetic compound.

Restrictions and Adverse Effects: Toxic. Irritant for some individuals. It is limited to 0.1 percent of the finished, rinse-off products only, and must not be used in cosmetics that stay in contact with the skin. Capable of interacting with amine-ingredients, forming carcinogens. (See *A–Z of Cosmetic Terms – Nitrosamines.*)

Usage: EU/USA

5-Chloro-3-methyl-4-isothiazolin-3-one

(Chloromethylisotiazolinone. See – *Methylchloroisotiazolinone.*)

5-Methoxypsoralen

Function: Tanning agent.

Origin: Synthetic compound.

Restrictions and Adverse Effects: Phototoxin. Photocarcinogen (can cause cancer under the influence of sunlight).

Usage: USA/Banned from cosmetics in the EU except for normal content in natural essences.

6-Methylcoumarin

Function: Oral care agent / Fragrance.

Origin: Restrictions and Adverse Effects: Harmful. Skin sensitizer. Causes photosensitivity and photoallergies. In 1978 the FDA asked manufacturers of sunscreen products not to use 6-methylcoumarin. Maximum allowed content in products sold in the EU is 0.003 percent of the finished product.

Usage: EU/USA

6-Methylquinophthalone

Function: Hair dye.

Origin: Synthetic compound.

Restrictions and Adverse Effects: Can cause dermatitis.

Usage: USA/Not currently on the EU inventory of cosmetic ingredients.

7-Ethylbicyclooxazolidine

Function: Preservative.

Origin: Synthetic compound.

Restrictions and Adverse Effects: Harmful. It is limited to 0.3 percent of the finished product and is prohibited from oral hygiene products and any preparation that may come into contact with the mucous membranes (mouth, nose, genitals, and eyelids).

Usage: EU/USA

7-Methylpyrido[3,4, c]psoralen

Function: Tanning agent.

Origin: Semisynthetic or synthetic compound.

Restrictions and Adverse Effects: Phototoxin.

Usage: USA/Not currently on the EU inventory of cosmetic ingredients.

8-Methoxypsoralen

(Methoxsalen)

Function: Tanning agent.

Origin: Synthetic compound.

Restrictions and Adverse Effects: Phototoxin.

Usage: USA/Banned from cosmetics in the EU except for normal content in natural essences.

Acetone

(Propanone)

Function: Denaturant / Solvent.

Origin: Synthetic compound prepared from petroleum.

Restrictions and Adverse Effects: No currently known adverse effects, but is highly flammable.

Usage: EU/USA

Acetonitrile

Function: Solvent, especially for artificial nails.

Origin: Synthetic compound.

Restrictions and Adverse Effects: Fatal if swallowed (causes cyanide poisoning).

Usage: USA/Banned from cosmetics in the EU.

Acetylated lanolin alcohol

Function: Antistatic agent / Emollient / Moisturizer / Emulsifier.

Claimed to be a hypoallergenic lanolin-derived emollient with a smooth, velvety feel. Acetylated lanolin forms a protective coating on the skin's surface and prevents moisture loss.

Origin: Lanolin (extract of sheep's wool) derivative.

Restrictions and Adverse Effects: No currently known adverse effects.

Usage: EU/USA

Acetylmethionyl methylsilanol elastinate

Function: Antistatic agent.

Origin: A semisynthetic compound derived from elastin, a flexible protein extracted from the layers of skin and artery walls of mammals.

Restrictions and Adverse Effects: No currently known adverse effects. For BSE precautions see *Chapter 17 – Animal Products and Animal Testing.*

Usage: EU/USA

Acid Black 52

(CI 15711)

Function: Hair dye.

Origin: Synthetic azo dye.

Restrictions and Adverse Effects: See *A–Z of Cosmetic Terms – Azo Dyes.*

Usage: EU/USA

Acid Blue 1

(CI 42045)

Function: Hair dye.

Origin: Synthetic coal tar dye.

Restrictions and Adverse Effects: Harmful or irritant if in contact with the mucous membranes of the eyelids, mouth, nose, respiratory tract, or genitals. This dye is not allowed in any product intended for use on or near these areas.

Usage: EU/USA

Acid Blue 3

(CI 42051)

Function: Hair dye.

Origin: Synthetic coal tar dye.

Restrictions and Adverse Effects: Allowed in all products.

Usage: EU/USA

Acid Blue 9

(CI 42090)

Function: Hair dye.

Origin: Synthetic coal tar dye.

Restrictions and Adverse Effects: Allowed in all products.

Usage: EU/USA

Acid Blue 62
(CI 62045)
Function: Hair dye.
Origin: Synthetic coal tar dye.
Restrictions and Adverse Effects: Harmful or irritant by prolonged contact with the skin. Allowed only in products that are rinsed off immediately after use.
Usage: EU/USA

Acid Blue 74
(CI 73015)
Function: Hair dye.
Origin: Synthetic coal tar dye.
Restrictions and Adverse Effects: Allowed in all products.
Usage: EU/USA

Acid Green 1
(CI 10020)
Function: Hair dye.
Origin: Synthetic coal tar dye.
Restrictions and Adverse Effects: Harmful or irritant if in contact with the mucous membranes of the eyelids, mouth, nose, respiratory tract, or genitals. This dye is not allowed in any product intended for use on or near these areas.
Usage: EU/USA

Acid Green 25 (D&C Green #5)
(CI 61570)
Function: Hair dye.
Origin: Synthetic coal tar dye.
Restrictions and Adverse Effects: Allowed in all products.
Usage: EU/USA

Acid Green 50
(CI 44090)
Function: Hair dye.
Origin: Synthetic coal tar dye.
Restrictions and Adverse Effects: Allowed in all products.
Usage: EU/USA

Acid Orange 6
(CI 14270)
Function: Hair dye.
Origin: Synthetic azo dye.
Restrictions and Adverse Effects: Allowed in all products. See *A–Z of Cosmetic Terms – Azo Dyes*.
Usage: EU/USA

Acid Orange 7
(CI 15510)
Function: Hair dye.
Origin: Synthetic azo dye.
Restrictions and Adverse Effects: Harmful or irritant to eyes. This dye is not allowed in any product intended for use on or near the eyes. See *A–Z of Cosmetic Terms – Azo Dyes*.
Usage: EU/USA

Acid Orange 24
(CI 20170)
Function: Hair dye.
Origin: Synthetic azo dye.
Restrictions and Adverse Effects: Harmful or irritant if in contact with the mucous membranes of the eyelids, mouth, nose, respiratory tract, or genitals. This dye is not allowed in any product intended for use on or near these areas. See *A–Z of Cosmetic Terms – Azo Dyes*.
Usage: EU/USA

Acid Red 14
(CI 14720)
Function: Hair dye.
Origin: Synthetic azo dye.
Restrictions and Adverse Effects: Allowed in all products. See *A–Z of Cosmetic Terms – Azo Dyes*.
Usage: EU/USA

Acid Red 18
(CI 16255)
Function: Hair dye.
Origin: Synthetic azo dye.
Restrictions and Adverse Effects: Allowed in all products. See *A–Z of Cosmetic Terms – Azo Dyes*.
Usage: EU/USA

Acid Red 27

(CI 16185)

Function: Hair dye.

Origin: Synthetic azo dye.

Restrictions and Adverse Effects: Allowed in all products. See *A–Z of Cosmetic Terms – Azo Dyes*.

Usage: EU/USA

Acid Red 33 (D&C Red #33)

(CI 17200)

Function: Hair dye / Red colorant.

Origin: Synthetic azo dye.

Restrictions and Adverse Effects: Allowed in all products sold in the EU. FDA regulations allow it in all externally applied cosmetics but limit it to 3 percent of the finished product in oral care preparations and lip cosmetics. See *A–Z of Cosmetic Terms – Azo Dyes*.

Usage: EU/USA

Acid Red 35

(CI 18065)

Function: Hair dye.

Origin: Synthetic azo dye.

Restrictions and Adverse Effects: See *A–Z of Cosmetic Terms – Azo Dyes*.

Usage: EU/USA

Acid Red 51

(CI 45430, Erythrosine)

Function: Hair dye.

Origin: Synthetic coal tar dye.

Restrictions and Adverse Effects: Allowed in all products. This colorant is known to contain two harmful impurities which must be reduced to EU-specified levels before use.

Usage: EU/USA

Acid Red 52

(CI 45100)

Function: Hair dye.

Origin: Synthetic coal tar dye.

Restrictions and Adverse Effects: Harmful or irritant by prolonged contact with the skin. This dye is only allowed in products that are rinsed off immediately after use.

Usage: EU/USA

Acid Red 73

(CI 27290)

Function: Hair dye.

Origin: Synthetic azo dye.

Restrictions and Adverse Effects: Harmful or irritant by prolonged contact with the skin. This dye is only allowed in products that are rinsed off immediately after use. See *A–Z of Cosmetic Terms – Azo Dyes*.

Usage: EU/USA

Acid Red 87

(CI 45380, Eosin)

Function: Hair dye.

Origin: Synthetic dye.

Restrictions and Adverse Effects: Allowed in all products. This colorant is known to contain two harmful impurities which must be reduced to EU-specified levels before use. May cause photosensitivity.

Usage: EU/USA

Acid Red 92 (D&C Red #28)

(CI 45410)

Function: Hair dye.

Origin: Synthetic dye.

Restrictions and Adverse Effects: Allowed in all products. This colorant is known to contain two harmful impurities which must be reduced to EU-specified levels before use. FDA regulations allow this dye in any externally applied cosmetic except eye products.

Usage: EU/USA

Acid Red 95

(CI 45380)

Function: Hair dye.

Origin: Synthetic coal tar dye.

Restrictions and Adverse Effects: Allowed in all products. This colorant is known to contain two harmful impurities which must be reduced to EU-specified levels before use.

Usage: EU/USA

Acid Red 195

Function: Red colorant.

Origin: Synthetic azo dye.

Restrictions and Adverse Effects: Harmful or irritant if in contact with the mucous membranes of the eyelids, mouth, nose, respiratory tract, or genitals. This dye is not allowed in any product intended for use on or near these areas. See *A–Z of Cosmetic Terms – Azo Dyes.*

Usage: EU/USA

Acid Violet 43 (Ext. D&C Violet #2)

(CI 60730)

Function: Hair dye.

Origin: Synthetic coal tar dye.

Restrictions and Adverse Effects: Harmful or irritant if in contact with the mucous membranes of the eyelids, mouth, nose, respiratory tract, or genitals. EU regulations prohibit it from any product intended for use on or near these areas. FDA regulations allow its use in any externally applied cosmetic except eye products.

Usage: EU/USA

Acid Yellow 1 (Ext D&C Yellow #7)

(CI 10316)

Function: Hair dye.

Origin: Synthetic coal tar dye.

Restrictions and Adverse Effects: Harmful or irritant to eyes. EU regulations prohibit this dye in any product intended for use on or near the eyes. FDA regulations allow this dye in any externally applied cosmetic except eye products.

Usage: EU/USA

Acid Yellow 23

(CI 19140)

Function: Hair dye.

Origin: Synthetic azo dye.

Restrictions and Adverse Effects: Allowed in all products. See *A–Z of Cosmetic Terms – Azo Dyes.*

Usage: EU/USA

Acid Yellow 73 – Sodium salt (D&C Yellow #8)

(CI 45350, Fluorescein sodium)

Function: Hair dye.

Origin: Synthetic coal tar dye.

Restrictions and Adverse Effects: Allowed in all products. This dye is limited to 6 percent of the finished product. FDA regulations allow this dye in any externally applied cosmetic except eye products.

Usage: EU/USA

Acrylates / C10-30 alkyl acrylate crosspolymer

Function: Film former.

Origin: Synthetic compound derived from petroleum.

Restrictions and Adverse Effects: No currently known adverse effects.

Usage: EU/USA

Acrylates copolymer

Function: Antistatic agent / Binding agent / Film former.

Origin: Synthetic compound derived from petroleum.

Restrictions and Adverse Effects: No currently known adverse effects.

Usage: EU/USA

Acrylates dimethicone crosspolymer

Function: Film former.

Origin: Synthetic silicone polymer.

Restrictions and Adverse Effects: No currently known adverse effects.

Usage: USA/Not currently on the EU inventory of cosmetic ingredients under this name.

Adeps bovis

Function: Emollient / Moisturizer.

Origin: Animal fat.

Restrictions and Adverse Effects: No currently known adverse effects. For BSE precautions see *Chapter 17 – Animal Products and Animal Testing*.

Usage: EU/USA

Alcohol
(Ethanol)

Function: Solvent / Carrier for fragrance chemicals.

Origin: Prepared by the fermentation of carbohydrates or synthetically from petroleum.

Restrictions and Adverse Effects: Can cause systemic, eczematous contact dermatitis.

Usage: EU/USA

Alcohol denat.
(Denatured alcohol, Ethanol, Alcohol)

Function: Solvent / Carrier for fragrance chemicals.

Origin: Prepared by the fermentation of carbohydrates or synthetically from petroleum. It contains additives, such as benzyl alcohol, to impart an unpleasant taste, making it undrinkable.

Restrictions and Adverse Effects: Can cause systemic, eczematous contact dermatitis.

Usage: EU/USA

Almondamide DEA

Function: Surfactant.

Origin: Semisynthetic compound derived from almond oil.

Restrictions and Adverse Effects: DEA residues are cancer suspects currently under investigation. See *A–Z of Cosmetic Terms – DEA*.

Usage: EU/USA

Aloe barbadensis
(Aloe extract, Aloe juice, Aloe vera oil, Aloe vera gel)

Function: Emollient / Demulcent.

Said to have hydrating and soothing properties, therefore is used in after-sun lotions, for example. It is a natural plant extract widely used in cosmetics to produce a soothing effect, but the therapeutic dose required for this far exceeds the amount normally found in these products.

Origin: An oil-soluble extract of the aloe vera plant (usually the leaves) or any other member of the aloe family (a member of the lily family).

Restrictions and Adverse Effects: Irritant for some individuals.

Usage: EU/USA

Alpha hydroxy and botanical complexes

Function: Exfoliating agents.

Origin: A mixture of natural fruit extracts and synthetic compounds.

Restrictions and Adverse Effects: Alpha-hydroxy acids (AHAs) are used to exfoliate skin. They are also known as skin peelers because they dissolve and remove the outer layer of skin. They can cause increased sensitivity to the sun due to loss of the protective outer layer of skin cells. Do not expose skin to the sun immediately following treatment with AHAs. Test a small area before use and discontinue use if skin irritation, redness, bleeding, or pain is experienced. Not recommended for use on children. May cause exfoliative dermatitis.

Usage: USA/Not currently on the EU inventory of cosmetic ingredients.

Alpha-hydroxy ethanoic acid

Function: Exfoliating agent.

Origin: Synthetic compound.

Restrictions and Adverse Effects: Alpha-hydroxy acids (AHAs) are used to exfoliate skin. They are also known as skin peelers because they dissolve and remove the outer layer of skin. They can cause increased sensitivity to the sun due to loss of the protective outer layer of skin cells. Do not expose skin to the sun immediately following treatment with AHAs. Test a small area before use and discontinue use if skin irritation, redness, bleeding, or pain is experienced. Not recommended for use on children. May cause exfoliative dermatitis.

Usage: USA/Not currently on the EU inventory of cosmetic ingredients.

Alpha-hydroxy octanoic acid

(Hydroxyoctanoic Acid, Alpha-Hydroxycaprylic Acid, Hydroxycaprylic Acid)

Function: Exfoliating agent.

Origin: Semisynthetic or synthetic compound.

Restrictions and Adverse Effects: Alpha-hydroxy acids (AHAs) are used to exfoliate skin. They are also known as skin peelers because they dissolve and remove the outer layer of skin. They can cause increased sensitivity to the sun due to loss of the protective outer layer of skin cells. Do not expose skin to the sun immediately following treatment with AHAs. Test a small area before use and discontinue use if skin irritation, redness, bleeding, or pain is experienced. Not recommended for use on children. May cause exfoliative dermatitis.

Usage: USA/Not currently on the EU inventory of cosmetic ingredients.

Alpha-pinene

Function: Additive / Fragrance.

Origin: A natural terpene related to camphor, extracted from coniferous trees.

Restrictions and Adverse Effects: Can cause contact dermatitis.

Usage: USA/Not currently on the EU inventory of cosmetic ingredients.

Aluminum chlorohydrate

Function: Antiperspirant / Deodorant.

This is the most commonly used material for antiperspirant preparations. It is considered to be the least irritating of the aluminum salts.

Origin: Synthetic compound.

Restrictions and Adverse Effects: Irritant for some individuals. Avoid inhaling the spray if it is present in an aerosol product.

Usage: EU/USA

Aluminum dimyristate

Function: Emulsion stabilizer / Opacifier / Viscosity adjuster.

Origin: Synthetic compound.

Restrictions and Adverse Effects: Some myristates are comedogenic (see *A–Z of Cosmetic Terms – Comedogen*).

Usage: EU/USA

Aluminum fluoride

Function: Oral care agent.

Origin: Synthetic compound.

Restrictions and Adverse Effects: Fluorides are toxic. They can discolor teeth (fluorosis). Children should only use a small quantity of toothpaste and be discouraged from swallowing it. The total amount of fluoride allowed by EU regulations is 0.15 percent of the finished product.

Usage: EU/USA

Aluminum isostearates / laurates / palmitates

Function: Emulsion stabilizer / Opacifier / Viscosity adjuster.

Origin: Synthetic compound.

Restrictions and Adverse Effects: Some palmitates have been linked to contact dermatitis.

Usage: EU/USA

Aluminum isostearates / myristates

Function: Emulsion stabilizer / Opacifier / Viscosity adjuster.

Origin: Synthetic compound.

Restrictions and Adverse Effects: Some myristates are comedogenic (see *A–Z of Cosmetic Terms – Comedogen*).

Usage: EU/USA

Aluminum isostearates / palmitates

Function: Emulsion stabilizer / Opacifier / Viscosity adjuster.

Origin: Synthetic compound.

Restrictions and Adverse Effects: Some palmitates have been linked to contact dermatitis.

Usage: EU/USA

Aluminum myristates / palmitates

Function: Emulsion stabilizer / Opacifier / Viscosity adjuster.
Origin: Synthetic compound.
Restrictions and Adverse Effects: Some myristates are comedogenic (see *A–Z of Cosmetic Terms – Comedogen*). Some palmitates have been linked to contact dermatitis.
Usage: EU/USA

Aluminum starch octenylsuccinate

Function: Absorbent / Viscosity adjuster.
Origin: Semisynthetic compound.
Restrictions and Adverse Effects: No currently known adverse effects.
Usage: EU/USA

Aluminum stearate

(Aluminum monostearate)
Function: White colorant.
Origin: Synthetic compound.
Restrictions and Adverse Effects: Allowed in all products.
Usage: EU/USA

Aluminum zirconium octachlorohydrate

Function: Antiperspirant / Deodorant.
Origin: Synthetic compound.
Restrictions and Adverse Effects: Harmful. Can cause lung damage and granulomas. Maximum allowed content is 20 percent, with no more than 5.4 percent zirconium. It is banned from use in aerosol dispensers and sprays in the EU and USA. The label must warn against using this product on damaged or irritated skin.
Usage: EU/USA

Aluminum zirconium octachlorohydrex gly

Function: Antiperspirant / Deodorant.
Origin: Synthetic compound.
Restrictions and Adverse Effects: Harmful. Can cause lung damage and granulomas. Maximum allowed content is 20 percent, with no more than 5.4 percent zirconium. It is banned from use in aerosol dispensers and sprays in the EU and USA. The label must warn against using this product on damaged or irritated skin.
Usage: EU/USA

Aluminum zirconium pentachlorohydrate

Function: Antiperspirant / Deodorant.
Origin: Synthetic compound.
Restrictions and Adverse Effects: Harmful. Can cause lung damage and granulomas. Maximum allowed content is 20 percent, with no more than 5.4 percent zirconium. It is banned from use in aerosol dispensers and sprays in the EU and USA. The label must warn against using this product on damaged or irritated skin.
Usage: EU/USA

Aluminum zirconium pentachlorohydrex gly

Function: Antiperspirant / Deodorant.
Origin: Synthetic compound.
Restrictions and Adverse Effects: Harmful. Can cause lung damage and granulomas. Maximum allowed content is 20 percent, with no more than 5.4 percent zirconium. It is banned from use in aerosol dispensers and sprays in the EU and USA. The label must warn against using this product on damaged or irritated skin.
Usage: EU/USA

Aluminum zirconium tetrachlorohydrate

Function: Antiperspirant / Deodorant.
Origin: Synthetic compound.
Restrictions and Adverse Effects: Harmful. Can cause lung damage and granulomas. Maximum allowed content is 20 percent, with no more than 5.4 percent zirconium. It is banned from use in aerosol dispensers and sprays in the EU and USA. The label must warn against using this product on damaged or irritated skin.
Usage: EU/USA

Aluminum zirconium tetrachlorohydrex gly

Function: Antiperspirant / Deodorant.

Origin: Synthetic compound.

Restrictions and Adverse Effects: Harmful. Can cause lung damage and granulomas. Maximum allowed content is 20 percent, with no more than 5.4 percent zirconium. It is banned from use in aerosol dispensers and sprays in the EU and USA. The label must warn against using this product on damaged or irritated skin.

Usage: EU/USA

Aluminum zirconium trichlorohydrate

Function: Antiperspirant / Deodorant.

Origin: Synthetic compound.

Restrictions and Adverse Effects: Harmful. Can cause lung damage and granulomas. Maximum allowed content is 20 percent, with no more than 5.4 percent zirconium. It is banned from use in aerosol dispensers and sprays in the EU and USA. The label must warn against using this product on damaged or irritated skin.

Usage: EU/USA

Aluminum zirconium trichlorohydrex gly

Function: Antiperspirant / Deodorant.

Origin: Synthetic compound.

Restrictions and Adverse Effects: Harmful. Can cause lung damage and granulomas. Maximum allowed content is 20 percent with no more than 5.4 percent zirconium. It is banned from use in aerosol dispensers and sprays in the EU and USA. The label must warn against using this product on damaged or irritated skin.

Usage: EU/USA

Ammonia

Function: pH control.

Origin: Synthetic compound.

Restrictions and Adverse Effects: Harmful vapor. Irritant. Maximum allowed content is 6 percent of the finished product and the label must carry a warning if it is above 2 percent.

Usage: EU/USA

Ammonium benzoate

Function: Preservative.

Origin: Synthetic compound of the benzoate family.

Restrictions and Adverse Effects: Benzoic acid and benzoates have been implicated in a large number of health issues. (See *A–Z of Cosmetic Terms – Benzoates*.) It is limited to 0.5 percent of the finished product if used as a preservative. It may be added in larger quantities for other stated purposes.

Usage: EU/USA

Ammonium bisulfite

Function: Preservative.

Origin: Synthetic compound.

Restrictions and Adverse Effects: Irritant. It is limited to 0.2 percent of the finished product if used as a preservative but it may be added in larger quantities for other stated purposes.

Usage: EU/USA

Ammonium chloride

Function: pH control / Viscosity adjuster.

Origin: Synthetic compound.

Restrictions and Adverse Effects: Skin and eye irritant for some individuals.

Usage: EU/USA

Ammonium fluoride

Function: Oral care agent.

Origin: Synthetic compound.

Restrictions and Adverse Effects: Fluorides are toxic. They can discolor teeth (fluorosis). Children should only use a small quantity of toothpaste and be discouraged from swallowing it. The total amount of fluoride allowed by EU regulations is 0.15 percent of the finished product.

Usage: EU/USA

Ammonium fluorosilicate

Function: Oral care agent.

Origin: Synthetic compound.

Restrictions and Adverse Effects: Fluorides are toxic. They can discolor teeth (fluorosis). Children should only use a small quantity of toothpaste and be discouraged from swallowing it. The total amount

of fluoride allowed by EU regulations is 0.15 percent of the finished product.
Usage: EU/USA

Ammonium glycolate

Function: Exfoliating agent.
Origin: Synthetic or semisynthetic alpha-hydroxy acid.
Restrictions and Adverse Effects: Ammonium glycolate is an alpha-hydroxy acid (AHA) which is used to exfoliate skin. AHAs are also known as skin peelers because they dissolve and remove the outer layer of skin. They can cause increased sensitivity to the sun due to loss of the protective outer layer of skin cells. Do not expose skin to the sun immediately following treatment with AHAs. Test a small area before use and discontinue use if skin irritation, redness, bleeding, or pain is experienced. Not recommended for use on children. May cause exfoliative dermatitis.
Usage: USA/Not currently on the EU inventory of cosmetic ingredients.

Ammonium laureth sulfate

Function: Surfactant.
Used as a surfactant for many shampoos, often in conjunction with other detergents. It is considered to be less irritating than other synthetic detergents.
Origin: Synthetic detergent.
Restrictions and Adverse Effects: No currently known adverse effects. This ethoxylated ingredient is made using ethylene oxide (oxirane), which can form 1,4-dioxane, a carcinogen, as a by-product of manufacture. See *A–Z of Cosmetic Terms – Dioxane.*
Usage: EU/USA

Ammonium lauryl sulfate

Function: Surfactant.
Used as a primary surfactant for many shampoos. Although it is an irritant itself, it is considered to be less irritating than other synthetic detergents such as sodium lauryl sulfate (SLS).
Origin: Synthetic compound.
Restrictions and Adverse Effects: Skin and eye irritant for some individuals.
Usage: EU/USA

Ammonium monofluorophosphate

Function: Oral care agent.
Origin: Synthetic compound.
Restrictions and Adverse Effects: Fluorides are toxic. They can discolor teeth (fluorosis). Children should only use a small quantity of toothpaste and be discouraged from swallowing it. The total amount of fluoride allowed by EU regulations is 0.15 percent of the finished product.
Usage: EU/USA

Ammonium palmitate

Function: Surfactant.
Origin: Synthetic detergent.
Restrictions and Adverse Effects: No currently known adverse effects.
Usage: USA/Not currently on the EU inventory of cosmetic ingredients.

Ammonium persulfate

(Ammonium peroxodisulfate, Diammonium peroxodisulfate)
Function: Bleaching agent.
Origin: Synthetic compound.
Restrictions and Adverse Effects: Linked to asthma in hairdressers.
Usage: EU/USA

Ammonium propionate

Function: Preservative.
Origin: Synthetic compound made by neutralizing propanoic acid with ammonia.
Restrictions and Adverse Effects: Propanoic acid and its salts are limited to 2 percent of the finished product if used as a preservative, but it may be added in larger quantities for other stated purposes.
Usage: EU/USA

Ammonium stearate

Function: Emulsifier / Surfactant.
Origin: Synthetic soapy detergent derived from animal or vegetable fats and oils.
Restrictions and Adverse Effects: No currently known adverse effects.
Usage: EU/USA

Ammonium sulfite

Function: Preservative.
Origin: Synthetic compound.
Restrictions and Adverse Effects: Irritant. It is limited to 0.2 percent of the finished product if used as a preservative, but it may be added in larger quantities for other stated purposes.
Usage: EU/USA

Ammonium thioglycolate

Function: Depilatory agent / Reducing agent.
Origin: Synthetic hair remover.
Restrictions and Adverse Effects: Harmful. May be alkaline (irritant and corrosive). In the EU its content is limited to 8 percent in hair perming preparations (11 percent for professional use), 5 percent in depilatories and 2 percent in rinse-off hair care products. The pH must be between 7 and 9.5 in hair care products and between 7 and 12.7 in depilatories. The label must clearly state "Contains Thioglycolate," and it must show the following mandatory warnings: "Follow the instructions. Keep out of reach of children. Avoid contact with eyes. In the event of contact with eyes, rinse with plenty of water and seek medical advice." Additionally, hair care products must state "Wear suitable gloves."
Usage: EU/USA

Amodimethicone

Function: Antistatic agent.
Origin: Synthetic silicone.
Restrictions and Adverse Effects: No currently known adverse effects.
Usage: EU/USA

Animal tissue extract

Function: Biological additive.
Origin: Extract of various animal tissues.
Restrictions and Adverse Effects: For BSE precautions see *Chapter 17 – Animal Products and Animal Testing*.
Usage: EU/USA

Anthocyanins

(E163)
Function: Red colorant.
Origin: Natural plant pigments.
Restrictions and Adverse Effects: Allowed in all products.
Usage: EU/USA

Aorta extract

Function: Biological additive.
Origin: Extract of animal tissues.
Restrictions and Adverse Effects: For BSE precautions *see Chapter 17 – Animal Products and Animal Testing*.
Usage: EU/USA

Apricotamide DEA

Function: Surfactant / Foaming agent / Viscosity adjuster.
Origin: Semisynthetic compound derived from apricot oil.
Restrictions and Adverse Effects: DEA residues are cancer suspects currently under investigation. See *A–Z of Cosmetic Terms – DEA*.
Usage: EU/USA

Aqua

(Water)
Function: Solvent.
Origin: Purified (distilled or deionised) water is used as the main ingredient in many cosmetics and toiletries. Occasionally water from other sources is used, e.g., spring water, mineral water, sea water, Dead Sea water.
Restrictions and Adverse Effects: None, but the finished product must meet the required standards for microbial infection.
Usage: EU/USA

Arachidyl behenate

Function: Emollient / Moisturizer.
Origin: Synthetic compound.
Restrictions and Adverse Effects: No currently known adverse effects.
Usage: EU/USA

Aroma

Function: Flavor.
Origin: A mixture of natural and synthetic flavor compounds.
Restrictions and Adverse Effects: May be responsible for allergies.
Usage: The term "aroma" is used in the EU; in America the word used is "flavor."

Ascorbyl dipalmitate

Function: Antioxidant.
Origin: Semisynthetic or synthetic compound derived from ascorbic acid (vitamin C).
Restrictions and Adverse Effects: Some palmitates have been linked to contact dermatitis.
Usage: EU/USA

Ascorbyl palmitate

Function: Antioxidant.
Origin: Semisynthetic or synthetic compound derived from ascorbic acid (vitamin C).
Restrictions and Adverse Effects: Some palmitates have been linked to contact dermatitis.
Usage: EU/USA

Avocadamide DEA

Function: Emulsifier / Emulsion stabilizer / Surfactant / Viscosity adjuster.
Origin: Semisynthetic compound derived from avocado oil.
Restrictions and Adverse Effects: DEA residues are cancer suspects currently under investigation. See *A–Z of Cosmetic Terms – DEA*.
Usage: EU/USA

Babassuamide DEA

Function: Surfactant.
Origin: Semisynthetic or synthetic compound.
Restrictions and Adverse Effects: DEA residues are cancer suspects currently under investigation. See *A–Z of Cosmetic Terms – DEA*.
Usage: EU/USA

Barium sulfide

Function: Depilatory agent.
Origin: Synthetic compound.
Restrictions and Adverse Effects: Sulfides are toxic. Irritant. May be alkaline (irritant and corrosive). The maximum allowed content is 6 percent of the finished product. The label must carry warnings to avoid contact with the eyes and to keep the product out of the reach of children.
Usage: EU/USA

Basic Blue 26

(CI 44045)
Function: Hair dye.
Origin: Synthetic coal tar dye.
Restrictions and Adverse Effects: Harmful or irritant if in contact with the mucous membranes of the eyelids, mouth, nose, respiratory tract, or genitals. It is not allowed in any product intended for use on or near these areas.
Usage: EU/USA

Basic Blue 41

(CI 11154)
Function: Hair dye.
Origin: Synthetic azo dye.
Restrictions and Adverse Effects: See *A–Z of Cosmetic Terms – Azo Dyes*.
Usage: EU/USA

Basic Brown 4

(CI 21010)
Function: Hair dye.
Origin: Synthetic azo dye.
Restrictions and Adverse Effects: See *A–Z of Cosmetic Terms – Azo Dyes*.
Usage: EU/USA

Basic Brown 16

(CI 12250)
Function: Hair dye.
Origin: Synthetic azo dye.
Restrictions and Adverse Effects: See *A–Z of Cosmetic Terms – Azo Dyes*.
Usage: EU/USA

Basic Brown 17

(CI 12251)

Function: Hair dye.

Origin: Synthetic azo dye.

Restrictions and Adverse Effects: See *A–Z of Cosmetic Terms – Azo Dyes.*

Usage: EU/USA

Basic Red 22

Function: Hair dye.

Origin: Synthetic azo dye.

Restrictions and Adverse Effects: See *A–Z of Cosmetic Terms – Azo Dyes.*

Usage: EU/USA

Basic Red 76

(CI 12245)

Function: Hair dye.

Origin: Synthetic azo dye.

Restrictions and Adverse Effects: See *A–Z of Cosmetic Terms – Azo Dyes.*

Usage: EU/USA

Basic Violet 14

(CI 42510)

Function: Hair dye.

Origin: Synthetic coal tar dye.

Restrictions and Adverse Effects: Harmful or irritant if in contact with the mucous membranes of the eyelids, mouth, nose, respiratory tract, or genitals. It is not allowed in any product intended for use on or near these areas.

Usage: EU/USA

Basic Yellow 57

(CI 12719)

Function: Hair dye.

Origin: Synthetic azo dye.

Restrictions and Adverse Effects: See *A–Z of Cosmetic Terms – Azo Dyes.*

Usage: EU/USA

Beeswax

(Cera alba, Cera flava)

Function: Emulsifier / Emollient / Moisturizer / Film former.

Origin: Natural beeswax, purified wax from the honeycomb of the bee.

Restrictions and Adverse Effects: Beeswax contains palmitates, which have been linked to contact dermatitis.

Usage: EU/USA

Behenamide DEA

Function: Surfactant.

Origin: Synthetic compound.

Restrictions and Adverse Effects: DEA residues are cancer suspects currently under investigation. See *A–Z of Cosmetic Terms – DEA.*

Usage: EU/USA

Behentrimonium chloride

Function: Preservative.

Origin: Synthetic compound.

Restrictions and Adverse Effects: This ingredient is harmful and is limited to 0.1 percent of the finished product if it is used as a preservative, but it may be added in larger quantities for other stated purposes.

Usage: EU/USA

Benzalkonium bromide

Function: Preservative.

Origin: Synthetic compound.

Restrictions and Adverse Effects: The safety of this substance was uncertain and its use in cosmetics was only provisionally permitted in the EU, until June 30, 1998. On September 3, 1998, following further scientific tests, the provisional status was removed and this ingredient was permitted for use in cosmetics. It is limited to a maximum of 0.1 percent of the finished product if it is used as a preservative, but it may be added in larger quantities if it is used for other stated purposes. The label must state, "Avoid contact with the eyes."

Usage: EU/USA

Benzalkonium chloride

Function: Preservative.

Origin: Synthetic compound.

Restrictions and Adverse Effects: The safety of this substance was uncertain and its use in cosmetics was only provisionally permitted in the EU, until June 30, 1998. On September 3, 1998, following further scientific tests, the provisional status was removed and this ingredient was permitted for use in cosmetics. It is limited to a maximum of 0.1 percent of the finished product if it is used as a preservative, but it may be added in larger quantities if it is used for other stated purposes. The label must state, "Avoid contact with the eyes."

Usage: EU/USA

Benzalkonium saccharinate

Function: Preservative.

Origin: Synthetic compound.

Restrictions and Adverse Effects: The safety of this substance was uncertain and its use in cosmetics was only provisionally permitted in the EU, until June 30, 1998. On September 3, 1998, following further scientific tests, the provisional status was removed and this ingredient was permitted for use in cosmetics. It is limited to a maximum of 0.1 percent of the finished product if it is used as a preservative, but it may be added in larger quantities if it is used for other stated purposes. The label must state, "Avoid contact with the eyes."

Usage: EU/USA

Benzethonium chloride

Function: Preservative.

Origin: Synthetic compound.

Restrictions and Adverse Effects: The safety of this substance was uncertain and its use in cosmetics was only provisionally permitted in the EU, until June 30, 1998. Following further scientific tests, the provisional status was removed and this preservative was permitted for use in cosmetics. It is limited to a maximum of 0.1 percent of the finished product and its use is restricted to rinse-off products only, as prolonged contact with the skin may be harmful.

Usage: EU/USA

Benzocaine

(Ethyl-p-aminobenzoate)

Function: Local anesthetic / Pain control.

This painkiller is mainly used in medicinal ointments and creams but occasionally it has been used in other cosmetics and toiletries to offset the irritant effect of other ingredients.

Origin: Synthetic compound.

Restrictions and Adverse Effects: Toxic by ingestion. Can cause contact dermatitis.

Usage: USA/Not currently on the EU inventory of cosmetic ingredients.

Benzoic acid

Function: Preservative.

Origin: Synthetic compound.

Restrictions and Adverse Effects: Benzoic acid and benzoates have been implicated in a large number of health issues. (See *A–Z of Cosmetic Terms – Benzoates*.) It is limited to 0.5 percent of the finished product if used as a preservative, but it may be added in larger quantities for other stated purposes.

Usage: EU/USA

Benzoic acid / Phthalic anhydride / Pentaerythritol / Neopentyl glycol / Palmitic acid copolymer

Function: Film former.

Origin: Synthetic compound.

Restrictions and Adverse Effects: Phthalic acid and phthalate residues may be present. These have been linked with testicular cancer and cell mutation.

Usage: EU/USA

Benzoin

(Benzoylphenyl carbinol, Phenylbenzoyl carbinol, 2-hydroxy-2-phenylacetophenone)

Function: UV absorber.

Origin: Synthetic compound.

Restrictions and Adverse Effects: Toxic. Can cause contact dermatitis.

Usage: USA/Not currently on the EU inventory of cosmetic ingredients.

Benzophenone

Function: UV absorber.

Origin: Synthetic compound.

Restrictions and Adverse Effects: May cause contact dermatitis and photosensitivity in some people.

Usage: EU/USA

Benzophenone-1

Function: UV absorber.

Origin: Synthetic compound.

Restrictions and Adverse Effects: May cause contact dermatitis and photosensitivity in some people.

Usage: EU/USA

Benzophenone-2

Function: UV absorber.

Origin: Synthetic compound.

Restrictions and Adverse Effects: May cause contact dermatitis and photosensitivity in some people.

Usage: EU/USA

Benzophenone-3

(Oxybenzone)

Function: UV absorber.

Origin: Synthetic compound.

Restrictions and Adverse Effects: Irritant. May cause contact dermatitis and photosensitivity in some people. This ingredient is restricted to a maximum of 10 percent of the finished sunscreen product. If used in a sunscreen, the label must state: "Contains oxybenzone."

Usage: EU/USA

Benzophenone-4

(Sulisobenzone)

Function: UV absorber.

Origin: Synthetic compound.

Restrictions and Adverse Effects: Can cause severe contact dermatitis and photosensitivity. The safety of this substance was uncertain and its use in sunscreens was only provisionally permitted in the EU, until June 30, 1998. On February 29, 2000, following further scientific tests, the provisional status was removed and this ingredient was permitted for use in cosmetics. It is limited to a maximum of 5 percent of the finished product. It may be used to protect the ingredients of other cosmetics and toiletries from the detrimental effects of sunlight.

Usage: EU/USA

Benzophenone-5

Function: UV absorber.

Origin: Synthetic compound.

Restrictions and Adverse Effects: Can cause severe contact dermatitis and photosensitivity. The safety of this substance was uncertain and its use in sunscreens was only provisionally permitted in the EU, until June 30, 1998. On February 29, 2000, following further scientific tests, the provisional status was removed and this ingredient was permitted for use in cosmetics. It is limited to a maximum of 5 percent of the finished product. It may be used to protect the ingredients of other cosmetics and toiletries from the detrimental effects of sunlight.

Usage: EU/USA

Benzophenone-6

Function: UV absorber.

Origin: Synthetic compound.

Restrictions and Adverse Effects: May cause contact dermatitis and photosensitivity in some people.

Usage: EU/USA

Benzophenone-7

Function: UV absorber.

Origin: Synthetic compound.

Restrictions and Adverse Effects: May cause contact dermatitis and photosensitivity in some people.

Usage: EU/USA

Benzophenone-8

(Dioxybenzone)

Function: UV absorber.

Origin: Synthetic compound.

Restrictions and Adverse Effects: May cause contact dermatitis and photosensitivity in some people.

Usage: EU/USA

Benzophenone-9

Function: UV absorber.

Origin: Synthetic compound.

Restrictions and Adverse Effects: May cause contact dermatitis and photosensitivity in some people.

Usage: EU/USA

Benzophenone-10

(Mexenone)

Function: UV absorber.

Origin: Synthetic compound.

Restrictions and Adverse Effects: May cause contact dermatitis and photosensitivity in some people.

Usage: EU/USA

Benzophenone-11

Function: UV absorber.

Origin: Synthetic compound.

Restrictions and Adverse Effects: May cause contact dermatitis and photosensitivity in some people.

Usage: EU/USA

Benzophenone-12

(Octabenzone)

Function: UV absorber.

Origin: Synthetic compound.

Restrictions and Adverse Effects: May cause contact dermatitis and photosensitivity in some people.

Usage: EU/USA

Benzoyl peroxide

Function: Acne treatment.

Origin: Synthetic compound derived from benzoic acid.

Restrictions and Adverse Effects: Corrosive. Harmful.

Usage: USA/Now banned in the EU.

Benzyl alcohol

Function: Preservative / Solvent / Fragrance. Benzyl alcohol is a solvent with a faint, sweet odor used in many perfumes as both a fragrance chemical and a carrier (solvent for other fragrance chemicals). It is also used to denature ethanol (alcohol), giving it an unpleasant taste, thus rendering it undrinkable.

Origin: Synthetic alcohol derived from petroleum or coal tar.

Restrictions and Adverse Effects: Toxic. Can cause contact dermatitis. It is limited to 1 percent of the finished product if used as a preservative, but it may be added in larger quantities for other stated purposes.

Usage: EU/USA

Benzyl cinnamate

Function: Additive. UV absorber used to protect a product from the detrimental effects of sunlight.

Origin: Synthetic compound.

Restrictions and Adverse Effects: Cinnamates have been reported to cause a stinging sensation in some people.

Usage: EU/USA

Benzylhemiformal

Function: Preservative.

Origin: Synthetic compound.

Restrictions and Adverse Effects: The safety of this substance was uncertain and its use in cosmetics was only provisionally permitted in the EU, until June 30, 1998. After this date its safety was still unproven and its provisional status was extended. It is limited to a maximum of 0.03 percent of the finished product and is restricted to rinse-off products only, as prolonged contact with the skin may be harmful.

Usage: EU/USA

Benzylidene camphor sulfonic acid

Function: UV absorber.

Origin: Synthetic compound.

Restrictions and Adverse Effects: Irritant. This ingredient is restricted to a maximum of 6 percent of the finished product.

Usage: EU/USA

Beta hydroxy complex

Function: Exfoliating agent.

Origin: Mixture containing chemically modified natural extracts, synthetic and semisynthetic compounds.

Restrictions and Adverse Effects: Beta-hydroxy acids (BHAs) are used to exfoliate skin. They are also known as skin peelers because they dissolve and remove the outer layer of skin. They can cause increased sensitivity to the sun due to loss of the protective outer layer of skin cells. Do not expose skin to the sun immediately following treatment with BHAs. Test a small area before use and discontinue use if skin irritation, redness, bleeding, or pain is experienced. Not recommended for use on children. May cause exfoliative dermatitis.

Usage: USA/Not currently on the EU inventory of cosmetic ingredients.

Beta vulgaris

(E162, Beetroot red)

Function: Red colorant.

Origin: Natural plant color.

Restrictions and Adverse Effects: Allowed in all products.

Usage: EU/USA

Beta-carotene

(Pro-vitamin A)

Function: Additive.

A pro-vitamin that is converted by the body into vitamin A (Retinol) and gives a yellow to orange-red color to cosmetics and toiletries.

Origin: Found primarily in carrots.

Restrictions and Adverse Effects: Can cause reduced red blood cell production and damage to the retina. May cause hypersensitivity. Its use in suntan

pills is banned in the USA and these tablets are not licensed in the UK.

Usage: EU/USA

Beta-hydroxybutanoic acid

(2-Hydroxybutanoic acid)

Function: Exfoliating agent.

Origin: Synthetic compound.

Restrictions and Adverse Effects: This ingredient is a beta-hydroxy acid (BHA) which is used to exfoliate skin. BHAs are also known as skin peelers because they dissolve and remove the outer layer of skin. They can cause increased sensitivity to the sun due to loss of the protective outer layer of skin cells. Do not expose skin to the sun immediately following treatment with BHAs. Test a small area before use and discontinue use if skin irritation, redness, bleeding, or pain is experienced. Not recommended for use on children. May cause exfoliative dermatitis.

Usage: USA/Not currently on the EU inventory of cosmetic ingredients.

BHA

(E320, Butylated hydroxyanisole)

Function: Antioxidant.

Origin: Synthetic compound.

Restrictions and Adverse Effects: Can cause contact allergies and contact dermatitis. If absorbed it can cause lipid and cholesterol levels to increase and encourage the breakdown of important nutrients such as vitamin D. It is a suspected endocrine disrupter chemical ("gender bender"). See *A–Z of Cosmetic Terms – Gender Bender.*

Usage: EU/USA

BHT

(E321, Butylated hydroxytoluene)

Function: Antioxidant.

Origin: Synthetic compound.

Restrictions and Adverse Effects: Can cause contact allergies and contact dermatitis. Cancer suspect. If absorbed it can encourage the breakdown of important nutrients such as vitamin D.

Usage: EU/USA

Bioflavonoids

Function: Additive.
Origin: Natural plant extract from a variety of sources including lemons.
Restrictions and Adverse Effects: Extracts from lemon juice can cause dermatitis.
Usage: EU/USA

Biotin

(Vitamin B complex)
Function: Biological additive.
Biotin is part of the Vitamin B complex.
Origin: Natural extract.
Restrictions and Adverse Effects: No currently known adverse effects.
Usage: EU/USA

Bis-diglyceryl caprylate / Caprate / Isostearate / Stearate / Hydroxystearate adipate

Function: Emollient / Moisturizer.
Origin: Semisynthetic or synthetic mixed compound.
Restrictions and Adverse Effects: No currently known adverse effects.
Usage: EU/USA

Bis-(8-hydroxy-quinolinium) sulfate

Function: Stabilizer for Hydrogen peroxide.
Origin: Synthetic compound.
Restrictions and Adverse Effects: Irritant. Harmful. This ingredient is limited to 0.3 percent in rinse-off hair care preparations and to 0.03 percent in non-rinse off preparations.
Usage: EU/USA

Bisabolol

Function: Demulcent / Anti-inflammatory agent.
Origin: Synthetic forms exist but it is the essential oil of *Chamomilla recutita*, which is grown mainly in central and eastern Europe, Egypt, and Argentina. Camomile oil is a deep blue or bluish-green liquid that turns green, then brown when exposed to light and air. Bisabolol contributes to the anti-inflammatory properties of camomile oil and is used in shampoos, including baby shampoos, moisturizing creams, and skincare lotions.

Restrictions and Adverse Effects: Can cause contact allergies and contact dermatitis.
Usage: EU/USA

Bismuth citrate

Function: pH control / Chelating agent / Progressive hair dye.
Origin: Semisynthetic compound derived from citric acid, a fruit extract.
Restrictions and Adverse Effects: Bismuth compounds are toxic, causing intellectual impairment, memory loss, confusion, loss of coordination (clumsiness), trembling, convulsions, and difficulty in walking.
Usage: EU/USA

Bismuth oxychloride

(CI 77163, Bismuth chloride oxide)
Function: Colorant.
Origin: Synthetic compound.
Restrictions and Adverse Effects: Bismuth compounds are toxic, causing intellectual impairment, memory loss, confusion, loss of coordination (clumsiness), trembling, convulsions, and difficulty in walking.
Usage: EU/USA

Bismuth subnitrate

Function: Absorbent / Opacifier.
Origin: Synthetic compound.
Restrictions and Adverse Effects: Bismuth compounds are toxic, causing intellectual impairment, memory loss, confusion, loss of coordination (clumsiness), trembling, convulsions, and difficulty in walking.
Usage: EU/USA

Boric acid

Function: Antimicrobial / Oral care agent.
Origin: Synthetic compound.
Restrictions and Adverse Effects: Toxic, Irritant. Boric acid and borates have been linked to fetal malformations. It is limited to 5 percent in body powders, 0.5 percent in oral care products, and 3 percent in other preparations. It must not be used in products for children under the age of 3.
Usage: EU/USA

Bornelone

Function: UV absorber.
Origin: Synthetic compound.
Restrictions and Adverse Effects: May cause contact allergies in some individuals.
Usage: EU/USA

Brilliant black 1

Function: Hair dye.
Origin: Synthetic azo dye.
Restrictions and Adverse Effects: See *A–Z of Cosmetic Terms – Azo Dyes*.
Usage: EU/USA

Bromochlorophene

Function: Preservative.
Origin: Synthetic compound.
Restrictions and Adverse Effects: This ingredient is limited to 0.1 percent of the finished product if used as a preservative, but it may be added in larger quantities if used for other stated purposes.
Usage: EU/USA

Bromocresol green

Function: Green colorant.
Origin: Synthetic coal tar dye.
Restrictions and Adverse Effects: Harmful or irritant by prolonged contact with the skin. It is only allowed in products that are rinsed off immediately after use.
Usage: EU/USA

Bromothymol blue

Function: Blue colorant.
Origin: Synthetic coal tar dye.
Restrictions and Adverse Effects: Harmful or irritant by prolonged contact with the skin. It is only allowed in products that are rinsed off immediately after use.
Usage: EU/USA

Butadiene / Acrylonitrile copolymer

Function: Film former / Viscosity adjuster.
Origin: Synthetic compound.
Restrictions and Adverse Effects: Some nitriles have been linked to allergic reactions and contact eczema.
Usage: EU/USA

Butane

Function: Propellant for aerosol sprays. (Often used in combination with Propane and Isobutane.)
Origin: Petroleum product.
Restrictions and Adverse Effects: A flammable hydrocarbon gas that is used as an alternative to CFCs, which are known to damage the ozone layer. It is a powerful greenhouse gas (contributes to the greenhouse effect causing global warming) and is inhaled by solvent abusers. It is harmless if inhaled in small concentrations. There is a danger of fire or explosion if used near a source of ignition.
Usage: EU/USA

Butyl acetate

Function: Solvent.
Origin: Synthetic compound.
Restrictions and Adverse Effects: Skin irritant for some individuals. Respiratory irritant.
Usage: EU/USA

Butyl benzoate

Function: Preservative.
Origin: Synthetic compound of the benzoate family.
Restrictions and Adverse Effects: Benzoic acid and benzoates have been implicated in a large number of health issues. (See *A–Z of Cosmetic Terms – Benzoates*.) It is limited to 0.5 percent of the finished product if used as a preservative, but it may be added in larger quantities if used for other stated purposes.
Usage: EU/USA

Butyl benzoic acid / Phthalic anhydride / Trimethylolethane copolymer

Function: Film former.
Origin: Synthetic compound.
Restrictions and Adverse Effects: Phthalic acid and phthalate residues may be present. These have been linked with testicular cancer and cell mutation.
Usage: EU/USA

Butyl benzyl phthalate

Function: Film former.
Origin: Synthetic compound.
Restrictions and Adverse Effects: Phthalic acid and phthalates have been linked with testicular cancer and cell mutation.
Usage: EU/USA

Butyl methoxydibenzoylmethane

(t-Butyl-4-methoxydibenzoylmethane, Avobenzone)
Function: UV absorber.
Origin: Synthetic compound.
Restrictions and Adverse Effects: Irritant for some individuals. This ingredient is restricted to a maximum of 5 percent of the finished product.
Usage: EU/USA

Butyl myristate

Function: Emollient / Moisturizer.
Origin: Semisynthetic compound.
Restrictions and Adverse Effects: Some myristates are comedogenic (acne promoting, see *A–Z of Cosmetic Terms – Comedogen*).
Usage: EU/USA

Butyl phthalyl butyl glycolate

Function: Film former.
Origin: Semisynthetic or synthetic compound.
Restrictions and Adverse Effects: Phthalic acid and phthalates have been linked with testicular cancer and cell mutation.
Usage: EU/USA

Butyl stearate

Function: Emollient / Moisturizer.
Origin: Semisynthetic or synthetic compound.
Restrictions and Adverse Effects: Comedogenic (acne promoting, see *A–Z of Cosmetic Terms – Comedogen*).
Usage: EU/USA

Butyl thioglycolate

Function: Additive.
Origin: Synthetic compound.

Restrictions and Adverse Effects: EU regulations require the following mandatory warnings: "May cause sensitization in the event of skin contact. Avoid contact with eyes. In the event of contact with eyes, rinse with plenty of water and seek medical advice. Wear suitable gloves. Follow the instructions. Keep out of reach of children." The label must also state "Contains Thioglycolate." It is limited to 8 percent for general use or 11 percent for professional use, and the pH must be between 6 and 9.5.
Usage: EU/USA

Butylene glycol

Function: Humectant / Solvent.
Origin: Synthetic compound.
Restrictions and Adverse Effects: No currently known adverse effects.
Usage: EU/USA

Butylene glycol dicaprylate / Dicaprate

Function: Emollient / Moisturizer.
Origin: Semisynthetic or synthetic compound.
Restrictions and Adverse Effects: No currently known adverse effects.
Usage: EU/USA

Butylparaben

Function: Preservative.
Origin: Synthetic compound of the benzoate family.
Restrictions and Adverse Effects: Benzoic acid, benzoates and parabens have been implicated in a large number of health issues. (See *A–Z of Cosmetic Terms – Benzoates*.) It is limited to 0.4 percent of the finished product if used on its own as a preservative, or 0.8 percent in total if used in combination with other parabens. Parabens may be added in larger quantities if used for other stated purposes.
Usage: EU/USA

Cnumber-number Pareth – Family

Examples include C11-15 Pareth-28 and C12-15 Pareth-12 oleate.

Function: Mainly emulsifiers and surfactants.

Origin: A range of synthetic ingredients manufactured from ethylene oxide. These ethoxylated compounds may be combined with a variety of other molecules to produce a wide range of cosmetic materials. Higher numbers mean higher ethoxylation (bigger molecules), usually resulting in a greater solubility in water.

Restrictions and Adverse Effects: Ethoxylated ingredients are made using ethylene oxide (oxirane) which can form 1,4-dioxane, a carcinogen, as a by-product of manufacture. See *A–Z of Cosmetic Terms – Dioxane*.

Usage: EU/USA

C10-30 cholesterol / Lanosterol esters

Function: Emulsifier.

Origin: Mixture of semisynthetic compounds.

Restrictions and Adverse Effects: No currently known adverse effects.

Usage: EU/USA

C12-15 alkyl benzoate

(C12-15 Alcohols Benzoate)

Function: Emollient / Moisturizer /Preservative.

Origin: Mixture of synthetic compounds.

Restrictions and Adverse Effects: No currently known adverse effects.

Usage: EU/USA

C14-16 glycol palmitate

Function: Emulsifier.

Origin: Mixture of semisynthetic or synthetic compounds.

Restrictions and Adverse Effects: Some palmitates have been linked to contact dermatitis.

Usage: EU/USA

C18-36 acid glycol ester

Function: Emollient / Moisturizer.

Origin: Mixture of synthetic compounds.

Restrictions and Adverse Effects: No currently known adverse effects.

Usage: EU/USA

Calcium benzoate

Function: Preservative.

Origin: Synthetic compound of the benzoate family.

Restrictions and Adverse Effects: Benzoic acid and benzoates have been implicated in a large number of health issues. (See *A–Z of Cosmetic Terms – Benzoates*.) It is limited to 0.5 percent of the finished product if used as a preservative, but it may be added in larger quantities if used for other stated purposes.

Usage: EU/USA

Calcium fluoride

Function: Oral care agent.

Origin: Synthetic compound.

Restrictions and Adverse Effects: Fluorides are toxic. They can discolor teeth (fluorosis). Children should only use a small quantity of toothpaste and be discouraged from swallowing it. The total amount of fluoride allowed by EU regulations is 0.15 percent of the finished product.

Usage: EU/USA

Calcium monofluorophosphate

Function: Oral care agent.

Origin: Synthetic compound.

Restrictions and Adverse Effects: Fluorides are toxic. They can discolor teeth (fluorosis). Children should only use a small quantity of toothpaste and be discouraged from swallowing it. The total amount of fluoride allowed by EU regulations is 0.15 percent of the finished product.

Usage: EU/USA

Calcium myristate

Function: Surfactant.

Origin: Semisynthetic or synthetic compound.

Restrictions and Adverse Effects: Some myristates are comedogenic (acne promoting, see *A–Z of Cosmetic Terms – Comedogen*).

Usage: EU/USA

Calcium paraben

Function: Preservative.

Origin: Synthetic compound of the benzoate family.

Restrictions and Adverse Effects: Benzoic acid, benzoates and parabens have been implicated in a large number of health issues. (See *A–Z of Cosmetic Terms – Benzoates.*) It is limited to 0.4 percent of the finished product if used on its own as a preservative, or 0.8 percent in total if used in combination with other parabens. Parabens may be added in larger quantities if used for other stated purposes.

Usage: EU/USA

Calcium propionate

Function: Preservative.

Origin: Synthetic compound.

Restrictions and Adverse Effects: Propanoic acid and its salts are limited to 2 percent of the finished product if used as a preservative, but may be added in larger quantities for other stated purposes.

Usage: EU/USA

Calcium salicylate

Function: Preservative.

Origin: Synthetic compound.

Restrictions and Adverse Effects: Limited to 0.5 percent of the finished product if used as a preservative, but may be added in larger quantities for other stated purposes. With the exception of shampoo, it must not be used in preparations intended for children under the age of 3 and must clearly state this restriction on the label.

Usage: EU/USA

Calcium sorbate

Function: Preservative.

Origin: Semisynthetic compound.

Restrictions and Adverse Effects: Limited to 0.6 percent of the finished product if used as a preservative, but may be added in larger quantities for other stated purposes.

Usage: EU/USA

Calcium stearate

Function: White colorant often used as an opacifier in liquid formulations such as shampoos and conditioners, or as a colorant in thicker preparations.

Origin: Semisynthetic or synthetic compound.

Restrictions and Adverse Effects: Allowed in all products. No known adverse effects.

Usage: EU/USA

Calcium sulfide

Function: Depilatory agent.

Origin: Synthetic compound.

Restrictions and Adverse Effects: Sulfides are toxic. Irritant. May be alkaline (irritant and corrosive). Maximum allowed content is 6 percent of the finished product. The label must carry warnings to avoid contact with the eyes and to keep the product out of the reach of children.

Usage: EU/USA

Calcium thioglycolate

Function: Depilatory agent / Reducing agent.

Origin: Synthetic compound.

Restrictions and Adverse Effects: Harmful. May be alkaline (irritant and corrosive). In the EU its content is limited to 8 percent in hair perming preparations (11 percent for professional use), 5 percent in depilatories and 2 percent in rinse-off hair care products. The pH must be between 7 and 9.5 in hair care products and between 7 and 12.7 in depilatories. The label must clearly state "Contains Thioglycolate," and it must show the following mandatory warnings: "Follow the instructions. Keep out of reach of children. Avoid contact with eyes. In the event of contact with eyes, rinse with plenty of water and seek medical advice." Additionally, hair care products must state "Wear suitable gloves."

Usage: EU/USA

Calcium undecylenate

Function: Preservative.
Origin: Semisynthetic or synthetic compound.
Restrictions and Adverse Effects: Limited to 0.2 percent of the finished product if used as a preservative, but may be added in larger quantities for other stated purposes.
Usage: EU/USA

Calendula officinalis

(Calendula extract)
Function: Emollient / Moisturizer.
Origin: Natural plant extract.
Restrictions and Adverse Effects: Can cause skin irritation and contact dermatitis.
Usage: EU/USA

Calgon

(Calgon S)
Function: Water softener.
Origin: Synthetic compound.
Restrictions and Adverse Effects: No currently known adverse effects.
Usage: EU/USA

Calomel

(Mercurous chloride, Mercury (I) chloride)
Function: White pigment with some antimicrobial properties.
Origin: Synthetic compound of mercury and chlorine.
Restrictions and Adverse Effects: Highly toxic.
Usage: Banned from use in cosmetics in both the EU and the USA. This ingredient has been found in face creams manufactured in Mexico in concentrations up to 10 percent by weight. This is a thousand times higher than the allowed levels of mercury-based preservatives, which are restricted to eye make-up and eye make-up removers.

Camphor benzalkonium methosulfate

Function: UV absorber.
Origin: Synthetic compound.
Restrictions and Adverse Effects: Irritant for some individuals. This ingredient is restricted to a maximum of 6 percent of the finished product.
Usage: EU/USA

Canthaxanthin

(E161g, CI 75135)
Function: Orange colorant used in cosmetics and food products.
Origin: A natural orange pigment extracted from flamingo feathers and some fungi.
Restrictions and Adverse Effects: Can cause loss of night vision and hypersensitivity. Its use in suntan pills is banned in the USA and these tablets are not licensed in the UK.
Usage: USA/Not currently on the EU inventory of cosmetic ingredients.

Capramide DEA

Function: Antistatic agent / Viscosity adjuster.
Origin: Semisynthetic or synthetic compound.
Restrictions and Adverse Effects: DEA residues are cancer suspects currently under investigation. See *A–Z of Cosmetic Terms – DEA*.
Usage: EU/USA

Caprylic / Capric / Stearic triglyceride

Function: Emollient / Moisturizer / Solvent.
Origin: Mixed semisynthetic or synthetic compounds.
Restrictions and Adverse Effects: No currently known adverse effects.
Usage: EU/USA

Capsanthin / Capsorubin

(E160c)
Function: Orange colorant.
Origin: Natural plant colorant.
Restrictions and Adverse Effects: Allowed in all products. No known adverse effects.
Usage: EU/USA

Caramel

(E150)

Function: Brown colorant.

Origin: Semi-natural colorant.

Restrictions and Adverse Effects: Allowed in all products. Some types of caramel have been shown to cause a deficiency of vitamin B_6 in rats.

Usage: EU/USA

Carba-mix

Function: Preservative.

Origin: Mixture of synthetic compounds – Diphenylguanidine, Zincdibutyldithiocarbamate and Zincdiethyldithiocarbamate.

Restrictions and Adverse Effects: May cause contact dermatitis in some individuals.

Usage: USA/Not currently on the EU inventory of cosmetic ingredients.

Carbomer

Function: Emulsion stabilizer / Viscosity adjuster.

Origin: Synthetic compound. A high molecular weight crosslinked polymer (plastic) of acrylic acid.

Restrictions and Adverse Effects: No currently known adverse effects.

Usage: EU/USA

Carnauba

(Carnauba wax, Cera carnauba)

Function: Emollient / Moisturizer / Film former.

Origin: A natural wax obtained from the leaves of the Brazilian Wax Palm. There is also a synthetic form of Carnauba derived from petroleum.

Restrictions and Adverse Effects: No currently known adverse effects.

Usage: EU/USA

Carotene

(Pro-vitamin A (synthetic))

Function: A pro-vitamin that is converted by the body into vitamin A. Carotene gives a yellow to orange-red color to formulations.

Origin: Synthetic compound.

Restrictions and Adverse Effects: Can cause reduced red blood cell production and damage to the retina. May cause hypersensitivity.

Usage: USA/Not currently on the EU inventory of cosmetic ingredients.

Carum petroselinum

(Parsley seed oil, Parsley extract)

Function: Botanical additive.

Origin: Plant extract.

Restrictions and Adverse Effects: Irritant for some individuals. Can cause allergic contact dermatitis.

Usage: EU/USA

Cellulose gum

(Carboxymethyl cellulose sodium, Carmellose)

Function: Binding agent / Emulsion stabilizer / Film former / Viscosity adjuster.

Origin: Semisynthetic compound.

Restrictions and Adverse Effects: No currently known adverse effects.

Usage: EU/USA

Cera alba

(Beeswax, Cera flava)

Function: Emollient / Moisturizer / Emulsifier / Film former.

Origin: Natural beeswax from the honeycomb of the bee.

Restrictions and Adverse Effects: Beeswax contains palmitates, which have been linked to contact dermatitis.

Usage: EU/USA

Cera microcristallina

Function: Binding agent / Emulsion stabilizer / Opacifier / Viscosity adjuster.

Origin: A mixture of waxy hydrocarbons purified from petroleum.

Restrictions and Adverse Effects: No currently known adverse effects.

Usage: EU/USA

Ceresin

Function: Antistatic agent / Binding agent / Emulsion stabilizer / Opacifier / Viscosity adjuster.

Origin: A complex combination of waxy hydrocarbons produced by the purification of ozocerite, a waxy compound obtained from petroleum, with sulfuric acid followed by filtration through animal charcoal.

Restrictions and Adverse Effects: No currently known adverse effects.

Usage: EU/USA

Cetalkonium chloride

Function: Preservative.

Origin: Synthetic compound.

Restrictions and Adverse Effects: The safety of this substance was uncertain and its use in cosmetics was only provisionally permitted in the EU, until June 30, 1998. On September 3, 1998, following further scientific tests, the provisional status was removed and this ingredient was permitted for use in cosmetics. It is limited to a maximum of 0.1 percent of the finished product if it is used as a preservative, but it may be added in larger quantities if it is used for other stated purposes. The label must state, "Avoid contact with the eyes."

Usage: EU/USA

Cetearalkonium bromide

Function: Preservative.

Origin: Synthetic compound.

Restrictions and Adverse Effects: The safety of this substance was uncertain and its use in cosmetics was only provisionally permitted in the EU, until June 30, 1998. On September 3, 1998, following further scientific tests, the provisional status was removed and this ingredient was permitted for use in cosmetics. It is limited to a maximum of 0.1 percent of the finished product if it is used as a preservative, but it may be added in larger quantities if it is used for other stated purposes. The label must state, "Avoid contact with the eyes."

Usage: EU/USA

Ceteareth – Family

Examples include Ceteareth-15 and Ceteareth-25 carboxylic acid

Function: Mainly emulsifiers and surfactants.

Origin: A range of synthetic ingredients manufactured from ethylene oxide. These ethoxylated compounds may be combined with a variety of other molecules to produce a wide range of cosmetic materials. Higher numbers mean higher ethoxylation (bigger molecules), usually resulting in a greater solubility in water.

Restrictions and Adverse Effects: Ethoxylated ingredients are made using ethylene oxide (oxirane), which can form 1,4-dioxane, a carcinogen, as a by-product of manufacture. See *A–Z of Cosmetic Terms – Dioxane*.

Usage: EU/USA

Ceteareth-2 phosphate

Function: Surfactant.

Origin: Synthetic compound derived from cetearyl alcohol by ethoxylation with ethylene oxide.

Restrictions and Adverse Effects: No currently known adverse effects. This ethoxylated ingredient is made using ethylene oxide (oxirane), which can form 1,4-dioxane, a carcinogen, as a by-product of manufacture. See *A–Z of Cosmetic Terms – Dioxane*.

Usage: EU/USA

Ceteareth-20

Function: Emulsifier / Surfactant / Viscosity adjuster. Derived from cetearyl alcohol by ethoxylation with ethylene oxide. Used with the parent alcohol or with other fatty alcohols, it functions as a primary emulsifier and thickening agent.

Origin: Synthetic compound.

Restrictions and Adverse Effects: No currently known adverse effects. This ethoxylated ingredient is made using ethylene oxide (oxirane), which can form 1,4-dioxane, a carcinogen, as a by-product of manufacture. See *A–Z of Cosmetic Terms – Dioxane*.

Usage: EU/USA

Cetearyl alcohol

Function: Emollient / Moisturizer / Emulsifier / Emulsion stabilizer / Opacifier / Viscosity adjuster.

Origin: Semisynthetic or synthetic compound.

Restrictions and Adverse Effects: May cause contact dermatitis and contact sensitivity in some individuals.

Usage: EU/USA

Cetearyl isononanoate

Function: Emollient / Moisturizer.
Origin: Semisynthetic or synthetic compound.
Restrictions and Adverse Effects: No currently known adverse effects.
Usage: EU/USA

Cetearyl palmitate

Function: Emollient / Moisturizer.
Origin: Semisynthetic or synthetic compound.
Restrictions and Adverse Effects: Some palmitates have been linked to contact dermatitis.
Usage: EU/USA

Ceteth-20

Function: Emulsifier / Surfactant.
Origin: Synthetic compound.
Restrictions and Adverse Effects: No currently known adverse effects. This ethoxylated ingredient is made using ethylene oxide (oxirane), which can form 1,4-dioxane, a carcinogen, as a by-product of manufacture. See *A–Z of Cosmetic Terms – Dioxane*.
Usage: EU/USA

Cetrimonium bromide

Function: Preservative.
Origin: Synthetic compound.
Restrictions and Adverse Effects: Limited to 0.1 percent of the finished product if used as a preservative, but may be added in larger quantities for other stated purposes.
Usage: EU/USA

Cetrimonium chloride

Function: Preservative.
Origin: Synthetic compound.
Restrictions and Adverse Effects: Limited to 0.1 percent of the finished product if used as a preservative, but may be added in larger quantities for other stated purposes.
Usage: EU/USA

Cetyl acetate

Function: Emollient / Moisturizer.
Origin: Semisynthetic or synthetic compound.
Restrictions and Adverse Effects: No currently known adverse effects.
Usage: EU/USA

Cetyl alcohol

(Hexadecanol, Palmityl alcohol)
Function: Emollient / Moisturizer / Emulsifier / Opacifier / Viscosity adjuster.
Origin: Semisynthetic or synthetic compound.
Restrictions and Adverse Effects: May cause contact dermatitis in some individuals.
Usage: EU/USA

Cetyl betaine

Function: Antistatic agent / Surfactant.
Origin: Semisynthetic or synthetic compound.
Restrictions and Adverse Effects: No currently known adverse effects.
Usage: EU/USA

Cetyl dimethicone copolyol

Function: Emulsifier.
Origin: Synthetic compound related to silicones.
Restrictions and Adverse Effects: No currently known adverse effects.
Usage: EU/USA

Cetyl esters

Function: Emollient / Moisturizer.
Origin: Mixture of semisynthetic or synthetic compounds.
Restrictions and Adverse Effects: Contains cetyl palmitate. Some palmitates have been linked to contact dermatitis.
Usage: EU/USA

Cetyl myristate

Function: Emollient / Moisturizer.
Origin: Semisynthetic or synthetic compounds.
Restrictions and Adverse Effects: Some myristates are comedogenic (acne promoting, see *A–Z of Cosmetic Terms – Comedogen*).
Usage: EU/USA

Cetyl palmitate

Function: Emollient / Moisturizer.
Origin: Semisynthetic or synthetic compounds.
Restrictions and Adverse Effects: Some palmitates have been linked to contact dermatitis.
Usage: EU/USA

Cetylamine hydrofluoride

(Hetaflur)
Function: Oral care agent.
Origin: Synthetic compound.
Restrictions and Adverse Effects: Fluorides are toxic. They can discolor teeth (fluorosis). Children should only use a small quantity of toothpaste and be discouraged from swallowing it. The total amount of fluoride allowed by EU regulations is 0.15 percent of the finished product.
Usage: EU/USA

Chamomilla recutita

(Camomile Extract. See also – Bisabolol)
Function: Emollient / Moisturizer / Demulcent.
Origin: Plant extract containing Bisabolol, a natural anti-inflammatory agent.
Restrictions and Adverse Effects: May cause contact allergies and contact dermatitis in some individuals.
Usage: EU/USA

Chloramine-T

(Tosylchloramide sodium)
Function: Antimicrobial.
Origin: Synthetic compound.
Restrictions and Adverse Effects: Harmful. Maximum allowed content is 0.2 percent of the finished product.
Usage: EU/USA

Chloramphenicol

Function: Antibiotic.
Synthetic antibiotic used mainly to treat eye infections.
Origin: Synthetic compound.
Restrictions and Adverse Effects: Can cause contact dermatitis. May have deleterious side effects and is regulated by the FDA in the USA. It is available only with a doctor's prescription in the UK.
Usage: USA/Antibiotics are banned from cosmetics in the EU.

Chlorhexidine

Function: Preservative.
Origin: Synthetic compound.
Restrictions and Adverse Effects: Limited to 0.3 percent of the finished product if used as a preservative, but may be added in larger quantities for other stated purposes.
Usage: EU/USA

Chlorhexidine diacetate

Function: Preservative.
Origin: Synthetic compound.
Restrictions and Adverse Effects: Limited to 0.3 percent of the finished product if used as a preservative, but may be added in larger quantities for other stated purposes.
Usage: EU/USA

Chlorhexidine digluconate

Function: Preservative.
Origin: Synthetic compound.
Restrictions and Adverse Effects: Limited to 0.3 percent of the finished product if used as a preservative, but may be added in larger quantities for other stated purposes.
Usage: EU/USA

Chlorhexidine dihydrochloride

Function: Preservative.
Origin: Synthetic compound.
Restrictions and Adverse Effects: Limited to 0.3 percent of the finished product if used as a preservative, but may be added in larger quantities for other stated purposes.
Usage: EU/USA

Chlorinated phenols

(TCP)

Function: Antiseptic.

Seldom used in cosmetics but frequently found in antiseptic creams, lotions, cleaning fluids, and throat lozenges.

Origin: Synthetic compounds, often a mixture including bromo and iodophenols.

Restrictions and Adverse Effects: Skin and mucous membrane irritant.

Usage: EU/USA

Chloroacetamide

Function: Preservative.

Origin: Synthetic compound.

Restrictions and Adverse Effects: Can cause contact dermatitis and contact allergies. Limited to 0.3 percent of the finished product, and the label must clearly state the name of this substance separately from the list of ingredients.

Usage: EU/USA

Chlorobutanol

Function: Preservative.

Origin: Synthetic compound.

Restrictions and Adverse Effects: Harmful by inhalation. Prohibited from use in aerosol dispensers and sprays and limited to 0.5 percent of the finished product. The label must clearly state the name of this substance separately from the list of ingredients.

Usage: EU/USA

Chlorophene

Function: Preservative.

Origin: Synthetic compound.

Restrictions and Adverse Effects: This ingredient is limited to 0.2 percent of the finished product.

Usage: EU/USA

Chloroxylenol

Function: Preservative.

Origin: Synthetic compound.

Restrictions and Adverse Effects: Limited to 0.5 percent of the finished product if used as a preservative, but it may be added in larger quantities for other stated purposes.

Usage: EU/USA

Chlorphenesin

Function: Preservative.

Origin: Synthetic compound.

Restrictions and Adverse Effects: This substance is restricted to 0.3 percent of the finished product.

Usage: EU/USA

CI 10006

Function: Green colorant.

Origin: Synthetic coal tar dye.

Restrictions and Adverse Effects: Harmful or irritant by prolonged contact with the skin. It is only allowed in products that are rinsed off immediately after use.

Usage: EU/USA

CI 10020

Function: Green colorant.

Origin: Synthetic coal tar dye.

Restrictions and Adverse Effects: Harmful or irritant if in contact with the mucous membranes of the eyelids, mouth, nose, respiratory tract, or genitals. It is not allowed in any product intended for use on or near these areas.

Usage: EU/USA

CI 10316 (Ext. D&C Yellow #7)

(Acid Yellow #1)

Function: Yellow colorant.

Origin: Synthetic coal tar dye.

Restrictions and Adverse Effects: Harmful or irritant to eyes. EU regulations prohibit this dye in any product intended for use on or near the eyes. FDA regulations allow this dye in any externally applied cosmetic except eye products.

Usage: EU/USA

CI 11680

Function: Yellow colorant.

Origin: Synthetic azo dye.

Restrictions and Adverse Effects: Harmful or irritant if in contact with the mucous membranes of the eyelids, mouth, nose, respiratory tract, or genitals.

It is not allowed in any product intended for use on or near these areas. See *A–Z of Cosmetic Terms – Azo Dyes*.

Usage: EU/USA

CI 11710

Function: Yellow colorant.

Origin: Synthetic azo dye.

Restrictions and Adverse Effects: Harmful or irritant if in contact with the mucous membranes of the eyelids, mouth, nose, respiratory tract, or genitals. It is not allowed in any product intended for use on or near these areas. See *A–Z of Cosmetic Terms – Azo Dyes*.

Usage: EU/USA

CI 11725

Function: Orange colorant.

Origin: Synthetic azo dye.

Restrictions and Adverse Effects: Harmful or irritant by prolonged contact with the skin. It is only allowed in products that are rinsed off immediately after use. See *A–Z of Cosmetic Terms – Azo Dyes*.

Usage: EU/USA

CI 11920

Function: Orange colorant.

Origin: Synthetic azo dye.

Restrictions and Adverse Effects: Allowed in all products. See *A–Z of Cosmetic Terms – Azo Dyes*.

Usage: EU/USA

CI 12010

Function: Red colorant.

Origin: Synthetic azo dye.

Restrictions and Adverse Effects: Harmful or irritant if in contact with the mucous membranes of the eyelids, mouth, nose, respiratory tract, or genitals. It is not allowed in any product intended for use on or near these areas. See *A–Z of Cosmetic Terms – Azo Dyes*.

Usage: EU/USA

CI 12085 (D&C Red #36)

(Pigment Red 4)

Function: Red colorant.

Origin: Synthetic azo dye.

Restrictions and Adverse Effects: Allowed in all products sold in the EU up to a maximum of 3 percent of the finished product. FDA regulations allow its use in all externally applied cosmetics (except eye products) and lip cosmetics, again limiting it to 3 percent of the finished product. See *A–Z of Cosmetic Terms – Azo Dyes*.

Usage: EU/USA

CI 12120

Function: Red colorant.

Origin: Synthetic azo dye.

Restrictions and Adverse Effects: Harmful or irritant by prolonged contact with the skin. It is only allowed in products that are rinsed off immediately after use. See *A–Z of Cosmetic Terms – Azo Dyes*.

Usage: EU/USA

CI 12150

Function: Red colorant.

Origin: Synthetic azo dye.

Restrictions and Adverse Effects: Allowed in all products. See *A–Z of Cosmetic Terms – Azo Dyes*.

Usage: EU/USA

CI 12370

Function: Red colorant.

Origin: Synthetic azo dye.

Restrictions and Adverse Effects: Harmful or irritant by prolonged contact with the skin. It is only allowed in products that are rinsed off immediately after use. See *A–Z of Cosmetic Terms – Azo Dyes*.

Usage: EU/USA

CI 12420

Function: Red colorant.

Origin: Synthetic azo dye.

Restrictions and Adverse Effects: Harmful or irritant by prolonged contact with the skin. It is only allowed in products that are rinsed off immediately after use. See *A–Z of Cosmetic Terms – Azo Dyes*.

Usage: EU/USA

CI 12480

Function: Brown colorant.
Origin: Synthetic azo dye.
Restrictions and Adverse Effects: Harmful or irritant by prolonged contact with the skin. It is only allowed in products that are rinsed off immediately after use. See *A–Z of Cosmetic Terms – Azo Dyes*.
Usage: EU/USA

CI 12490

Function: Red colorant.
Origin: Synthetic azo dye.
Restrictions and Adverse Effects: Allowed in all products. See *A–Z of Cosmetic Terms – Azo Dyes*.
Usage: EU/USA

CI 12700

Function: Yellow colorant.
Origin: Synthetic azo dye.
Restrictions and Adverse Effects: Harmful or irritant by prolonged contact with the skin. It is only allowed in products that are rinsed off immediately after use. See *A–Z of Cosmetic Terms – Azo Dyes*.
Usage: EU/USA

CI 13015

(E105)
Function: Yellow colorant.
Origin: Synthetic azo dye.
Restrictions and Adverse Effects: Allowed in all products. See *A–Z of Cosmetic Terms – Azo Dyes*.
Usage: EU/USA

CI 14270

Function: Orange colorant.
Origin: Synthetic azo dye.
Restrictions and Adverse Effects: Allowed in all products. See *A–Z of Cosmetic Terms – Azo Dyes*.
Usage: EU/USA

CI 14700 (FD&C Red #4)

(Ponceau SX)
Function: Red colorant.
Origin: Synthetic azo dye.
Restrictions and Adverse Effects: Allowed in all products in the EU. Allowed in all externally applied cosmetics sold in the USA except eye products. See *A–Z of Cosmetic Terms – Azo Dyes*.
Usage: EU/USA

CI 14720

(E122)
Function: Red colorant.
Origin: Synthetic azo dye.
Restrictions and Adverse Effects: Allowed in all products. See *A–Z of Cosmetic Terms – Azo Dyes*.
Usage: EU/USA

CI 14815

(E125)
Function: Red colorant.
Origin: Synthetic azo dye.
Restrictions and Adverse Effects: Allowed in all products. See *A–Z of Cosmetic Terms – Azo Dyes*.
Usage: EU/USA

CI 15510 (D&C Orange #4)

Function: Orange colorant.
Origin: Synthetic azo dye.
Restrictions and Adverse Effects: Harmful or irritant to eyes. EU regulations prohibit its use in any product intended for use on or near the eyes. FDA regulations allow it to be used in all externally applied cosmetics except eye products. See *A–Z of Cosmetic Terms – Azo Dyes*.
Usage: EU/USA

CI 15525

Function: Red colorant.
Origin: Synthetic azo dye.
Restrictions and Adverse Effects: Allowed in all products. See *A–Z of Cosmetic Terms – Azo Dyes*.
Usage: EU/USA

CI 15580

Function: Red colorant.
Origin: Synthetic azo dye.
Restrictions and Adverse Effects: Allowed in all products. See *A–Z of Cosmetic Terms – Azo Dyes*.
Usage: EU/USA

CI 15620

Function: Red colorant.

Origin: Synthetic azo dye.

Restrictions and Adverse Effects: Harmful or irritant by prolonged contact with the skin. It is only allowed in products that are rinsed off immediately after use. See *A–Z of Cosmetic Terms – Azo Dyes*.

Usage: EU/USA

CI 15630

Function: Red colorant.

Origin: Synthetic azo dye.

Restrictions and Adverse Effects: Allowed in all products up to a maximum of 3 percent of the finished product. See *A–Z of Cosmetic Terms – Azo Dyes*.

Usage: EU/USA

CI 15800 (D&C Red #31)

(Pigment Red 64:1)

Function: Red colorant.

Origin: Synthetic azo dye.

Restrictions and Adverse Effects: Harmful or irritant if in contact with the mucous membranes of the eyelids, mouth, nose, respiratory tract, or genitals. EU regulations prohibit its use in any product intended for use on or near these areas. FDA regulations allow it to be used in any externally applied cosmetic except eye products. See *A–Z of Cosmetic Terms – Azo Dyes*.

Usage: EU/USA

CI 15850 (D&C Red #6 and D&C Red #7)

D&C Red #6 is the disodium salt of this azo dye (Pigment Red 57), while D&C Red #7 is the lake (insoluble calcium salt – Pigment Red 57:1)

Function: Red colorant.

Origin: Synthetic azo dye.

Restrictions and Adverse Effects: Allowed in all products except eye products sold in the USA. See *A–Z of Cosmetic Terms – Azo Dyes*.

Usage: EU/USA

CI 15865

Function: Red colorant.

Origin: Synthetic azo dye.

Restrictions and Adverse Effects: Allowed in all products. See *A–Z of Cosmetic Terms – Azo Dyes*.

Usage: EU/USA

CI 15865:4

Function: Red colorant.

Origin: Synthetic azo dye.

Restrictions and Adverse Effects: Allowed in all products. See *A–Z of Cosmetic Terms – Azo Dyes*.

Usage: EU/USA

CI 15880 (D&C Red #34)

(Pigment Red 63:1)

Function: Red colorant.

Origin: Synthetic azo dye.

Restrictions and Adverse Effects: Allowed in all products sold in the EU. FDA regulations allow it in all externally applied cosmetics except eye products. See *A–Z of Cosmetic Terms – Azo Dyes*.

Usage: EU/USA

CI 15980

(E111)

Function: Orange colorant.

Origin: Synthetic azo dye.

Restrictions and Adverse Effects: Allowed in all products. See *A–Z of Cosmetic Terms – Azo Dyes*.

Usage: EU/USA

CI 15985 (FD&C Yellow #6)

(E110, Sunset Yellow)

Function: Yellow colorant.

Origin: Synthetic azo dye.

Restrictions and Adverse Effects: Allowed in all products except eye products sold in the USA. See *A–Z of Cosmetic Terms – Azo Dyes*.

Usage: EU/USA

CI 15985:1

Function: Red colorant.

Origin: Synthetic azo dye.

Restrictions and Adverse Effects: Allowed in all products. See *A–Z of Cosmetic Terms – Azo Dyes*.

Usage: EU/USA

CI 16035 (FD&C Red #40)

(Allura Red, Food Red 17)

Function: Red colorant.

Origin: Synthetic azo dye.

Restrictions and Adverse Effects: Allowed in all products. See *A–Z of Cosmetic Terms – Azo Dyes*.

Usage: EU/USA

CI 16185

(E123, Amaranth)

Function: Red colorant.

Origin: Synthetic azo dye.

Restrictions and Adverse Effects: Allowed in all products. See *A–Z of Cosmetic Terms – Azo Dyes*.

Usage: EU/USA

CI 16185:1

(E123, Amaranth)

Function: Red colorant.

Origin: Synthetic azo dye.

Restrictions and Adverse Effects: Allowed in all products. See *A–Z of Cosmetic Terms – Azo Dyes*.

Usage: EU/USA

CI 16230

Function: Orange colorant.

Origin: Synthetic azo dye.

Restrictions and Adverse Effects: Harmful or irritant if in contact with the mucous membranes of the eyelids, mouth, nose, respiratory tract, or genitals. It is not allowed in any product intended for use on or near these areas. See *A–Z of Cosmetic Terms – Azo Dyes*.

Usage: EU/USA

CI 16255

(E124)

Function: Red colorant.

Origin: Synthetic azo dye.

Restrictions and Adverse Effects: Allowed in all products. See *A–Z of Cosmetic Terms – Azo Dyes*.

Usage: EU/USA

CI 16290

(E126)

Function: Red colorant.

Origin: Synthetic azo dye.

Restrictions and Adverse Effects: Allowed in all products. See *A–Z of Cosmetic Terms – Azo Dyes*.

Usage: EU/USA

CI 17200 (D&C Red #31)

(Acid Red 33)

Function: Red colorant.

Origin: Synthetic azo dye.

Restrictions and Adverse Effects: Allowed in all products sold in the EU. FDA regulations allow it in all externally applied cosmetics except eye products, but limit it to 3 percent of the finished product in oral care preparations and lip cosmetics. See *A–Z of Cosmetic Terms – Azo Dyes*.

Usage: EU/USA

CI 18050

Function: Red colorant.

Origin: Synthetic azo dye.

Restrictions and Adverse Effects: Harmful or irritant if in contact with the mucous membranes of the eyelids, mouth, nose, respiratory tract, or genitals. It is not allowed in any product intended for use on or near these areas. See *A–Z of Cosmetic Terms – Azo Dyes*.

Usage: EU/USA

CI 18130

Function: Red colorant.

Origin: Synthetic azo dye.

Restrictions and Adverse Effects: Harmful or irritant by prolonged contact with the skin. It is only allowed in products that are rinsed off immediately after use. See *A–Z of Cosmetic Terms – Azo Dyes*.

Usage: EU/USA

CI 18690

Function: Yellow colorant.

Origin: Synthetic azo dye containing chromates.

Restrictions and Adverse Effects: Harmful or irritant by prolonged contact with the skin. Chromates cause contact allergies and contact dermatitis. It is

only allowed in products that are rinsed off immediately after use. See *A–Z of Cosmetic Terms – Azo Dyes*.
Usage: EU/USA

CI 18736

Function: Red colorant.
Origin: Synthetic azo dye containing chromates.
Restrictions and Adverse Effects: Harmful or irritant by prolonged contact with the skin. Chromates cause contact allergies and contact dermatitis. It is only allowed in products that are rinsed off immediately after use. See *A–Z of Cosmetic Terms – Azo Dyes*.
Usage: EU/USA

CI 18820

Function: Yellow colorant.
Origin: Synthetic azo dye.
Restrictions and Adverse Effects: Harmful or irritant by prolonged contact with the skin. It is only allowed in products that are rinsed off immediately after use. See *A–Z of Cosmetic Terms – Azo Dyes*.
Usage: EU/USA

CI 18965

Function: Yellow colorant.
Origin: Synthetic azo dye.
Restrictions and Adverse Effects: Allowed in all products. See *A–Z of Cosmetic Terms – Azo Dyes*.
Usage: EU/USA

CI 19140 (FD&C Yellow #5)

(E102, Tartrazine)
Function: Yellow colorant.
Origin: Synthetic azo dye.
Restrictions and Adverse Effects: Allowed in all products except eye products sold in the USA. See *A–Z of Cosmetic Terms – Azo Dyes*.
Usage: EU/USA

CI 19140:1

Function: Yellow colorant.
Origin: Synthetic azo dye.
Restrictions and Adverse Effects: Allowed in all products. See *A–Z of Cosmetic Terms – Azo Dyes*.
Usage: EU/USA

CI 20040

Function: Yellow colorant.
Origin: Synthetic azo dye.
Restrictions and Adverse Effects: Harmful or irritant by prolonged contact with the skin. It is only allowed in products that are rinsed off immediately after use. It is known to contain a harmful impurity (3,3'-dimethylbenzidine), which must be reduced to 5 ppm or less, before use. See *A–Z of Cosmetic Terms – Azo Dyes*.
Usage: EU/USA

CI 20170

Function: Orange colorant.
Origin: Synthetic azo dye.
Restrictions and Adverse Effects: Harmful or irritant if in contact with the mucous membranes of the eyelids, mouth, nose, respiratory tract, or genitals. It is not allowed in any product intended for use on or near these areas. See *A–Z of Cosmetic Terms – Azo Dyes*.
Usage: EU/USA

CI 20470

Function: Black colorant.
Origin: Synthetic azo dye.
Restrictions and Adverse Effects: Harmful or irritant by prolonged contact with the skin. It is only allowed in products that are rinsed off immediately after use. See *A–Z of Cosmetic Terms – Azo Dyes*.
Usage: EU/USA

CI 21100

Function: Yellow colorant.
Origin: Synthetic azo dye.
Restrictions and Adverse Effects: Harmful or irritant by prolonged contact with the skin. It is only allowed in products that are rinsed off immediately after use. It is known to contain a harmful impurity (3,3'-dimethylbenzidine), which must be reduced to 5 ppm or less, before use. See *A–Z of Cosmetic Terms – Azo Dyes*.
Usage: EU/USA

CI 21108

Function: Yellow colorant.

Origin: Synthetic azo dye.

Restrictions and Adverse Effects: Harmful or irritant if in contact with the mucous membranes of the eyelids, mouth, nose, respiratory tract, or genitals. It is not allowed in any product intended for use on or near these areas. It is known to contain a harmful impurity (3,3'-dimethylbenzidine), which must be reduced to 5 ppm or less, before use. See *A–Z of Cosmetic Terms – Azo Dyes.*

Usage: EU/USA

CI 21230

Function: Yellow colorant.

Origin: Synthetic azo dye.

Restrictions and Adverse Effects: Harmful or irritant if in contact with the mucous membranes of the eyelids, mouth, nose, respiratory tract, or genitals. It is not allowed in any product intended for use on or near these areas. See *A–Z of Cosmetic Terms – Azo Dyes.*

Usage: EU/USA

CI 24790

Function: Red colorant.

Origin: Synthetic azo dye.

Restrictions and Adverse Effects: Harmful or irritant if in contact with the mucous membranes of the eyelids, mouth, nose, respiratory tract, or genitals. It is not allowed in any product intended for use on or near these areas. See *A–Z of Cosmetic Terms – Azo Dyes.*

Usage: EU/USA

CI 26100 (D&C Red #17)

(Solvent Red 23)

Function: Red colorant.

Origin: Synthetic azo dye.

Restrictions and Adverse Effects: Harmful or irritant to eyes. EU regulations prohibit its use in any product intended for use on or near the eyes. FDA regulations allow this colorant to be used in any externally applied cosmetic except eye products. This colorant is known to contain five harmful impurities

which must be reduced to EU-specified levels before use. See *A–Z of Cosmetic Terms – Azo Dyes.*

Usage: EU/USA

CI 27290

Function: Red colorant.

Origin: Synthetic azo dye.

Restrictions and Adverse Effects: Harmful or irritant by prolonged contact with the skin. It is only allowed in products that are rinsed off immediately after use. See *A–Z of Cosmetic Terms – Azo Dyes.*

Usage: EU/USA

CI 27755

(E152)

Function: Black colorant.

Origin: Synthetic azo dye.

Restrictions and Adverse Effects: Allowed in all products. See *A–Z of Cosmetic Terms – Azo Dyes.*

Usage: EU/USA

CI 28440

(E151)

Function: Black colorant.

Origin: Synthetic azo dye.

Restrictions and Adverse Effects: Harmful or irritant by prolonged contact with the skin. It is only allowed in products that are rinsed off immediately after use. See *A–Z of Cosmetic Terms – Azo Dyes.*

Usage: EU/USA

CI 40215

Function: Orange colorant.

Origin: Synthetic azo dye.

Restrictions and Adverse Effects: Harmful or irritant by prolonged contact with the skin. It is only allowed in products that are rinsed off immediately after use. See *A–Z of Cosmetic Terms – Azo Dyes.*

Usage: EU/USA

CI 40800

(Beta-carotene)

Function: Orange colorant.

Origin: Natural plant colorant.

Restrictions and Adverse Effects: Allowed in all products. No known adverse effects.
Usage: EU/USA

CI 40820
(E160e)
Function: Orange colorant.
Origin: Natural plant colorant.
Restrictions and Adverse Effects: Allowed in all products. No known adverse effects.
Usage: EU/USA

CI 40825
(E160f)
Function: Orange colorant.
Origin: Natural plant colorant.
Restrictions and Adverse Effects: Allowed in all products. No known adverse effects.
Usage: EU/USA

CI 40850
(E160g)
Function: Orange colorant.
Origin: Natural plant colorant.
Restrictions and Adverse Effects: Allowed in all products. No known adverse effects.
Usage: EU/USA

CI 42045
Function: Blue colorant.
Origin: Synthetic coal tar dye.
Restrictions and Adverse Effects: Harmful or irritant if in contact with the mucous membranes of the eyelids, mouth, nose, respiratory tract, or genitals. It is not allowed in any product intended for use on or near these areas.
Usage: EU/USA

CI 42051
(E131, Patent Blue V)
Function: Blue colorant.
Origin: Synthetic coal tar dye.
Restrictions and Adverse Effects: Allowed in all products. Can cause skin sensitivity, itching, urticaria (nettle rash or hives), breathing difficulties, nausea, lowered blood pressure and shock. This colorant should be avoided by people with a history of allergies.
Usage: EU/USA

CI 42053 (FD&C Green #3)
(Fast Green FCF)
Function: Green colorant.
Origin: Synthetic coal tar dye.
Restrictions and Adverse Effects: Allowed in all products except eye products sold in the USA.
Usage: EU/USA

CI 42080
Function: Blue colorant.
Origin: Synthetic coal tar dye.
Restrictions and Adverse Effects: Harmful or irritant by prolonged contact with the skin. It is only allowed in products that are rinsed off immediately after use.
Usage: EU/USA

CI 42090 (FD&C Blue #1)
(E133, Brilliant Blue FCF)
Function: Blue colorant.
Origin: Synthetic coal tar dye.
Restrictions and Adverse Effects: Allowed in all products.
Usage: EU/USA

CI 42100
Function: Green colorant.
Origin: Synthetic coal tar dye.
Restrictions and Adverse Effects: Harmful or irritant by prolonged contact with the skin. It is only allowed in products that are rinsed off immediately after use.
Usage: EU/USA

CI 42170
Function: Green colorant.
Origin: Synthetic coal tar dye.
Restrictions and Adverse Effects: Harmful or irritant by prolonged contact with the skin. It is only allowed in products that are rinsed off immediately after use.
Usage: EU/USA

CI 42510

(Fuchsin)

Function: Violet colorant.

Origin: Synthetic coal tar dye.

Restrictions and Adverse Effects: Harmful or irritant if in contact with the mucous membranes of the eyelids, mouth, nose, respiratory tract, or genitals. It is not allowed in any product intended for use on or near these areas.

Usage: EU/USA

CI 42520

Function: Violet colorant.

Origin: Synthetic coal tar dye.

Restrictions and Adverse Effects: Harmful or irritant by prolonged contact with the skin. It is only allowed in products that are rinsed off immediately after use, and is limited to a maximum of 5 ppm in the finished product.

Usage: EU/USA

CI 42735

Function: Blue colorant.

Origin: Synthetic coal tar dye.

Restrictions and Adverse Effects: Harmful or irritant if in contact with the mucous membranes of the eyelids, mouth, nose, respiratory tract, or genitals. It is not allowed in any product intended for use on or near these areas.

Usage: EU/USA

CI 44045

Function: Blue colorant.

Origin: Synthetic coal tar dye.

Restrictions and Adverse Effects: Harmful or irritant if in contact with the mucous membranes of the eyelids, mouth, nose, respiratory tract, or genitals. It is not allowed in any product intended for use on or near these areas.

Usage: EU/USA

CI 44090

(E142, Green S, Acid Brilliant Green BS, Lissamine Green)

Function: Green colorant.

Origin: Synthetic coal tar dye.

Restrictions and Adverse Effects: Allowed in all products. No known adverse effects.

Usage: EU/USA

CI 45100

Function: Red colorant.

Origin: Synthetic coal tar dye.

Restrictions and Adverse Effects: Harmful or irritant by prolonged contact with the skin. It is only allowed in products that are rinsed off immediately after use.

Usage: EU/USA

CI 45190

Function: Violet colorant.

Origin: Synthetic coal tar dye.

Restrictions and Adverse Effects: Harmful or irritant by prolonged contact with the skin. It is only allowed in products that are rinsed off immediately after use.

Usage: EU/USA

CI 45220

Function: Red colorant.

Origin: Synthetic coal tar dye.

Restrictions and Adverse Effects: Harmful or irritant by prolonged contact with the skin. It is only allowed in products that are rinsed off immediately after use.

Usage: EU/USA

CI 45350 (D&C Yellow #8)

(Fluorescein sodium, Acid Yellow 73)

Function: Yellow colorant.

Origin: Synthetic coal tar dye.

Restrictions and Adverse Effects: Allowed in all products sold in the EU up to a maximum content of 6 percent of the finished product. FDA regulations allow D&C Yellow #8 to be used in all externally applied cosmetics with no concentration limit except eye products.

Usage: EU/USA

CI 45350:1 (D&C Yellow #7)

(Fluorescein, Solvent Yellow 94)

Function: Yellow colorant.

Origin: Synthetic coal tar dye.

Restrictions and Adverse Effects: FDA regulations allow D&C Yellow #7 to be used in all externally applied cosmetics with no concentration limit except eye products.

Usage: USA/Not currently on the EU inventory of cosmetic ingredients.

CI 45370

Function: Orange colorant.
Origin: Synthetic coal tar dye.
Restrictions and Adverse Effects: Allowed in all products. This colorant is known to contain two harmful impurities which must be reduced to EU-specified levels before use.
Usage: EU/USA

CI 45370

Function: Orange colorant.
Origin: Synthetic coal tar dye containing zirconium, derived from CI 45370 above and given the same color index number.
Restrictions and Adverse Effects: This colorant is known to contain two harmful impurities which must be reduced to EU-specified levels before use. Zirconium salts cause lung damage and granulomas, and are prohibited from aerosols in the EU and USA.
Usage: EU/USA

CI 45380

(Acid Red 87, Eosin)
Function: Red colorant.
Origin: Synthetic dye.
Restrictions and Adverse Effects: Allowed in all products. This colorant is known to contain two harmful impurities which must be reduced to EU-specified levels before use. May cause photosensitivity.
Usage: EU/USA

CI 45380

Function: Red colorant.
Origin: Synthetic dye containing zirconium, derived from CI 45380 above and given the same color index number.
Restrictions and Adverse Effects: This colorant is known to contain two harmful impurities which must

be reduced to EU-specified levels before use. Zirconium salts cause lung damage and granulomas, and are prohibited from aerosols in the EU and USA.
Usage: EU/USA

CI 45396

Function: Orange colorant.
Origin: Synthetic coal tar dye.
Restrictions and Adverse Effects: Allowed in all products. This colorant is known to contain two harmful impurities which must be reduced to EU-specified levels before use.
Usage: EU/USA

CI 45405

Function: Red colorant.
Origin: Synthetic dye.
Restrictions and Adverse Effects: Harmful or irritant to eyes. It is not allowed in any product intended for use on or near the eyes. This colorant is known to contain two harmful impurities which must be reduced to EU-specified levels before use.
Usage: EU/USA

CI 45410 (D&C Red #27 and D&C Red #28)

D&C Red #27 is essentially CI 45410 (Solvent Red 28) while D&C Red #28 is the disodium salt of CI 45410 (Acid Red 92)
Function: Red colorant.
Origin: Synthetic dye.
Restrictions and Adverse Effects: Allowed in all products. This colorant is known to contain two harmful impurities which must be reduced to EU-specified levels before use. FDA regulations allow these in all cosmetics except eye products.
Usage: EU/USA

CI 45410

Function: Red colorant.
Origin: Synthetic dye containing zirconium, derived from CI 45410 above and given the same color index number.
Restrictions and Adverse Effects: This colorant is known to contain two harmful impurities which must be reduced to EU-specified levels before use.

Zirconium salts cause lung damage and granulomas, and are prohibited from aerosols in the EU and USA.
Usage: EU/USA

CI 45425

Function: Red colorant.
Origin: Synthetic coal tar dye.
Restrictions and Adverse Effects: Allowed in all products. This colorant is known to contain two harmful impurities which must be reduced to EU-specified levels before use.
Usage: EU/USA

CI 45430 (FD&C Red #3)

(E127, Erythrosine)
Function: Red colorant.
Origin: Synthetic coal tar dye.
Restrictions and Adverse Effects: Allowed in all products. This colorant is known to contain two harmful impurities which must be reduced to EU-specified levels before use.
Usage: EU/USA

CI 47000

Function: Yellow colorant.
Origin: Synthetic coal tar dye.
Restrictions and Adverse Effects: Harmful or irritant if in contact with the mucous membranes of the eyelids, mouth, nose, respiratory tract, or genitals. It is not allowed in any product intended for use on or near these areas.
Usage: EU/USA

CI 47005

(E105)
Function: Yellow colorant.
Origin: Synthetic coal tar dye.
Restrictions and Adverse Effects: Allowed in all products.
Usage: EU/USA

CI 50325

Function: Violet colorant.
Origin: Synthetic coal tar dye.

Restrictions and Adverse Effects: Harmful or irritant by prolonged contact with the skin. It is only allowed in products that are rinsed off immediately after use.
Usage: EU/USA

CI 50420

Function: Black colorant.
Origin: Synthetic coal tar dye.
Restrictions and Adverse Effects: Harmful or irritant if in contact with the mucous membranes of the eyelids, mouth, nose, respiratory tract, or genitals. It is not allowed in any product intended for use on or near these areas.
Usage: EU/USA

CI 51319

Function: Black colorant.
Origin: Synthetic coal tar dye.
Restrictions and Adverse Effects: Harmful or irritant by prolonged contact with the skin. It is only allowed in products that are rinsed off immediately after use.
Usage: EU/USA

CI 58000

Function: Red colorant.
Origin: Synthetic coal tar dye.
Restrictions and Adverse Effects: Allowed in all products.
Usage: EU/USA

CI 59040 (D&C Green #8)

(Solvent Green 7)
Function: Green colorant.
Origin: Synthetic coal tar dye.
Restrictions and Adverse Effects: Harmful or irritant if in contact with the mucous membranes of the eyelids, mouth, nose, respiratory tract, or genitals. EU regulations prohibit it from any product intended for use on or near these areas. FDA regulations limit it to 0.01 percent of the finished product, but allow its use in any externally applied preparation except eye products.
Usage: EU/USA

CI 60724

Function: Violet colorant.

Origin: Synthetic coal tar dye.

Restrictions and Adverse Effects: Harmful or irritant by prolonged contact with the skin. It is only allowed in products that are rinsed off immediately after use.

Usage: EU/USA

CI 60725

Function: Violet colorant.

Origin: Synthetic coal tar dye.

Restrictions and Adverse Effects: Allowed in all products.

Usage: EU/USA

CI 60730 (Ext. D&C Violet #2)

(Acid Violet 43)

Function: Violet colorant.

Origin: Synthetic coal tar dye.

Restrictions and Adverse Effects: Harmful or irritant if in contact with the mucous membranes of the eyelids, mouth, nose, respiratory tract, or genitals. EU regulations prohibit it from any product intended for use on or near these areas. FDA regulations allow its use in any externally applied cosmetic except eye products.

Usage: EU/USA

CI 61565 (D&C Green #6)

(Solvent Green 3)

Function: Green colorant.

Origin: Synthetic coal tar dye.

Restrictions and Adverse Effects: Allowed in all products sold in the EU. In the USA it is allowed in all externally applied cosmetics except eye products.

Usage: EU/USA

CI 61570 (D&C Green #5)

(Acid Green 25)

Function: Green colorant.

Origin: Synthetic coal tar dye.

Restrictions and Adverse Effects: Allowed in all products.

Usage: EU/USA

CI 61585

Function: Blue colorant.

Origin: Synthetic coal tar dye.

Restrictions and Adverse Effects: Harmful or irritant by prolonged contact with the skin. It is only allowed in products that are rinsed off immediately after use.

Usage: EU/USA

CI 62045

Function: Blue colorant.

Origin: Synthetic coal tar dye.

Restrictions and Adverse Effects: Harmful or irritant by prolonged contact with the skin. It is only allowed in products that are rinsed off immediately after use.

Usage: EU/USA

CI 69800

(E130)

Function: Blue colorant.

Origin: Synthetic coal tar dye.

Restrictions and Adverse Effects: Allowed in all products.

Usage: EU/USA

CI 69825 (D&C Blue #9)

Function: Blue colorant.

Origin: Synthetic coal tar dye.

Restrictions and Adverse Effects: Allowed in all products.

Usage: EU/USA

CI 71105

Function: Orange colorant.

Origin: Synthetic coal tar dye.

Restrictions and Adverse Effects: Harmful or irritant if in contact with the mucous membranes of the eyelids, mouth, nose, respiratory tract, or genitals. It is not allowed in any product intended for use on or near these areas.

Usage: EU/USA

CI 73000

Function: Blue colorant.

Origin: Synthetic coal tar dye.

Restrictions and Adverse Effects: Allowed in all products.

Usage: EU/USA

CI 73015 (FD&C Blue #2)

(E132, Indigo carmine, Indigotine)
Function: Blue colorant.
Origin: Synthetic coal tar dye.
Restrictions and Adverse Effects: Irritant. Can cause skin rashes and itching. Allowed in all products.
Usage: EU/USA

CI 73360 (D&C Red #30)

(Vat Red 1)
Function: Red colorant.
Origin: Synthetic coal tar dye.
Restrictions and Adverse Effects: Allowed in all products except eye products sold in the USA.
Usage: EU/USA

CI 73385

Function: Violet colorant.
Origin: Synthetic coal tar dye.
Restrictions and Adverse Effects: Allowed in all products.
Usage: EU/USA

CI 73900

Function: Violet colorant.
Origin: Synthetic coal tar dye.
Restrictions and Adverse Effects: Harmful or irritant by prolonged contact with the skin. It is only allowed in products that are rinsed off immediately after use.
Usage: EU/USA

CI 73915

Function: Red colorant.
Origin: Synthetic coal tar dye.
Restrictions and Adverse Effects: Harmful or irritant by prolonged contact with the skin. It is only allowed in products that are rinsed off immediately after use.
Usage: EU/USA

CI 74100

Function: Blue colorant.
Origin: Synthetic dye related to chlorophyll.
Restrictions and Adverse Effects: Harmful or irritant by prolonged contact with the skin. It is only allowed in products that are rinsed off immediately after use.
Usage: EU/USA

CI 74160

Function: Blue colorant.
Origin: Synthetic dye related to chlorophyll.
Restrictions and Adverse Effects: Allowed in all products.
Usage: EU/USA

CI 74180

Function: Blue colorant.
Origin: Synthetic dye related to chlorophyll.
Restrictions and Adverse Effects: Harmful or irritant by prolonged contact with the skin. It is only allowed in products that are rinsed off immediately after use.
Usage: EU/USA

CI 74260

Function: Green colorant.
Origin: Synthetic dye related to chlorophyll.
Restrictions and Adverse Effects: Harmful or irritant to eyes. It is not allowed in any product intended for use on or near the eyes.
Usage: EU/USA

CI 75100

(Saffron)
Function: Yellow colorant.
Origin: Natural plant (crocus) extract.
Restrictions and Adverse Effects: Allowed in all products.
Usage: EU/USA

CI 75120

(E160b, Annatto, Bixin, Norbixin)
Function: Orange colorant.
Origin: Natural plant dye present in the seed coats of the Annatto tree (Bixa orellana).
Restrictions and Adverse Effects: Allowed in all products.
Usage: EU/USA

CI 75125

(E160d, Lycopene)
Function: Yellow colorant.
Origin: Natural dye extracted from tomatoes.

Restrictions and Adverse Effects: Allowed in all products.
Usage: EU/USA

CI 75130

(E160a, Beta-carotene)
Function: Orange colorant.
Origin: Natural plant dye.
Restrictions and Adverse Effects: Allowed in all products.
Usage: EU/USA

CI 75135

(E161d, Rubixanthin)
Function: Yellow colorant.
Origin: Natural plant dye abundant in rose hips. It is closely related to the food colorant canthaxanthin, which is also color indexed as CI 75135.
Restrictions and Adverse Effects: Allowed in all products.
Usage: EU/USA

CI 75170

Function: White colorant.
Origin: Natural dye – Guanine, a natural substance which is called a base and is an essential component of the DNA molecule.
Restrictions and Adverse Effects: Allowed in all products.
Usage: EU/USA

CI 75300

(E100)
Function: Yellow colorant.
Origin: Natural dye extracted from the turmeric root.
Restrictions and Adverse Effects: Allowed in all products. No known adverse effects.
Usage: EU/USA

CI 75470

(E120, Cochineal, Carminic Acid, Carmine of Cochineal)
Function: Red colorant.
Origin: Modified natural dye.

Restrictions and Adverse Effects: Allowed in all products. Has been linked to hyperactivity in children.
Usage: EU/USA

CI 75810

(E140, Chlorophyll)
Function: Green colorant.
Origin: Natural dye, often impure due to the difficulties in removing other, mainly harmless plant materials.
Restrictions and Adverse Effects: Allowed in all products. No known adverse effects.
Usage: EU/USA

CI 77000

Function: White or silver colorant, often used to give a sparkle to decorative cosmetics.
Origin: Aluminum powder.
Restrictions and Adverse Effects: Allowed in all products.
Usage: EU/USA

CI 77002

Function: White colorant.
Origin: Synthetic compound – Aluminum hydroxide sulfate.
Restrictions and Adverse Effects: Allowed in all products.
Usage: EU/USA

CI 77004

Function: White colorant.
Origin: Purified natural mineral – Bentonite, a colloidal clay containing mainly montmorillonite.
Restrictions and Adverse Effects: Allowed in all products.
Usage: EU/USA

CI 77007

Function: Blue colorant.
Origin: Purified natural mineral.
Restrictions and Adverse Effects: Allowed in all products.
Usage: EU/USA

CI 77015

Function: Red colorant.
Origin: Purified natural mineral – Lazurite.
Restrictions and Adverse Effects: Allowed in all products.
Usage: EU/USA

CI 77120

(Barium sulfate)
Function: White colorant.
Origin: Purified natural mineral. Can be artificially produced.
Restrictions and Adverse Effects: Allowed in all products.
Usage: EU/USA

CI 77163

Function: White colorant.
Origin: Synthetic compound – Bismuth chloride oxide.
Restrictions and Adverse Effects: Allowed in all products. Bismuth compounds are toxic, causing intellectual impairment, memory loss, confusion, loss of coordination (clumsiness), trembling, convulsions, and difficulty in walking.
Usage: EU/USA

CI 77220

(E170, Calcium carbonate)
Function: White colorant.
Origin: Purified natural mineral – Chalk or Marble. Can be artificially produced.
Restrictions and Adverse Effects: Allowed in all products.
Usage: EU/USA

CI 77231

(Calcium Sulfate, Gypsum)
Function: White colorant.
Origin: Purified natural mineral – Gypsum. Can be artificially produced.
Restrictions and Adverse Effects: Allowed in all products.
Usage: EU/USA

CI 77266

(Carbon black)
Function: Black colorant.
Origin: Soot produced by burning hydrocarbons in a limited supply of air.
Restrictions and Adverse Effects: Allowed in all products. Carcinogens have been found in carbon black obtained by the combustion of petroleum products.
Usage: EU/USA

CI 77267

Function: Black colorant.
Origin: Bone charcoal. A fine black powder obtained by burning animal bones in a closed container. It consists primarily of calcium phosphate and carbon.
Restrictions and Adverse Effects: Allowed in all products.
Usage: EU/USA

CI 77268:1

(E153)
Function: Black colorant.
Origin: Finely ground coke or charcoal from animal origin (carbon).
Restrictions and Adverse Effects: Allowed in all products. Banned as a food additive in the USA as it has been linked to cancer.
Usage: EU/USA

CI 77288

(Dichromium trioxide, Chromium (III) oxide, Chromic oxide)
Function: Green colorant.
Origin: Synthetic compound containing chromium, closely related to CI 77289 below, but with different physical characteristics.
Restrictions and Adverse Effects: Allowed in all products. This dye must be free from chromate ions before use. Chromates cause contact allergies and contact dermatitis.
Usage: EU/USA

CI 77289

(Dichromium trioxide, Chromium (III) oxide, Chromic oxide)

Function: Green colorant.

Origin: Synthetic compound containing chromium, closely related to CI 77288 above, but with different physical characteristics.

Restrictions and Adverse Effects: Allowed in all products. This dye must be free from chromate ions before use. Chromates cause contact allergies and contact dermatitis.

Usage: EU/USA

CI 77346

Function: Green colorant.

Origin: Synthetic dye related to chlorophyll.

Restrictions and Adverse Effects: Allowed in all products.

Usage: EU/USA

CI 77400

Function: Brown colorant.

Origin: Finely ground copper.

Restrictions and Adverse Effects: Allowed in all products.

Usage: EU/USA

CI 77480

(E175)

Function: Brown colorant. Can give a gold sparkle to decorative cosmetics.

Origin: Finely ground gold.

Restrictions and Adverse Effects: Allowed in all products.

Usage: EU/USA

CI 77489

(E172 – Orange)

Function: Orange colorant.

Origin: Purified oxide of iron.

Restrictions and Adverse Effects: Allowed in all products.

Usage: EU/USA

CI 77491

(E172 – Red)

Function: Red colorant.

Origin: Purified oxide of iron.

Restrictions and Adverse Effects: Allowed in all products.

Usage: EU/USA

CI 77492

(E172 – Yellow)

Function: Yellow colorant.

Origin: Purified oxide of iron.

Restrictions and Adverse Effects: Allowed in all products.

Usage: EU/USA

CI 77499

(E172 – Black)

Function: Black colorant.

Origin: Purified oxide of iron.

Restrictions and Adverse Effects: Allowed in all products.

Usage: EU/USA

CI 77510

(Prussian Blue)

Function: Blue colorant.

Origin: Synthetic compound made from iron salts and cyanide.

Restrictions and Adverse Effects: Allowed in all products. Contains cyanide as a by-product of manufacture, which must be removed before use.

Usage: EU/USA

CI 77713

Function: White colorant.

Origin: Natural mineral – Magnesium carbonate, often produced artificially.

Restrictions and Adverse Effects: Allowed in all products.

Usage: EU/USA

CI 77742

Function: Violet colorant.

Origin: Ammonium manganese diphosphate, produced artificially.

Restrictions and Adverse Effects: Allowed in all products.
Usage: EU/USA

CI 77745

Function: Red colorant.
Origin: Natural mineral containing manganese phosphates, often produced artificially.
Restrictions and Adverse Effects: Allowed in all products.
Usage: EU/USA

CI 77820

(E174 – Silver)
Function: White or silver colorant used to give a sparkle to decorative cosmetics such as nail polish.
Origin: Finely ground silver.
Restrictions and Adverse Effects: Allowed in all products sold in the EU. FDA regulations limit it to 1 percent of the finished product.
Usage: EU/USA

CI 77891

(E171 – Titanium dioxide)
Function: White colorant.
Origin: Natural mineral (rutile), often produced artificially.
Restrictions and Adverse Effects: Allowed in all products.
Usage: EU/USA

CI 77947

(Zinc oxide)
Function: White colorant.
Origin: Synthetic compound.
Restrictions and Adverse Effects: Allowed in all products.
Usage: EU/USA

Cinnamal

(Cinnamaldehyde)
Function: Denaturant.
Origin: Synthetic compound.
Restrictions and Adverse Effects: Can cause contact dermatitis.
Usage: EU/USA

Cinoxate

(2-ethoxyethyl-p-methoxy cinnamate)
Function: UV absorber.
Origin: Synthetic compound.
Restrictions and Adverse Effects: Can cause photosensitivity. Cinnamates have been reported to cause a stinging sensation in some people.
Usage: EU/USA

Citric acid

Function: pH control / Chelating agent / Exfoliating agent.
Citric acid can enhance the effectiveness of some antioxidants, thereby reducing the amount of these chemicals added to cosmetics.
Origin: Natural extract of citrus fruits.
Restrictions and Adverse Effects: Citric acid is an alpha-hydroxy acid (AHA) used to exfoliate skin (a skin peeler that removes the outer layer of skin cells). AHAs can cause increased sensitivity to the sun. Do not expose skin to the sun immediately following treatment with AHAs. Test a small area before use and discontinue use if skin irritation, redness, bleeding, or pain is experienced. Not recommended for use on children. May cause exfoliative dermatitis.
Usage: EU/USA

Citrus bergamia

(Bergamot oil)
Function: Botanical additive / Aromatherapy oil.
Origin: Plant extract.
Restrictions and Adverse Effects: Can cause contact dermatitis in some individuals.
Usage: EU/USA

Citrus limonum

(Lemon oil)
Function: Botanical additive.
Origin: Plant extract.
Restrictions and Adverse Effects: Can cause dermatitis, phototoxicity and pigmented contact dermatitis.
Usage: EU/USA

Climbazole

Function: Preservative.
Origin: Synthetic compound.
Restrictions and Adverse Effects: Limited to 0.5 percent of the finished product if used as a preservative, but may be added in larger quantities for other stated purposes.
Usage: EU/USA

Coal tar

Function: Antidandruff agent.
Available in the UK from a qualified pharmacist.
Origin: Extract of coal.
Restrictions and Adverse Effects: Reported to have comedogenic properties (see *A–Z of Cosmetic Terms – Comedogen*). Long term, low level exposure to coal tar has been linked to cancer. For this reason regular use of coal tar shampoos and antidandruff treatments should be avoided.
Usage: USA/Crude and refined coal tar are both banned for general use in the EU.

Cobalt

Function: Colorant.
Origin: A heavy metal.
Restrictions and Adverse Effects: May cause contact dermatitis in some individuals.
Usage: USA/Not currently on the EU inventory of cosmetic ingredients.

Cocamide DEA

Function: Emulsifier / Emulsion stabilizer / Surfactant / Viscosity adjuster / Foaming agent.
Origin: Semisynthetic compound derived from coconut oil obtained from the kernels of palm trees.
Restrictions and Adverse Effects: May cause contact allergies and contact dermatitis in some individuals. DEA residues are cancer suspects currently under investigation. See *A–Z of Cosmetic Terms – DEA; Nitrosamines*.
Usage: EU/USA

Cocamide MEA

Function: Emulsifier / Emulsion stabilizer / Surfactant / Viscosity adjuster.
Origin: Semisynthetic compound derived from coconut oil obtained from the kernels of palm trees.
Restrictions and Adverse Effects: May cause contact allergies and contact dermatitis in some individuals. See *A–Z of Cosmetic Terms – Nitrosamines*.
Usage: EU/USA

Cocamide MIPA

Function: Emulsifier / Emulsion stabilizer / Surfactant / Viscosity adjuster.
Origin: Semisynthetic compound derived from coconut oil obtained from the kernels of palm trees.
Restrictions and Adverse Effects: May cause contact allergies and contact dermatitis in some individuals. See *A–Z of Cosmetic Terms – Nitrosamines*.
Usage: EU/USA

Cocamidoethyl betaine

Function: Surfactant / Foaming agent.
Origin: Semisynthetic compound derived from coconut oil obtained from the kernels of palm trees.
Restrictions and Adverse Effects: May cause contact allergies and reported to cause eyelid contact dermatitis in some individuals. See *A–Z of Cosmetic Terms – Nitrosamines*.
Usage: EU/USA

Cocamidopropyl betaine

Function: Surfactant / Foaming agent.
Origin: Semisynthetic compound derived from coconut oil obtained from the kernels of palm trees.
Restrictions and Adverse Effects: May cause contact allergies and contact dermatitis in some individuals. See *A–Z of Cosmetic Terms – Nitrosamines*.
Usage: EU/USA

Cocamidopropyl dimethylamine

Function: Antistatic agent / Emulsifier / Surfactant.
Origin: Semisynthetic compound derived from coconut oil obtained from the kernels of palm trees.
Restrictions and Adverse Effects: May cause contact allergies and contact dermatitis in some

individuals. See *A–Z of Cosmetic Terms – Nitrosamines*.
Usage: EU/USA

Cocamidopropyl dimethylamine dihydroxymethylpropionate

Function: Surfactant.
Origin: Semisynthetic compound derived from coconut oil obtained from the kernels of palm trees.
Restrictions and Adverse Effects: See *A–Z of Cosmetic Terms – Nitrosamines*.
Usage: EU/USA

Cocamidopropyl dimethylamine hydrolysed collagen

Function: Antistatic agent / Surfactant.
Origin: Semisynthetic compound derived from coconut oil obtained from the kernels of palm trees and collagen, a protein obtained from animals.
Restrictions and Adverse Effects: See *A–Z of Cosmetic Terms – Nitrosamines*.
Usage: EU/USA

Cocamidopropyl dimethylamine lactate

Function: Surfactant.
Origin: Semisynthetic compound derived from coconut oil obtained from the kernels of palm trees.
Restrictions and Adverse Effects: See *A–Z of Cosmetic Terms – Nitrosamines*.
Usage: EU/USA

Cocamidopropyl dimethylamine propionate

Function: Antistatic agent / Surfactant.
Origin: Semisynthetic compound derived from coconut oil obtained from the kernels of palm trees.
Restrictions and Adverse Effects: See *A–Z of Cosmetic Terms – Nitrosamines*.
Usage: EU/USA

Cocamidopropyl dimethylaminohydroxypropyl hydrolysed collagen

Function: Antistatic agent / Surfactant.

Origin: Semisynthetic compound derived from coconut oil obtained from the kernels of palm trees and collagen, a protein obtained from animals.
Restrictions and Adverse Effects: See *A–Z of Cosmetic Terms – Nitrosamines*.
Usage: EU/USA

Cocamidopropyl dimethylammonium C8-16 isoalkylsuccinyl lactoglobulin sulfonate

Function: Antistatic agent / Surfactant.
Origin: Semisynthetic compound derived from coconut oil obtained from the kernels of palm trees, petroleum, and milk proteins.
Restrictions and Adverse Effects: See *A–Z of Cosmetic Terms – Nitrosamines*.
Usage: EU/USA

Cocamidopropyl ethyldimonium ethosulfate

Function: Antistatic agent.
Origin: Semisynthetic compound derived from coconut oil obtained from the kernels of palm trees.
Restrictions and Adverse Effects: See *A–Z of Cosmetic Terms – Nitrosamines*.
Usage: EU/USA

Cocamidopropyl hydroxysultaine

Function: Surfactant.
Origin: Semisynthetic compound derived from coconut oil obtained from the kernels of palm trees.
Restrictions and Adverse Effects: See *A–Z of Cosmetic Terms – Nitrosamines*.
Usage: EU/USA

Cocamidopropyl lauryl ether

Function: Emulsifier / Emulsion stabilizer / Surfactant.
Origin: Semisynthetic compound derived from coconut oil obtained from the kernels of palm trees and other vegetable oils.
Restrictions and Adverse Effects: See *A–Z of Cosmetic Terms – Nitrosamines*.
Usage: EU/USA

Cocamidopropyl morpholine

Function: Antistatic agent.
Origin: Semisynthetic compound derived from coconut oil obtained from the kernels of palm trees.
Restrictions and Adverse Effects: See *A–Z of Cosmetic Terms – Nitrosamines.*
Usage: EU/USA

Cocamidopropyl morpholine lactate

Function: Antistatic agent.
Origin: Semisynthetic compound derived from coconut oil obtained from the kernels of palm trees.
Restrictions and Adverse Effects: See *A–Z of Cosmetic Terms – Nitrosamines.*
Usage: EU/USA

Cocamidopropyl PG-dimonium chloride

Function: Antistatic agent.
Origin: Semisynthetic compound derived from coconut oil obtained from the kernels of palm trees.
Restrictions and Adverse Effects: See *A–Z of Cosmetic Terms – Nitrosamines.*
Usage: EU/USA

Cocamidopropyl PG-dimonium chloride phosphate

Function: Antistatic agent.
Origin: Semisynthetic compound derived from coconut oil obtained from the kernels of palm trees.
Restrictions and Adverse Effects: See *A–Z of Cosmetic Terms – Nitrosamines.*
Usage: EU/USA

Cocamidopropylamine oxide

Function: Surfactant.
Origin: Semisynthetic compound derived from coconut oil obtained from the kernels of palm trees.
Restrictions and Adverse Effects: See *A–Z of Cosmetic Terms – Nitrosamines.*
Usage: EU/USA

Cocamidopropyldimonium hydroxypropyl hydrolysed collagen

Function: Antistatic agent / Surfactant.
Origin: Semisynthetic compound derived from coconut oil obtained from the kernels of palm trees and collagen, a protein derived from animals.
Restrictions and Adverse Effects: See *A–Z of Cosmetic Terms – Nitrosamines.*
Usage: EU/USA

Cocamidopropyltrimonium chloride

Function: Antistatic agent.
Origin: Semisynthetic compound derived from coconut oil obtained from the kernels of palm trees.
Restrictions and Adverse Effects: See *A–Z of Cosmetic Terms – Nitrosamines.*
Usage: EU/USA

Cocamine

Function: Emulsifier.
Origin: Semisynthetic compound derived from coconut oil obtained from the kernels of palm trees.
Restrictions and Adverse Effects: See *A–Z of Cosmetic Terms – Nitrosamines.*
Usage: EU/USA

Cocamine oxide

Function: Antistatic agent / Surfactant.
Origin: Semisynthetic compound derived from coconut oil obtained from the kernels of palm trees.
Restrictions and Adverse Effects: See *A–Z of Cosmetic Terms – Nitrosamines.*
Usage: EU/USA

Cocaminobutyric acid

Function: Emollient / Moisturizer / Surfactant.
Origin: Semisynthetic compound derived from coconut oil obtained from the kernels of palm trees.
Restrictions and Adverse Effects: See *A–Z of Cosmetic Terms – Nitrosamines.*
Usage: EU/USA

Cocaminopropionic acid

Function: Emollient / Moisturizer / Surfactant.
Origin: Semisynthetic compound derived from coconut oil obtained from the kernels of palm trees.
Restrictions and Adverse Effects: See *A–Z of Cosmetic Terms – Nitrosamines.*
Usage: EU/USA

Coco-betaine

Function: Surfactant.
Origin: Semisynthetic compound derived from coconut oil obtained from the kernels of palm trees.
Restrictions and Adverse Effects: No currently known adverse effects.
Usage: EU/USA

Cocodiethanolimide

Function: Emulsifier.
Origin: Semisynthetic compound derived from coconut oil obtained from the kernels of palm trees.
Restrictions and Adverse Effects: No currently known adverse effects.
Usage: USA/Not currently on the EU inventory of cosmetic ingredients.

Coconut acid

Function: Emollient / Moisturizer / Emulsifier / Surfactant.
Origin: Natural extract derived from coconut oil obtained from the kernels of palm trees.
Restrictions and Adverse Effects: Skin irritant in some people. Sensitive people are advised to have a patch test carried out or, at the very least, test the product on a small area before using it.
Usage: EU/USA

Cocos nucifera

(Coconut oil)
Function: Emollient / Moisturizer / Solvent.
Origin: Natural extract obtained from the kernels of palm trees.
Restrictions and Adverse Effects: Skin irritant in some people.
Usage: EU/USA

Cocoyl sarcosinamide DEA

Function: Surfactant.
Origin: Semisynthetic compound derived from coconut oil obtained from the kernels of palm trees.
Restrictions and Adverse Effects: DEA residues are cancer suspects currently under investigation. See *A–Z of Cosmetic Terms – DEA.*
Usage: EU/USA

Collagen / Elastin

Function: Moisture binder.
Credited with the ability to keep skin soft and supple.
Origin: An animal protein, extracted from the layers of skin and artery walls of mammals.
Restrictions and Adverse Effects: No currently known adverse effects. For BSE precautions see *Chapter 17 – Animal Products and Animal Testing.*
Usage: USA/Not currently on the EU inventory of cosmetic ingredients.

Cornflower extract

(Cornflower Distillate)
Function: Botanical additive.
Origin: Natural extract of the cornflower, *Centaurea cyanus.* (Not to be confused with cornflour or corn starch. See – *Zea mays.*)
Restrictions and Adverse Effects: Can cause allergic reactions and photosensitivity.
Usage: EU/USA

Coumarin

(Cumarin, Benzopyrone)
Function: Additive.
Origin: Synthetic compound.
Restrictions and Adverse Effects: Cancer suspect. Toxic by ingestion. Banned in food products in the USA.
Usage: EU/USA

Cycloheximide

Function: Additive.
Origin: Synthetic compound.
Restrictions and Adverse Effects: Toxic. Inhibits skin cell metabolism.
Usage: USA/Not currently on the EU inventory of cosmetic ingredients.

Cyclohexylamine

(Aminocyclohexane)
Function: Additive.
Origin: Synthetic compound.
Restrictions and Adverse Effects: Corrosive liquid causing skin burns. Irritant in low concentrations

Harmful by skin absorption, ingestion, and inhalation causing irreversible effects.
Usage: USA/Not currently on the EU inventory of cosmetic ingredients.

Cyclomethicone
Function: Antistatic agent / Emollient / Moisturizer / Humectant / Solvent / Viscosity adjuster.
A volatile silicone compound used to reduce the greasy feel of cosmetics.
Origin: Synthetic silicone oil.
Restrictions and Adverse Effects: No currently known adverse effects.
Usage: EU/USA

Cysteine
Function: Antioxidant / Antistatic agent / Reducing agent.
Origin: An amino acid obtained by the hydrolysis of plant and animal proteins.
Restrictions and Adverse Effects: No currently known adverse effects.
Usage: EU/USA

D&C Blue #4
Function: Blue colorant.
Origin: Synthetic coal tar dye.
Restrictions and Adverse Effects: Allowed in all externally applied cosmetics except eye products.
Usage: USA

D&C Brown #1
Function: Brown colorant.
Origin: Synthetic azo dye.
Restrictions and Adverse Effects: Allowed in all externally applied cosmetics except eye products.
See *A–Z of Cosmetic Terms – Azo Dyes*.
Usage: USA

D&C Orange #5
Function: Orange colorant.
Origin: Mixture of synthetic coal tar dyes including CI 45370 (Solvent Red 72) and CI 45380 (Solvent Red 43).
Restrictions and Adverse Effects: Allowed in all externally applied cosmetics except eye products.
Restricted to 5 percent in lip products.
Usage: USA

D&C Orange #10
Function: Orange colorant.
Origin: Mixture of synthetic coal tar dyes including CI 45425 (Solvent Red 73).
Restrictions and Adverse Effects: Allowed in all externally applied cosmetics except eye products.
Usage: USA

D&C Orange #11
Function: Orange colorant.
Origin: Mixture of synthetic coal tar dyes.
Restrictions and Adverse Effects: Allowed in all externally applied cosmetics except eye products.
Usage: USA

D&C Red #21
Function: Red colorant.
Origin: Mixture of synthetic coal tar dyes including CI 45380:2 (Solvent Red 43).
Restrictions and Adverse Effects: Allowed in all cosmetics except eye products.
Usage: USA

D&C Red #22
Function: Red colorant.
Origin: Mixture of synthetic coal tar dyes including CI 45380 (Acid Red 87).
Restrictions and Adverse Effects: Allowed in all cosmetics except eye products.
Usage: USA

D&C Red #39
Function: Red colorant.
Origin: Synthetic azo dye.
Restrictions and Adverse Effects: Allowed in all products. See *A–Z of Cosmetic Terms – Azo Dyes*.
Usage: USA

D&C Violet #2
Function: Violet colorant.
Origin: Synthetic coal tar dye.
Restrictions and Adverse Effects: Allowed in all externally applied cosmetics except eye products.
Usage: USA

D&C Yellow #10

Function: Yellow colorant.
Origin: Mixture of synthetic coal tar dyes including CI 47005 (Acid Yellow 3).
Restrictions and Adverse Effects: Allowed in all products except eye cosmetics.
Usage: USA

D&C Yellow #11

Function: Yellow colorant.
Origin: Synthetic coal tar dye.
Restrictions and Adverse Effects: Allowed in all externally applied cosmetics except eye products.
Usage: USA

DEA

(Diethanolamine)
Function: pH control (used to reduce acidity). DEA itself is used in very few cosmetics or toiletries, but DEA-related ingredients are widely used in a variety of products, e.g., Cocamide DEA is a common surfactant and foam booster in many toiletries.
Origin: Synthetic compound.
Restrictions and Adverse Effects: Toxic. DEA is a cancer suspect currently under investigation. See *A–Z of Cosmetic Terms – DEA*.
Usage: USA/Not currently on the EU inventory of cosmetic ingredients.

DEA-C12-15 alkyl sulfate

Function: Surfactant.
Origin: Synthetic compound.
Restrictions and Adverse Effects: DEA residues are cancer suspects currently under investigation. See *A–Z of Cosmetic Terms – DEA*.
Usage: EU/USA

DEA-ceteareth-2 phosphate

Function: Emulsifier.
Origin: Synthetic compound.
Restrictions and Adverse Effects: DEA residues are cancer suspects currently under investigation. This ethoxylated ingredient is made using ethylene oxide (oxirane) which can form 1,4-dioxane, a carcinogen,

as a by-product of manufacture. See *A–Z of Cosmetic Terms – Dioxane; DEA*.
Usage: EU/USA

DEA-cetyl phosphate

Function: Surfactant.
Origin: Synthetic compound.
Restrictions and Adverse Effects: DEA residues are cancer suspects currently under investigation. See *A–Z of Cosmetic Terms – DEA*.
Usage: EU/USA

DEA-cetyl sulfate

Function: Surfactant.
Origin: Synthetic compound.
Restrictions and Adverse Effects: DEA residues are cancer suspects currently under investigation. See *A–Z of Cosmetic Terms – DEA*.
Usage: EU/USA

DEA-cocoamphodipropionate

Function: Surfactant.
Origin: Semisynthetic compound derived from coconut oil obtained from the kernels of palm trees.
Restrictions and Adverse Effects: DEA residues are cancer suspects currently under investigation. See *A–Z of Cosmetic Terms – DEA*.
Usage: EU/USA

DEA-cyclocarboxypropyloleate

Function: Surfactant.
Origin: Synthetic compound.
Restrictions and Adverse Effects: DEA residues are cancer suspects currently under investigation. See *A–Z of Cosmetic Terms – DEA*.
Usage: EU/USA

DEA-dodecylbenzenesulfonate

Function: Surfactant.
Origin: Synthetic compound.
Restrictions and Adverse Effects: DEA residues are cancer suspects currently under investigation. See *A–Z of Cosmetic Terms – DEA*.
Usage: EU/USA

DEA-hydrolyzed lecithin

Function: Emulsifier.

Origin: Semisynthetic compound derived from lecithin, a phospholipid (fatty phosphate) obtained from several natural sources, especially soya beans.

Restrictions and Adverse Effects: Some soya beans grown in the USA are genetically modified (GM) and these are mixed with natural soya beans, resulting in nearly all soya products containing some GM ingredients. There is no scientific reason for these to have any different effects to natural soya ingredients but many consumers prefer to avoid GM products for a variety of reasons. DEA residues are cancer suspects currently under investigation. See *A–Z of Cosmetic Terms – DEA.*

Usage: EU/USA

DEA-isostearate

Function: Surfactant.

Origin: Semisynthetic or synthetic compound.

Restrictions and Adverse Effects: DEA residues are cancer suspects currently under investigation. See *A–Z of Cosmetic Terms – DEA.*

Usage: EU/USA

DEA-lauraminopropionate

Function: Antistatic agent.

Origin: Semisynthetic or synthetic compound.

Restrictions and Adverse Effects: DEA residues are cancer suspects currently under investigation. See *A–Z of Cosmetic Terms – DEA.*

Usage: EU/USA

DEA-laureth sulfate

Function: Surfactant.

Origin: Semisynthetic or synthetic compound.

Restrictions and Adverse Effects: DEA residues are cancer suspects currently under investigation. This ethoxylated ingredient is made using ethylene oxide (oxirane) which can form 1,4-dioxane, a carcinogen, as a by-product of manufacture. See *A–Z of Cosmetic Terms – Dioxane; DEA.*

Usage: EU/USA

DEA-lauryl sulfate

Function: Surfactant.

Origin: Semisynthetic or synthetic compound.

Restrictions and Adverse Effects: DEA residues are cancer suspects currently under investigation. See *A–Z of Cosmetic Terms – DEA.*

Usage: EU/USA

DEA-linoleate

Function: Antistatic agent / Viscosity adjuster.

Origin: Semisynthetic or synthetic compound.

Restrictions and Adverse Effects: DEA residues are cancer suspects currently under investigation. See *A–Z of Cosmetic Terms – DEA.*

Usage: EU/USA

DEA-methoxycinnamate

Function: UV absorber.

Origin: Synthetic compound.

Restrictions and Adverse Effects: Cinnamates have been reported to cause a stinging sensation in some people. Can form carcinogenic nitrosamines in sunlight. DEA residues are cancer suspects currently under investigation. See *A–Z of Cosmetic Terms – DEA; Nitrosamines.*

Usage: EU/USA

DEA-methyl myristate sulfonate

Function: Surfactant.

Origin: Synthetic compound.

Restrictions and Adverse Effects: Some myristates are comedogenic (acne promoting). DEA residues are cancer suspects currently under investigation. See *A–Z of Cosmetic Terms – DEA; Comedogen.*

Usage: EU/USA

DEA-myreth sulfate

Function: Surfactant.

Origin: Synthetic compound.

Restrictions and Adverse Effects: DEA residues are cancer suspects currently under investigation. This ethoxylated ingredient is made using ethylene oxide (oxirane) which can form 1,4-dioxane, a carcinogen, as a by-product of manufacture. See *A–Z of Cosmetic Terms – Dioxane; DEA.*

Usage: EU/USA

DEA-myristate

Function: Surfactant.

Origin: Semisynthetic or synthetic compound.

Restrictions and Adverse Effects: Some myristates are comedogenic (acne promoting). DEA residues are cancer suspects currently under investigation. See *A–Z of Cosmetic Terms– DEA; Comedogen.*

Usage: EU/USA

DEA-myristyl sulfate

Function: Surfactant.

Origin: Semisynthetic or synthetic compound.

Restrictions and Adverse Effects: DEA residues are cancer suspects currently under investigation. See *A–Z of Cosmetic Terms – DEA.*

Usage: EU/USA

DEA-oleth-3 phosphate

Function: Emulsifier / Surfactant.

Origin: Synthetic compound.

Restrictions and Adverse Effects: Can cause contact allergies. DEA residues are cancer suspects currently under investigation. This ethoxylated ingredient is made using ethylene oxide (oxirane) which can form 1,4-dioxane, a carcinogen, as a by-product of manufacture. See *A–Z of Cosmetic Terms – Dioxane; DEA.*

Usage: EU/USA

DEA-oleth-5 phosphate

Function: Emulsifier / Surfactant.

Origin: Synthetic compound.

Restrictions and Adverse Effects: Can cause contact allergies. DEA residues are cancer suspects currently under investigation. This ethoxylated ingredient is made using ethylene oxide (oxirane) which can form 1,4-dioxane, a carcinogen, as a by-product of manufacture. See *A–Z of Cosmetic Terms – Dioxane; DEA.*

Usage: EU/USA

DEA-oleth-10 phosphate

Function: Emulsifier / Surfactant.

Origin: Synthetic compound.

Restrictions and Adverse Effects: Can cause contact allergies. DEA residues are cancer suspects currently under investigation. This ethoxylated ingredient is made using ethylene oxide (oxirane) which can form 1,4-dioxane, a carcinogen, as a by-product of manufacture. See *A–Z of Cosmetic Terms – Dioxane; DEA.*

Usage: EU/USA

DEA-oleth-20 phosphate

Function: Emulsifier / Surfactant.

Origin: Synthetic compound.

Restrictions and Adverse Effects: Can cause contact allergies. DEA residues are cancer suspects currently under investigation. This ethoxylated ingredient is made using ethylene oxide (oxirane) which can form 1,4-dioxane, a carcinogen, as a by-product of manufacture. See *A–Z of Cosmetic Terms – Dioxane; DEA.*

Usage: EU/USA

DEA-styrene / Acrylates / DVB copolymer

Function: Opacifier.

Origin: Synthetic compound.

Restrictions and Adverse Effects: DEA residues are cancer suspects currently under investigation. See *A–Z of Cosmetic Terms – DEA.*

Usage: EU/USA

Decyl myristate

Function: Emollient / Moisturizer.

Origin: Semisynthetic or synthetic compound.

Restrictions and Adverse Effects: Some myristates are comedogenic (acne promoting, see *A–Z of Cosmetic Terms – Comedogen*).

Usage: EU/USA

Decyl oleate

Function: Emollient / Moisturizer.

Origin: Semisynthetic or synthetic compound.

Restrictions and Adverse Effects: Comedogenic (acne promoting, see *A–Z of Cosmetic Terms – Comedogen*).

Usage: EU/USA

Decyl polyglucose

Function: Surfactant.
Origin: Semisynthetic compound derived from glucose.
Restrictions and Adverse Effects: No currently known adverse effects.
Usage: EU/USA

DEDM hydantoin

Function: Antimicrobial.
Origin: Synthetic compound.
Restrictions and Adverse Effects: Hydantoins have been linked to contact dermatitis.
Usage: EU/USA

DEDM hydantoin dilaurate

Function: Antimicrobial.
Origin: Synthetic compound.
Restrictions and Adverse Effects: Hydantoins have been linked to contact dermatitis.
Usage: EU/USA

DEET

(See Diethyltoluamide)

Dehydroacetic acid

Function: Preservative
Origin: Synthetic compound.
Restrictions and Adverse Effects: Harmful by inhalation. Prohibited from use in aerosol dispensers and sprays and limited to 0.6 percent of the finished product.
Usage: EU/USA

Denatonium benzoate

Function: Denaturant.
Origin: Synthetic compound.
Restrictions and Adverse Effects: No currently known adverse effects.
Usage: EU/USA

Dextrin myristate

Function: Emulsifier.
Origin: Semisynthetic compound.
Restrictions and Adverse Effects: Some myristates are comedogenic (acne promoting, see *A–Z of Cosmetic Terms – Comedogen*).
Usage: EU/USA

Dextrin palmitate

Function: Emulsifier.
Origin: Semisynthetic compound.
Restrictions and Adverse Effects: Some palmitates have been linked to contact dermatitis.
Usage: EU/USA

Di-t-butylhydroquinone

Function: Antioxidant.
Origin: Synthetic compound.
Restrictions and Adverse Effects: Can cause contact dermatitis in lips.
Usage: EU/USA

Diamine

(Hydrazine)
Function: Preservative.
Origin: Synthetic compound.
Restrictions and Adverse Effects: Toxic by ingestion and skin absorption. Strong skin and eye irritant. Cancer suspect.
Usage: USA/Banned from cosmetics in the EU.

Diammonium dithiodiglycolate

Function: Reducing agent.
Origin: Synthetic compound.
Restrictions and Adverse Effects: Can cause contact eczema and contact dermatitis.
Usage: EU/USA

Diazolidinyl urea

Function: Preservative.
Origin: Semisynthetic or synthetic compound.
Restrictions and Adverse Effects: Can cause dermatitis. Limited to 0.5 percent of the finished product.
Usage: EU/USA

Dibromohexamidine isethionate

Function: Preservative.
Origin: Synthetic compound.
Restrictions and Adverse Effects: It is limited to 0.1 percent of the finished product.
Usage: EU/USA

Dibutyl oxalate
Function: Chelating agent.
Origin: Synthetic compound.
Restrictions and Adverse Effects: Oxalates are toxic. Maximum allowed content is 5 percent and is restricted to professional use only.
Usage: EU/USA

Dibutyl phthalate
Function: Film former / Solvent.
Origin: Synthetic compound.
Restrictions and Adverse Effects: Phthalic acid and phthalates have been linked with testicular cancer and cell mutation.
Usage: EU/USA

Dichlorobenzyl alcohol
Function: Preservative.
Origin: Synthetic compound.
Restrictions and Adverse Effects: Limited to 0.1 percent of the finished product if used as a preservative, but may be added in larger quantities for other stated purposes.
Usage: EU/USA

Dichloromethane
(Methylene Chloride)
Function: Solvent.
The main component of solvent-based paint removers.
Origin: Synthetic compound.
Restrictions and Adverse Effects: Harmful vapor. Harmful by skin absorption. Has been shown to cause cancer in animal tests. Total maximum content is 35 percent. If used in combination with 1,1,1-trichloroethane the total solvent content is restricted to 35 percent. Total allowed as an impurity is 2 percent.
Usage: EU/Banned in the USA

Dichlorophene
(Dichlorophen)
Function: Antimicrobial / Deodorant.
Origin: Synthetic compound.
Restrictions and Adverse Effects: Harmful. Can cause allergic reactions. Maximum allowed content

is 0.5 percent of the finished product. The label must clearly show the name of this substance separately from the list of ingredients.
Usage: EU/USA

Diethanolamine
(See – DEA)

Diethanolamine bisulfate
Function: pH control.
Origin: Synthetic compound.
Restrictions and Adverse Effects: DEA residues are cancer suspects currently under investigation. See *A–Z of Cosmetic Terms – DEA.*
Usage: EU/USA

Diethanolaminooleamide DEA
Function: Surfactant.
Origin: Synthetic compound.
Restrictions and Adverse Effects: DEA residues are cancer suspects currently under investigation. See *A–Z of Cosmetic Terms – DEA.*
Usage: EU/USA

Diethyl oxalate
Function: Chelating agent.
Origin: Synthetic compound.
Restrictions and Adverse Effects: Oxalates are toxic. Maximum allowed content is 5 percent and it is restricted to professional use only.
Usage: EU/USA

Diethyl phthalate
Function: Denaturant / Film former / Solvent.
Origin: Synthetic compound.
Restrictions and Adverse Effects: Phthalic acid and phthalates have been linked with testicular cancer and cell mutation.
Usage: EU/USA

Diethyl toluamide (DEET)
Function: Insect repellent, known as DEET in North America.
Origin: Synthetic compound.
Restrictions and Adverse Effects: Poisonous if swallowed. Harmful to eyes. May damage plastics,

e.g., cameras, sunglasses, and some synthetic fabrics. Labels carry voluntary warnings to stop using the product if a rash or soreness occurs. If using an aerosol product avoid inhaling the vapor. Despite these warnings, DEET is a highly effective insect repellent with an excellent safety record.
Usage: EU/USA

Diethylaminomethylcoumarin
Function: Additive.
Origin: Synthetic compound.
Restrictions and Adverse Effects: Skin sensitizer.
Usage: EU/USA

Diethyldicasinamide
Function: Additive.
Origin: Semisynthetic compound.
Restrictions and Adverse Effects: No currently known adverse effects.
Usage: USA/Not currently on the EU inventory of cosmetic ingredients.

Diethylhexyl-p-methoxycinnamate
Function: UV absorber.
Origin: Synthetic compound.
Restrictions and Adverse Effects: Cinnamates have been reported to cause a stinging sensation in some people.
Usage: USA/Not currently on the EU inventory of cosmetic ingredients.

Digalloyl trioleate
Function: Antioxidant.
Origin: Semisynthetic or synthetic compound.
Restrictions and Adverse Effects: May cause photosensitivity in some individuals.
Usage: EU/USA

Dihydrocoumarin
Function: Additive.
Origin: Synthetic compound.
Restrictions and Adverse Effects: Possible skin sensitizer.
Usage: EU/USA

Dihydrogenated tallow phthalate
Function: Emollient / Moisturizer / Surfactant.
Origin: Semisynthetic compound derived from animal fats (tallow).
Restrictions and Adverse Effects: Phthalic acid and phthalates have been linked with testicular cancer and cell mutation. See *Chapter 17 – Animal Products and Animal Testing* for BSE precautions.
Usage: EU/USA

Dihydrogenated tallow phthalic acid amide
Function: Emulsifier.
Origin: Semisynthetic compound derived from animal fats (tallow).
Restrictions and Adverse Effects: Phthalic acid and phthalates have been linked with testicular cancer and cell mutation. See *Chapter 17 – Animal Products and Animal Testing* for BSE precautions.
Usage: EU/USA

Dihydroxyacetone
(DHA)
Function: Tan extender.
Produces an artificial tanning effect that offers no protection from UV rays.
Origin: Synthetic compound.
Restrictions and Adverse Effects: May cause contact allergies in some individuals.
Usage: EU/USA

Diisobutyl adipate
Function: Emollient / Moisturizer.
Origin: Semisynthetic or synthetic compound.
Restrictions and Adverse Effects: No currently known adverse effects.
Usage: EU/USA

Diisobutyl oxalate
Function: Chelating agent.
Origin: Synthetic compound.
Restrictions and Adverse Effects: Oxalates are toxic. Maximum allowed content is 5 percent and it is restricted to professional use only.
Usage: EU/USA

Diisopropyl methyl cinnamate

Function: UV absorber.
Origin: Synthetic compound.
Restrictions and Adverse Effects: Cinnamates have been reported to cause a stinging sensation in some people.
Usage: EU/USA

Diisopropyl oxalate

Function: Chelating agent.
Origin: Synthetic compound.
Restrictions and Adverse Effects: Oxalates are toxic. Maximum allowed content is 5 percent and it is restricted to professional use only.
Usage: EU/USA

Diisopropyl sebacate

Function: Emollient / Moisturizer.
Origin: Semisynthetic or synthetic compound.
Restrictions and Adverse Effects: No currently known adverse effects.
Usage: EU/USA

Dilithium oxalate

Function: Chelating agent.
Origin: Synthetic compound.
Restrictions and Adverse Effects: Oxalates are toxic. Maximum allowed content is 5 percent and it is restricted to professional use only.
Usage: EU/USA

Dimethicone

(Dimethicon, Dimethyl polysiloxane, E900)
Function: Antifoaming agent / Emollient / Moisturizer.
Origin: Synthetic silicone polymer.
Restrictions and Adverse Effects: Cancer suspect. Has caused tumors and mutations in laboratory animals.
Usage: EU/USA

Dimethicone copolyol

Function: Antistatic agent / Emollient / Moisturizer.
Origin: Synthetic silicone polymer.
Restrictions and Adverse Effects: No currently known adverse effects.
Usage: EU/USA

Dimethicone copolyol phthalate

Function: Emollient / Moisturizer.
Origin: Synthetic silicone polymer.
Restrictions and Adverse Effects: Phthalic acid and phthalates have been linked with testicular cancer and cell mutation.
Usage: EU/USA

Dimethyl ether

(Methoxymethane)
Function: Propellant / Solvent.
Origin: Synthetic compound.
Restrictions and Adverse Effects: Highly flammable gas.
Usage: EU/USA

Dimethyl oxalate

Function: Chelating agent.
Origin: Synthetic compound.
Restrictions and Adverse Effects: Oxalates are toxic. Maximum allowed content is 5 percent and it is restricted to professional use only.
Usage: EU/USA

Dimethyl oxazolidine

Function: Preservative.
Origin: Synthetic compound.
Restrictions and Adverse Effects: Limited to 0.1 percent of the finished product and the pH must be lower than 6. It is dangerous to mix products containing this ingredient with preparations that contain alkalis.
Usage: EU/USA

Dimethyl phthalate

Function: Film former / Solvent.
Origin: Synthetic compound.
Restrictions and Adverse Effects: Phthalic acid and phthalates have been linked with testicular cancer and cell mutation.
Usage: EU/USA

Dimethylol ethylene thiourea

Function: Additive.
Origin: Synthetic compound.

Restrictions and Adverse Effects: Harmful vapor. This product is limited to a maximum of 2 percent of the finished product and is banned from use in aerosol dispensers and sprays. The label must clearly show the name of this substance separately from the list of ingredients.
Usage: EU/USA

Dioctyl phthalate
Function: Film former.
Origin: Synthetic compound.
Restrictions and Adverse Effects: Phthalic acid and phthalates have been linked with testicular cancer and cell mutation.
Usage: EU/USA

Dipotassium oxalate
Function: Chelating agent.
Origin: Synthetic compound.
Restrictions and Adverse Effects: Oxalates are toxic. Maximum allowed content is 5 percent and it is restricted to professional use only.
Usage: EU/USA

Dipropyl oxalate
Function: Chelating agent.
Origin: Synthetic compound.
Restrictions and Adverse Effects: Oxalates are toxic. Maximum allowed content is 5 percent and it is restricted to professional use only.
Usage: EU/USA

Dipropylene glycol
Function: Solvent.
Origin: Synthetic compound.
Restrictions and Adverse Effects: No currently known adverse effects.
Usage: EU/USA

Direct black 38
Function: Colorant.
Origin: Synthetic compound.
Restrictions and Adverse Effects: Cancer suspect.
Usage: USA/Not currently on the EU inventory of cosmetic ingredients.

Direct blue 6
Function: Colorant.
Origin: Synthetic compound.
Restrictions and Adverse Effects: Cancer suspect.
Usage: USA/Not currently on the EU inventory of cosmetic ingredients.

Disodium cocoamphodiacetate
Function: Surfactant.
Origin: Semisynthetic compound.
Restrictions and Adverse Effects: No currently known adverse effects.
Usage: EU/USA

Disodium cocoamphodipropionate
Function: Surfactant.
Origin: Semisynthetic compound.
Restrictions and Adverse Effects: No currently known adverse effects.
Usage: EU/USA

Disodium dimethicone
Function: Film former.
Origin: Synthetic silicone polymer.
Restrictions and Adverse Effects: No currently known adverse effects.
Usage: USA/Not currently on the EU inventory of cosmetic ingredients.

Disodium EDTA
(Disodium edetate)
Function: Chelating agent / Viscosity adjuster.
Origin: Synthetic compound.
Restrictions and Adverse Effects: No currently known adverse effects.
Usage: EU/USA

Disodium lauroamphodiacetate
Function: Antistatic agent / Surfactant / Viscosity adjuster.
Origin: Semisynthetic or synthetic compound.
Restrictions and Adverse Effects: No currently known adverse effects.
Usage: EU/USA

Disodium phosphate

(Sodium phosphate, dibasic)

Function: pH control.

Origin: Synthetic compound.

Restrictions and Adverse Effects: No currently known adverse effects.

Usage: EU/USA

DM hydantoin

Function: Viscosity adjuster.

Origin: Synthetic compound.

Restrictions and Adverse Effects: Hydantoins have been linked to contact dermatitis.

Usage: EU/USA

DMDM hydantoin

Function: Preservative.

Origin: Synthetic compound.

Restrictions and Adverse Effects: Can cause contact dermatitis. It is limited to 0.6 percent of the finished product if used as a preservative, but may be added in larger quantities for other stated purposes.

Usage: EU/USA

Drometrizole trisiloxane

Function: UV absorber.

Origin: Synthetic compound.

Restrictions and Adverse Effects: Restricted to 15 percent of the finished product.

Usage: EU/USA

Elastin

Function: Biological additive / Moisture binder. Credited with the ability to keep skin soft and supple.

Origin: An animal protein, extracted from the layers of skin and artery walls of mammals.

Restrictions and Adverse Effects: No currently known adverse effects. See *Chapter 17 – Animal Products and Animal Testing* for BSE precautions.

Usage: EU/USA

Elastin amino acids

Function: Biological additive.

Origin: Amino acids derived from elastin, a flexible protein extracted from the layers of skin and artery walls of mammals.

Restrictions and Adverse Effects: No currently known adverse effects. See *Chapter 17 – Animal Products and Animal Testing* for BSE precautions.

Usage: EU/USA

Ethanolamine

(MEA)

Function: pH control.

Origin: Synthetic compound.

Restrictions and Adverse Effects: Harmful. Skin irritant. Danger of nitrosamine contamination (see *A–Z of Cosmetic Terms – Nitrosamines*). This product must have a minimum purity of 99 percent, with a maximum secondary alkolamine contamination of 0.5 percent. The maximum allowed content is 0.5 percent of the finished product.

Usage: EU/USA

Ethanolamine thioglycolate

Function: Depilatory agent / Reducing agent.

Origin: Synthetic compound.

Restrictions and Adverse Effects: EU regulations require the following mandatory warnings: "May cause sensitization in the event of skin contact. Avoid contact with eyes. In the event of contact with eyes, rinse with plenty of water and seek medical advice. Wear suitable gloves. Follow the instructions. Keep out of reach of children." The label must also state "Contains Thioglycolate." It is limited to 8 percent for general use or 11 percent for professional use, and the pH must be between 6 and 9.5.

Usage: EU/USA

Ethyl acetate

Function: Solvent.

Origin: Synthetic compound.

Restrictions and Adverse Effects: No currently known adverse effects. It has a highly flammable vapor and is subject to solvent abuse.

Usage: EU/USA

Ethyl benzoate

Function: Preservative.

Origin: Synthetic compound of the benzoate family.

Restrictions and Adverse Effects: Benzoic acid and benzoates have been implicated in a large number of health issues. (See *A–Z of Cosmetic Terms – Benzoates*.) It is limited to 0.5 percent of the finished product if it is used as a preservative, but may be added in larger quantities for other stated purposes.

Usage: EU/USA

Ethyl brassylate

Function: Additive.

Origin: Semisynthetic or synthetic compound.

Restrictions and Adverse Effects: No currently known adverse effects.

Usage: USA/Not currently on the EU inventory of cosmetic ingredients.

Ethyl cinnamate

Function: UV absorber.

Origin: Synthetic compound.

Restrictions and Adverse Effects: Cinnamates have been reported to cause a stinging sensation in some people.

Usage: EU/USA

Ethyl diisopropylcinnamate

Function: UV absorber.

Origin: Synthetic compound.

Restrictions and Adverse Effects: Cinnamates have been reported to cause a stinging sensation in some people.

Usage: EU/USA

Ethyl methoxycinnamate

Function: UV absorber.

Origin: Synthetic compound.

Restrictions and Adverse Effects: Cinnamates have been reported to cause a stinging sensation in some people.

Usage: EU/USA

Ethyl minkate

Function: Emollient / Moisturizer.

Origin: A semisynthetic compound derived from mink oil obtained from the fatty, subcutaneous tissues of mink.

Restrictions and Adverse Effects: No currently known adverse effects.

Usage: EU/USA

Ethyl myristate

Function: Emollient / Moisturizer.

Origin: Semisynthetic or synthetic compound.

Restrictions and Adverse Effects: Some myristates are comedogenic (acne promoting, see *A–Z of Cosmetic Terms – Comedogen*).

Usage: EU/USA

Ethyl palmitate

Function: Emollient / Moisturizer.

Origin: Semisynthetic or synthetic compound.

Restrictions and Adverse Effects: Some palmitates have been linked to contact dermatitis.

Usage: EU/USA

Ethyl thioglycolate

Function: Depilatory agent / Reducing agent.

Origin: Semisynthetic or synthetic compound.

Restrictions and Adverse Effects: EU regulations require the following mandatory warnings: "May cause sensitization in the event of skin contact. Avoid contact with eyes. In the event of contact with eyes, rinse with plenty of water and seek medical advice. Wear suitable gloves. Follow the instructions. Keep out of reach of children." The label must also state "Contains Thioglycolate." It is limited to 8 percent for general use or 11 percent for professional use, and the pH must be between 6 and 9.5.

Usage: EU/USA

Ethyl urocanate

Function: UV absorber.

Origin: Synthetic compound.

Restrictions and Adverse Effects: This substance is considered harmful and is banned from use in cosmetics in the EU.

Usage: USA

Ethylene / Methacrylate copolymer

Function: Binding agent / Film former.

Origin: Synthetic compound.

Restrictions and Adverse Effects: No currently known adverse effects.

Usage: USA/Not currently on the EU inventory of cosmetic ingredients.

Ethylenediamine

(1,2-Diaminoethane)

Function: pH control.

Origin: Synthetic compound.

Restrictions and Adverse Effects: Toxic by inhalation and skin absorption. Severe skin and eye irritant. May cause contact dermatitis and contact sensitization.

Usage: USA/Not currently on the EU inventory of cosmetic ingredients.

Ethylhexyl-p-methoxycinnamate

Function: UV absorber.

Origin: Synthetic compound.

Restrictions and Adverse Effects: Cinnamates have been reported to cause a stinging sensation in some people.

Usage: USA/Not currently on the EU inventory of cosmetic ingredients.

Ethylparaben

Function: Preservative.

Origin: Synthetic compound of the benzoate family.

Restrictions and Adverse Effects: Benzoic acid, benzoates and parabens have been implicated in a large number of health issues. (See *A–Z of Cosmetic Terms – Benzoates*.) It is limited to 0.4 percent of the finished product if used on its own as a preservative, or 0.8 percent in total if used in combination with other parabens. Parabens may be added in larger quantities for other stated purposes.

Usage: EU/USA

Etidronic acid

Function: Chelating agent.

Origin: Synthetic compound.

Restrictions and Adverse Effects: Harmful. It is limited to 1.5 percent in hair care preparations and 0.2 percent in soap.

Usage: EU/USA

Eugenol

Function: Denaturant.

Origin: Synthetic compound.

Restrictions and Adverse Effects: No currently known adverse effects.

Usage: EU/USA

Formaldehyde

Function: Preservative / Nail hardener.

Origin: Synthetic compound.

Restrictions and Adverse Effects: Irritant. Harmful. Cancer suspect. Prohibited from use in aerosol dispensers and sprays. If used as a preservative it is limited to 0.2 percent, or 0.1 percent in oral hygiene preparations, but it may be used in nail hardeners up to a maximum of 5 percent of the finished product. If the nail hardener contains more than 0.05 percent of this substance the label must clearly state "Contains formaldehyde. Protect cuticles with grease or oil."

Usage: EU/USA. Banned in Sweden and Japan.

Formic acid

Function: Preservative.

Origin: Synthetic compound.

Restrictions and Adverse Effects: Skin irritant, eye irritant. It is limited to 0.5 percent of the finished product if used as a preservative, but it may be added in larger quantities for other stated purposes.

Usage: EU/USA

Fragrance

(Parfum)

Function: Fragrance.

Origin: A mixture of many synthetic and natural fragrance chemicals, often dissolved in a carrier solvent, e.g., ethanol or benzyl alcohol.

Restrictions and Adverse Effects: May cause contact dermatitis and contact allergies.

Usage: EU/USA

Geraniol

Function: Additive.
Origin: Plant extract.
Restrictions and Adverse Effects: Can cause contact dermatitis, often discoloring the affected area.
Usage: EU/USA

Geranium

(Geranium extract)
Function: Botanical additive.
Origin: Plant extract.
Restrictions and Adverse Effects: Can cause contact dermatitis and skin irritation.
Usage: EU/USA

Geranium maculatum

Function: Botanical additive.
Origin: Plant extract.
Restrictions and Adverse Effects: Can cause contact dermatitis and skin irritation.
Usage: EU/USA

Geranium robertianum

Function: Botanical additive.
Origin: Plant extract.
Restrictions and Adverse Effects: Can cause contact dermatitis and skin irritation.
Usage: EU/USA

Glutaral

Function: Preservative.
Origin: Synthetic compound.
Restrictions and Adverse Effects: Harmful by inhalation. Prohibited from use in aerosol dispensers and sprays and limited to 0.1 percent of the finished product. If it exceeds 0.05 percent, the name of this substance must be clearly stated on the label separately from the list of ingredients.
Usage: EU/USA

Glycereth – Family

Examples include Glycereth-12, Glycereth-20 stearate and Glycereth-26 phosphate.
Function: Mainly emulsifiers.

Origin: A range of synthetic ingredients manufactured from glycerine and ethylene oxide. These ethoxylated compounds may be combined with a variety of other molecules to produce a wide range of cosmetic materials. Higher numbers mean higher ethoxylation (bigger molecules), usually resulting in a greater solubility in water.
Restrictions and Adverse Effects: Ethoxylated ingredients are made using ethylene oxide (oxirane), which can form 1,4-dioxane, a carcinogen, as a by-product of manufacture. See *A–Z of Cosmetic Terms – Dioxane*.
Usage: EU/USA

Glycerin

(Glycerol, Glycerine, Propan-1,2,3-triol)
Function: Denaturant / Humectant / Solvent.
A naturally derived skin-friendly humectant prepared by the hydrolysis of fats and oils, commonly used in a large variety of cosmetics and toiletries. The less expensive Sorbitol is rapidly taking the place of glycerin in many preparations.
Origin: Can be processed from natural fats and oils of plant or animal origin. A by-product of the soap manufacturing industry.
Restrictions and Adverse Effects: Skin irritant in some people.
Usage: EU/USA

Glyceryl – Family

Function: Glyceryl esters are widely used in cosmetics as emollients, moisturizers, film formers, and emulsifiers. Examples include Glyceryl adipate, Glyceryl alginate, Glyceryl caprylate, Glyceryl linoleate and Glyceryl hydrogenated rosinate.
Origin: Semisynthetic or synthetic compounds derived from glycerin and a variety of fatty acids.
Restrictions and Adverse Effects: Some glyceryl monoesters have been linked to contact dermatitis.
Usage: EU/USA

Glyceryl cocoate

Function: Emollient / Moisturizer / Emulsifier.
Origin: Semisynthetic compound derived from coconut oil extracted from the kernels of palm trees.

Restrictions and Adverse Effects: Glyceryl monoesters have been linked to contact dermatitis.
Usage: EU/USA

Glyceryl collagenate

Function: Additive.
Origin: Semisynthetic compound derived from collagen, a protein obtained from animal sources.
Restrictions and Adverse Effects: Glyceryl monoesters have been linked to contact dermatitis.
Usage: EU/USA

Glyceryl diisopalmitate

Function: Emollient / Moisturizer.
Origin: Semisynthetic or synthetic compound.
Restrictions and Adverse Effects: Both glyceryl esters and palmitates have been linked to contact dermatitis.
Usage: EU/USA

Glyceryl diisostearate

Function: Emollient / Moisturizer / Emulsifier / Opacifier.
Origin: Semisynthetic or synthetic compound.
Restrictions and Adverse Effects: Glyceryl esters have been linked to contact dermatitis.
Usage: EU/USA

Glyceryl dimyristate

Function: Emollient / Moisturizer.
Origin: Semisynthetic or synthetic compound.
Restrictions and Adverse Effects: Glyceryl esters have been linked to contact dermatitis. Some myristates are comedogenic (acne promoting, see A–Z of Cosmetic Terms – Comedogen).
Usage: EU/USA

Glyceryl dipalmitate

Function: Emollient / Moisturizer / Emulsifier.
Origin: Semisynthetic or synthetic compound.
Restrictions and Adverse Effects: Both glyceryl esters and palmitates have been linked to contact dermatitis.
Usage: EU/USA

Glyceryl distearate

Function: Antistatic agent / Emollient / Moisturizer.
Origin: Semisynthetic or synthetic compound.
Restrictions and Adverse Effects: Glyceryl esters have been linked to contact dermatitis.
Usage: EU/USA

Glyceryl lanolate

Function: Antistatic agent / Emollient / Moisturizer / Emulsifier.
Origin: Semisynthetic or synthetic compound.
Restrictions and Adverse Effects: Glyceryl monoesters have been linked to contact dermatitis.
Usage: EU/USA

Glyceryl laurate

(Glyceryl monolaurate)
Function: Emollient / Moisturizer / Emulsifier.
Origin: Semisynthetic or synthetic compound.
Restrictions and Adverse Effects: Glyceryl monoesters have been linked to contact dermatitis. Skin irritant for some individuals.
Usage: EU/USA

Glyceryl myristate

Function: Emollient / Moisturizer / Emulsifier.
Origin: Semisynthetic or synthetic compound.
Restrictions and Adverse Effects: Glyceryl monoesters have been linked to contact dermatitis. Some myristates are comedogenic (acne promoting, see A–Z of Cosmetic Terms – Comedogen).
Usage: EU/USA

Glyceryl octanoate dimethoxycinnamate

Function: UV absorber.
Origin: Semisynthetic or synthetic compound.
Restrictions and Adverse Effects: Cinnamates have been reported to cause a stinging sensation in some people. Glyceryl monoesters have been linked to contact dermatitis.
Usage: EU/USA

Glyceryl oleate

Function: Emollient / Moisturizer / Emulsifier.
Origin: Semisynthetic or synthetic compound.
Restrictions and Adverse Effects: Glyceryl monoesters have been linked to contact dermatitis. May cause skin allergies in some individuals.
Usage: EU/USA

Glyceryl PABA

Function: UV absorber.
Origin: Synthetic compound.
Restrictions and Adverse Effects: Glyceryl monoesters have been linked to contact dermatitis. May cause photosensitivity in some individuals.
Usage: EU/USA

Glyceryl palmitate

Function: Emollient / Moisturizer.
Origin: Semisynthetic or synthetic compound.
Restrictions and Adverse Effects: Both glyceryl esters and palmitates have been linked to contact dermatitis.
Usage: EU/USA

Glyceryl palmitate / Stearate

Function: Emollient / Moisturizer.
Origin: Semisynthetic or synthetic compound.
Restrictions and Adverse Effects: Both glyceryl esters and palmitates have been linked to contact dermatitis.
Usage: EU/USA

Glyceryl palmitate lactate

Function: Emollient / Moisturizer / Emulsifier.
Origin: Semisynthetic or synthetic compound.
Restrictions and Adverse Effects: Both glyceryl esters and palmitates have been linked to contact dermatitis.
Usage: EU/USA

Glyceryl polymethacrylate

Function: Viscosity adjuster.
Origin: Semisynthetic or synthetic compound.
Restrictions and Adverse Effects: Glyceryl monoesters have been linked to contact dermatitis.
Usage: EU/USA

Glyceryl starch

Function: Absorbent / Binding agent.
Origin: Semisynthetic compound.
Restrictions and Adverse Effects: Glyceryl monoesters have been linked to contact dermatitis.
Usage: EU/USA

Glyceryl stearate

(Glyceryl monostearate)
Function: Emollient / Moisturizer / Emulsifier.
Origin: Semisynthetic or synthetic compound.
Restrictions and Adverse Effects: Glyceryl monoesters have been linked to contact dermatitis. May cause skin allergies in some individuals.
Usage: EU/USA

Glyceryl thioglycolate

Function: Depilatory agent / Reducing agent.
Origin: Synthetic compound.
Restrictions and Adverse Effects: EU regulations require the following mandatory warnings: "May cause sensitization in the event of skin contact. Avoid contact with eyes. In the event of contact with eyes, rinse with plenty of water and seek medical advice. Wear suitable gloves. Follow the instructions. Keep out of reach of children." The label must also state "Contains Thioglycolate." It is limited to 8 percent for general use or 11 percent for professional use, and the pH must be between 6 and 9.5.
Usage: EU/USA

Glyceryl thiopropionate

Function: Reducing agent.
Origin: Semisynthetic or synthetic compound.
Restrictions and Adverse Effects: Glyceryl monoesters have been linked to contact dermatitis.
Usage: EU/USA

Glyceryl triacetyl hydroxystearate

Function: Emollient / Moisturizer / Solvent / Viscosity adjuster.
Origin: Semisynthetic or synthetic compound.
Restrictions and Adverse Effects: Glyceryl esters have been linked to contact dermatitis.
Usage: EU/USA

Glyceryl triacetyl ricinoleate

Function: Emollient / Moisturizer / Solvent / Viscosity adjuster.
Origin: Semisynthetic or synthetic compound.
Restrictions and Adverse Effects: Glyceryl esters have been linked to contact dermatitis.
Usage: EU/USA

Glycol

(Ethylene glycol, Ethan-1,2-diol)
Function: Solvent.
Origin: Synthetic compound derived from petroleum. Manufactured in vast quantities as its main use is antifreeze for car radiators.
Restrictions and Adverse Effects: Toxic if ingested. May cause contact allergies, contact dermatitis, and contact eczema.
Usage: EU/USA

Glycol palmitate

Function: Emulsifier.
Origin: Semisynthetic or synthetic compound.
Restrictions and Adverse Effects: Some palmitates have been linked to contact dermatitis.
Usage: EU/USA

Glycolic acid

Function: pH control / Exfoliating agent.
Origin: Synthetic compound.
Restrictions and Adverse Effects: Glycolic acid is an alpha-hydroxy acid (AHA) used to exfoliate skin. They are also known as skin peelers because they dissolve and remove the outer layer of skin. They can cause increased sensitivity to the sun due to loss of the protective outer layer of skin cells. Do not expose skin to the sun immediately following treatment with AHAs. Test a small area before use and discontinue use if skin irritation, redness, bleeding, or pain is experienced. Not recommended for use on children. May cause exfoliative dermatitis.
Usage: EU/USA

Glycomer in crosslinked fatty acids alpha natrium

Function: Exfoliating agent.
Origin: Semisynthetic or synthetic compound.

Restrictions and Adverse Effects: This ingredient contains alpha-hydroxy acids (AHAs), which are used to exfoliate skin. They are also known as skin peelers because they dissolve and remove the outer layer of skin. They can cause increased sensitivity to the sun due to loss of the protective outer layer of skin cells. Do not expose skin to the sun immediately following treatment with AHAs. Test a small area before use and discontinue use if skin irritation, redness, bleeding, or pain is experienced. Not recommended for use on children. May cause exfoliative dermatitis.
Usage: USA/Not currently on the EU inventory of cosmetic ingredients.

Glyoxal

Function: Antimicrobial.
Glyoxal is gradually replacing formaldehyde, a cancer suspect, as an inexpensive preservative.
Origin: Synthetic compound.
Restrictions and Adverse Effects: Irritant for some individuals.
Usage: EU/USA

Hedra helix

(Ivy extract)
Function: Stimulant / Toning agent.
A mild irritant believed to stimulate blood circulation to the areas on which it is applied and known for its toning and tightening properties.
Origin: Extract of the ivy plant.
Restrictions and Adverse Effects: Irritant. May cause contact dermatitis in some individuals.
Usage: EU/USA

Hexachlorophene

Function: Preservative.
Origin: Synthetic compound.
Restrictions and Adverse Effects: Hexachlorophene can penetrate the skin and has a neurotoxic effect. It is normally banned from cosmetics in both the EU and USA but FDA regulations allow its use when it has been shown to be more effective than an alternative preservative. In this case it is limited to 0.1 percent of the finished product and must not be used in products that come into contact with the mucous membranes.

Usage: Banned in the EU. Generally prohibited in the USA

Hexamidine

Function: Preservative.

Origin: Synthetic compound.

Restrictions and Adverse Effects: Limited to 0.1 percent of the finished product if used as a preservative, but may be added in larger quantities for other stated purposes.

Usage: EU/USA

Hexamidine diisethionate

Function: Preservative.

Origin: Synthetic compound.

Restrictions and Adverse Effects: Can cause contact dermatitis. Limited to 0.1 percent of the finished product if used as a preservative, but may be added in larger quantities for other stated purposes.

Usage: EU/USA

Hexamidine paraben

Function: Preservative.

Origin: Synthetic compound of the benzoate family.

Restrictions and Adverse Effects: Benzoic acid, benzoates and parabens have been implicated in a large number of health issues. (See *A–Z of Cosmetic Terms – Benzoates*.) It is limited to 0.4 percent of the finished product if used on its own as a preservative, or 0.8 percent in total if used in combination with other parabens. Parabens may be added in larger quantities for other stated purposes.

Usage: EU/USA

Hexetidine

Function: Preservative.

Origin: Synthetic compound.

Restrictions and Adverse Effects: Limited to 0.1 percent of the finished product.

Usage: EU/USA

Hexylene glycol

Function: Solvent.

Origin: Synthetic compound.

Restrictions and Adverse Effects: Toxic by inhalation and ingestion. Can cause contact dermatitis and irritation to skin, eyes, and mucous membranes.

Usage: EU/USA

Homosalate

(Homomenthyl salicylate)

Function: UV absorber.

Origin: Synthetic or semisynthetic compound.

Restrictions and Adverse Effects: Irritant. Can cause follicular eruptions (rash or pustules in the hair follicles). This ingredient is restricted to a maximum amount of 10 percent of the finished product.

Usage: EU/USA

Hydrogen peroxide

Function: Oxidizing agent.

Origin: Synthetic compound.

Restrictions and Adverse Effects: Corrosive. Harmful to skin. Harmful to eyes. Causes bleaching of hair and fabrics. Possible cancer suspect. Maximum allowed content: 12 percent in hair care products (protective gloves should be worn), 4 percent in skin preparations, 2 percent in nail hardeners, and 0.1 percent in oral hygiene products. The label must clearly show the name of this ingredient, and warn the user to avoid contact with the eyes and to rinse eyes with cold water in the event of accidental contact. When used as a contact lens cleaning agent care should be taken to allow sufficient time to ensure it is completely neutralized by the neutralizing agent supplied with the product.

Usage: EU/USA

Hydrogenated mink oil

Function: Emollient / Moisturizer.

Origin: A semisynthetic compound derived from mink oil obtained from the fatty, subcutaneous tissues of mink.

Restrictions and Adverse Effects: No currently known adverse effects.

Usage: EU/USA

Hydrogenated tallowamide DEA

Function: Surfactant.

Origin: Semisynthetic compound derived from animal fat (tallow).

Restrictions and Adverse Effects: DEA residues are cancer suspects currently under investigation. See *A–Z of Cosmetic Terms – DEA*. See *Chapter 17 – Animal Products and Animal Testing* for BSE precautions.

Usage: EU/USA

Hydrolyzed elastin

Function: Antistatic agent / Film former / Humectant.

Origin: Amino acids and protein fragments derived from elastin, a flexible protein extracted from the layers of skin and artery walls of mammals.

Restrictions and Adverse Effects: No currently known adverse effects. See *Chapter 17 – Animal Products and Animal Testing* for BSE precautions.

Usage: EU/USA

Hydroquinone

Function: Hair dye / Bleaching agent / Skin lightener.

Origin: Synthetic compound.

Restrictions and Adverse Effects: Harmful. Irritant. Toxic by ingestion and inhalation. Can cause hyperpigmentation (brown patches on the skin). Before February 29, 2000 it was limited to 2 percent of the finished product. After this date its use in skin lightening products was prohibited in the EU, and its use in hair dyes was further restricted to a maximum of 0.3 percent of the finished product. Labels must carry the following warnings: "Contains Hydroquinone. Do not use to dye eyelashes or eyebrows. Rinse the eyes immediately if the product comes into contact with them." Before its use in skin lightening products was prohibited the following warnings were required: "Avoid contact with the eyes. Apply to small areas only. Do not use on children under the age of 12. If irritation develops discontinue use."

Usage: EU/USA

Hydroquinone PCA

Function: Additive.

Origin: Synthetic compound.

Restrictions and Adverse Effects: Can cause hyperpigmentation (brown patches on the skin) and contact dermatitis.

Usage: EU/USA

Hydroxycitronella

(Citronellal Hydrate, 3,7-Dimethyl-7-hydroxyoctenal)

Function: Additive.

Origin: Semisynthetic or synthetic compound.

Restrictions and Adverse Effects: Can cause contact dermatitis, pigmented contact dermatitis and contact allergies in some individuals.

Usage: USA/Not currently on the EU inventory of cosmetic ingredients.

Hydroxycitronellal

Function: Additive.

Origin: Synthetic compound.

Restrictions and Adverse Effects: Linked to facial psoriasis.

Usage: EU/USA

Hydroxypropyl methylcellulose

Function: Binding agent / Emulsion stabilizer / Film former / Viscosity adjuster.

Origin: Synthetic compound.

Restrictions and Adverse Effects: Mild eye and skin irritant.

Usage: EU/USA

Imidazolidinyl urea

Function: Preservative.

Origin: Synthetic compound.

Restrictions and Adverse Effects: Can cause dermatitis. Limited to 0.6 percent of the finished product if used as a preservative, but may be added in larger quantities for other stated purposes.

Usage: EU/USA

Iodopropynyl butylcarbamate

Function: Preservative.

Origin: Synthetic compound.

Restrictions and Adverse Effects: The safety of this substance was uncertain and its use in cosmetics was only provisionally permitted in the EU, until June 30, 1998. After this date its safety was still unproven and its provisional status was extended. It is limited to a maximum of 0.1 percent of the finished product and is banned from oral care products and lip products.
Usage: EU/USA

Isoamyl p-methoxycinnamate
Function: UV absorber.
Origin: Synthetic compound.
Restrictions and Adverse Effects: The safety of this substance was uncertain and its use in cosmetics was only provisionally permitted in the EU, until June 30, 1998. Following further scientific tests, the provisional status was removed and this ingredient was permitted for use in cosmetics. It is limited to a maximum of 10 percent of the finished product. It may be used to protect the ingredients of other cosmetics and toiletries from the detrimental effects of sunlight. Cinnamates have been reported to cause a stinging sensation in some people.
Usage: EU/USA

Isobutane
Function: Propellant for aerosol sprays. (Often used in combination with Propane and Butane.)
Origin: Petroleum product.
Restrictions and Adverse Effects: A flammable hydrocarbon gas that is used as an alternative to CFCs, which are known to damage the ozone layer. It is a powerful greenhouse gas (it contributes to the greenhouse effect causing global warming) and is inhaled by solvent abusers. It is harmless if inhaled in small concentrations. There is a danger of fire or explosion if used near a source of ignition.
Usage: EU/USA

Isobutyl benzoate
Function: Preservative.
Origin: Synthetic compound of the benzoate family.
Restrictions and Adverse Effects: Benzoic acid and benzoates have been implicated in a large number of

health issues. (See *A–Z of Cosmetic Terms – Benzoates*.) It is limited to 0.5 percent of the finished product if used as a preservative. It may be added in larger quantities for other stated purposes.
Usage: EU/USA

Isobutyl myristate
Function: Emollient / Moisturizer.
Origin: Semisynthetic or synthetic compound.
Restrictions and Adverse Effects: Some myristates are comedogenic (acne promoting, see *A–Z of Cosmetic Terms – Comedogen*).
Usage: EU/USA

Isobutyl palmitate
Function: Emollient / Moisturizer.
Origin: Semisynthetic or synthetic compound.
Restrictions and Adverse Effects: Some palmitates have been linked to contact dermatitis.
Usage: EU/USA

Isobutylparaben
Function: Preservative.
Origin: Synthetic compound of the benzoate family.
Restrictions and Adverse Effects: Benzoic acid, benzoates and parabens have been implicated in a large number of health issues. (See *A–Z of Cosmetic Terms – Benzoates*.) It is limited to 0.4 percent of the finished product if used on its own as a preservative, or 0.8 percent in total if used in combination with other parabens. Parabens may be added in larger quantities for other stated purposes.
Usage: EU/USA

Isoceteth – Family
Examples include Isoceteth-20 and Isoceteth-10 stearate.
Function: Mainly emulsifiers.
Origin: A range of synthetic ingredients manufactured from ethylene oxide. These ethoxylated compounds may be combined with a variety of other molecules to produce a wide range of cosmetic materials. Higher numbers mean higher ethoxylation (bigger molecules), usually resulting in a greater solubility in water.

Restrictions and Adverse Effects: Ethoxylated ingredients are made using ethylene oxide (oxirane), which can form 1,4-dioxane, a carcinogen, as a by-product of manufacture. See *A–Z of Cosmetic Terms – Dioxane*.
Usage: EU/USA

Isocetyl myristate

Function: Emollient / Moisturizer.
Origin: Semisynthetic or synthetic compound.
Restrictions and Adverse Effects: Some myristates are comedogenic (acne promoting, see *A–Z of Cosmetic Terms – Comedogen*).
Usage: EU/USA

Isocetyl palmitate

Function: Emollient / Moisturizer.
Origin: Semisynthetic or synthetic compound.
Restrictions and Adverse Effects: Some palmitates have been linked to contact dermatitis.
Usage: EU/USA

Isocetyl stearate

Function: Emollient / Moisturizer.
Origin: Semisynthetic or synthetic compound.
Restrictions and Adverse Effects: Comedogenic (acne promoting, see *A–Z of Cosmetic Terms – Comedogen*).
Usage: EU/USA

Isodecyl myristate

Function: Emollient / Moisturizer.
Origin: Semisynthetic or synthetic compound.
Restrictions and Adverse Effects: Some myristates are comedogenic (acne promoting, see *A–Z of Cosmetic Terms – Comedogen*).
Usage: EU/USA

Isodecyl palmitate

Function: Emollient / Moisturizer.
Origin: Semisynthetic or synthetic compound.
Restrictions and Adverse Effects: Some palmitates have been linked to contact dermatitis.
Usage: EU/USA

Isoeugenol

Function: Additive.
Origin: Semisynthetic compound.
Restrictions and Adverse Effects: May cause contact dermatitis in some individuals.
Usage: EU/USA

Isohexyl palmitate

Function: Emollient / Moisturizer.
Origin: Semisynthetic or synthetic compound.
Restrictions and Adverse Effects: Some palmitates have been linked to contact dermatitis.
Usage: EU/USA

Isolaureth – Family

Examples include Isolaureth-10, Isolaureth-3 and Isolaureth-6.
Function: Mainly emulsifiers.
Origin: A range of synthetic ingredients manufactured from ethylene oxide. These ethoxylated compounds may be combined with a variety of other molecules to produce a wide range of cosmetic materials. Higher numbers mean higher ethoxylation (bigger molecules), usually resulting in a greater solubility in water.
Restrictions and Adverse Effects: Ethoxylated ingredients are made using ethylene oxide (oxirane), which can form 1,4-dioxane, a carcinogen, as a by-product of manufacture. See *A–Z of Cosmetic Terms – Dioxane*.
Usage: EU/USA

Isooctyl thioglycolate

Function: Depilatory agent / Reducing agent.
Origin: Semisynthetic or synthetic compound.
Restrictions and Adverse Effects: EU regulations require the following mandatory warnings: "May cause sensitization in the event of skin contact. Avoid contact with eyes. In the event of contact with eyes, rinse with plenty of water and seek medical advice. Wear suitable gloves. Follow the instructions. Keep out of reach of children." The label must also state "Contains Thioglycolate." It is limited to 8 percent for general use or 11 percent for professional use, and the pH must be between 6 and 9.5.
Usage: EU/USA

Isopropanolamine
(MIPA)

Function: pH control.

Origin: Synthetic compound.

Restrictions and Adverse Effects: Harmful. Severe eye and skin irritant. Can cause contact allergies and contact dermatitis. Danger of nitrosamine contamination (see *A–Z of Cosmetic Terms – Nitrosamines*). This product must have a minimum purity of 99 percent, with a maximum secondary alkolamine contamination of 0.5 percent. The maximum allowed content is 0.5 percent of the finished product.

Usage: EU/USA

Isopropyl benzoate

Function: Preservative.

Origin: Synthetic compound of the benzoate family.

Restrictions and Adverse Effects: Benzoic acid and benzoates have been implicated in a large number of health issues. (See *A–Z of Cosmetic Terms – Benzoates*.) It is limited to 0.5 percent of the finished product if used as a preservative. It may be added in larger quantities for other stated purposes.

Usage: EU/USA

Isopropyl cresols

Function: Preservative.

Origin: Synthetic mixture of compounds.

Restrictions and Adverse Effects: Irritant. It is limited to 0.1 percent of the finished product.

Usage: EU/USA

Isopropyl hydroxypalmityl ether

Function: Surfactant / Emulsifier.

Origin: Semisynthetic or synthetic compound.

Restrictions and Adverse Effects: May cause contact allergies in some individuals.

Usage: USA/Not currently on the EU inventory of cosmetic ingredients.

Isopropyl isostearate

Function: Emollient / Moisturizer.

Origin: Semisynthetic or synthetic compound.

Restrictions and Adverse Effects: Comedogenic (acne promoting, see *A–Z of Cosmetic Terms – Comedogen*).

Usage: EU/USA

Isopropyl methoxycinnamate

Function: UV absorber.

Origin: Synthetic compound.

Restrictions and Adverse Effects: Cinnamates have been reported to cause a stinging sensation in some people.

Usage: EU/USA

Isopropyl myristate

Function: Binding agent / Emollient / Moisturizer / Solvent.

Origin: Semisynthetic or synthetic compound.

Restrictions and Adverse Effects: Comedogenic (acne promoting, see *A–Z of Cosmetic Terms – Comedogen*).

Usage: EU/USA

Isopropyl palmitate

Function: Antistatic agent / Binding agent / Emollient / Moisturizer / Solvent.

Origin: Semisynthetic or synthetic compound.

Restrictions and Adverse Effects: Comedogenic (acne promoting, see *A–Z of Cosmetic Terms – Comedogen*). Some palmitates have been linked to contact dermatitis.

Usage: EU/USA

Isopropyl thioglycolate

Function: Depilatory agent / Reducing agent.

Origin: Synthetic compound.

Restrictions and Adverse Effects: EU regulations require the following mandatory warnings: "May cause sensitization in the event of skin contact. Avoid contact with eyes. In the event of contact with eyes, rinse with plenty of water and seek medical advice. Wear suitable gloves. Follow the instructions. Keep out of reach of children." The label must also state "Contains Thioglycolate." It is limited to 8 percent for general use or 11 percent for professional use, and the pH must be between 6 and 9.5.

Usage: EU/USA

Isopropylbenzyl salicylate

Function: UV absorber.

Origin: Synthetic compound.

Restrictions and Adverse Effects: The safety of this substance was uncertain and its use in cosmetics was only provisionally permitted in the EU, until June 30, 1998. After this date its safety was still unproven and its provisional status was extended. It is limited to a maximum of 4 percent of the finished product. It may be used to protect the ingredients of other cosmetics and toiletries from the detrimental effects of sunlight.

Usage: EU/USA

Isopropylparaben

Function: Preservative.

Origin: Synthetic compound of the benzoate family.

Restrictions and Adverse Effects: Benzoic acid, benzoates and parabens have been implicated in a large number of health issues. (See *A–Z of Cosmetic Terms – Benzoates*.) It is limited to 0.4 percent of the finished product if used on its own as a preservative, or 0.8 percent in total if used in combination with other parabens. Parabens may be added in larger quantities for other stated purposes.

Usage: EU/USA

Isostearamide DEA

Function: Antistatic agent / Viscosity adjuster / Foaming agent.

Origin: Semisynthetic or synthetic compound.

Restrictions and Adverse Effects: DEA residues are cancer suspects currently under investigation. See *A–Z of Cosmetic Terms – DEA*.

Usage: EU/USA

Isosteareth – Family

Examples include Isosteareth-10 stearate and Isosteareth-20.

Function: Mainly emulsifiers and surfactants.

Origin: A range of synthetic ingredients manufactured from ethylene oxide. These ethoxylated compounds may be combined with a variety of other molecules to produce a wide range of cosmetic materials. Higher numbers mean higher ethoxylation (bigger molecules), usually resulting in a greater solubility in water.

Restrictions and Adverse Effects: Ethoxylated ingredients are made using ethylene oxide (oxirane), which can form 1,4-dioxane, a carcinogen, as a by-product of manufacture. See *A–Z of Cosmetic Terms – Dioxane*.

Usage: EU/USA

Isostearyl myristate

Function: Emollient / Moisturizer.

Origin: Semisynthetic or synthetic compound.

Restrictions and Adverse Effects: Some myristates are comedogenic (acne promoting, see *A–Z of Cosmetic Terms – Comedogen*).

Usage: EU/USA

Isostearyl neopentanoate

Function: Emollient / Moisturizer.

Origin: Synthetic compound.

Restrictions and Adverse Effects: Comedogenic (acne promoting, see *A–Z of Cosmetic Terms – Comedogen*).

Usage: EU/USA

Isostearyl palmitate

Function: Emollient / Moisturizer.

Origin: Semisynthetic or synthetic compound.

Restrictions and Adverse Effects: Some palmitates have been linked to contact dermatitis.

Usage: EU/USA

Isothiazolinone

Function: Preservative.

Origin: Synthetic compound.

Restrictions and Adverse Effects: May cause contact dermatitis in some individuals.

Usage: USA/Not currently on the EU inventory of cosmetic ingredients.

Isotridecyl myristate

Function: Emollient / Moisturizer.

Origin: Semisynthetic or synthetic compound.

Restrictions and Adverse Effects: Some myristates are comedogenic (acne promoting, see *A–Z of Cosmetic Terms – Comedogen*).
Usage: EU/USA

Ivy
(Ivy extract, see *Hedera helix*)

l-Alpha hydroxy acids
(Alpha hydroxy acids)
Function: Exfoliating agents.
Origin: Various origins.
Restrictions and Adverse Effects: Alpha-hydroxy acids (AHAs) are used to exfoliate skin (a skin peeler to remove outer layer of skin cells). AHAs can cause increased sensitivity to the sun due to loss of the protective outer layer of skin cells. Do not expose skin to the sun immediately following treatment with AHAs. Test a small area before use and discontinue use if skin irritation, redness, bleeding, or pain is experienced. Not recommended for use on children. May cause exfoliative dermatitis.
Usage: USA/Not currently on the EU inventory of cosmetic ingredients.

Lactic acid
Function: pH control / Humectant / Exfoliating agent.
Origin: Natural extract formed by the bacterial oxidation of milk lactose.
Restrictions and Adverse Effects: Lactic acid is an alpha-hydroxy acid (AHA), which is used to exfoliate skin (a skin peeler to remove outer layer of skin cells). AHAs can cause increased sensitivity to the sun due to loss of the protective outer layer of skin cells. Do not expose skin to the sun immediately following treatment with AHAs. Test a small area before use and discontinue use if skin irritation, redness, bleeding, or pain is experienced. Not recommended for use on children. May cause exfoliative dermatitis.
Usage: EU/USA

Lactoflavin
(E101)
Function: Yellow colorant.
Origin: Natural plant extract.
Restrictions and Adverse Effects: Allowed in all products.
Usage: EU/USA

Lactoyl methylsilanol elastinate
Function: Antistatic agent.
Origin: A semisynthetic compound derived from elastin, a flexible protein extracted from the layers of skin and artery walls of mammals.
Restrictions and Adverse Effects: No currently known adverse effects. For BSE precautions see *Chapter 17 – Animal Products and Animal Testing*.
Usage: EU/USA

Laneth – Family
Examples include Laneth-10, Laneth-15, Laneth-10 acetate and Laneth-4 phosphate.
Function: Mainly emulsifiers, viscosity adjusters, emollients and surfactants.
Origin: A range of synthetic ingredients manufactured from ethylene oxide and lanolin. Higher numbers mean higher ethoxylation (bigger molecules), usually resulting in a greater solubility in water.
Restrictions and Adverse Effects: The Laneth group have comedogenic (acne promoting) properties. Some Laneth ingredients can cause contact dermatitis in some individuals. These ethoxylated ingredients are made using ethylene oxide (oxirane), which can form 1,4-dioxane, a carcinogen, as a by-product of manufacture. See *A–Z of Cosmetic Terms – Comedogen; Dioxane*.
Usage: EU/USA

Lanolin
(Wool fat)
Function: Antistatic agent / Emollient / Lubricant / Moisturizer.
Origin: Lanolin is extracted from the wool of sheep. It is secreted by the sebaceous glands to waterproof and protect the wool. Cosmetic quality lanolin

consists of a highly complex mixture of esters of high molecular weight aliphatic, steroid or triterpenoid alcohols and fatty acids. It is an excellent emollient, skin lubricant and barrier cream, capable of absorbing up to 50 percent of its own weight of water. It is rich in cholesterol and other skin-friendly sterols.

Restrictions and Adverse Effects: Comedogenic (acne promoting). May cause contact dermatitis in some individuals. See *A–Z of Cosmetic Terms – Comedogen.*

Usage: EU/USA

Lanolin alcohol

Function: Antistatic agent / Emollient / Moisturizer / Emulsifier.

Origin: An extract of lanolin, obtained from the wool of sheep.

Restrictions and Adverse Effects: Comedogenic (acne promoting, see *A–Z of Cosmetic Terms – Comedogen*).

Usage: EU/USA

Lanolinamide DEA

Function: Emulsifier / Emulsion stabilizer / Surfactant / Viscosity adjuster / Foaming agent.

Origin: Semisynthetic compound derived from lanolin.

Restrictions and Adverse Effects: DEA residues are cancer suspects currently under investigation. See *A–Z of Cosmetic Terms – DEA.*

Usage: EU/USA

Lauralkonium bromide

Function: Preservative.

Origin: Synthetic compound.

Restrictions and Adverse Effects: The safety of this substance was uncertain and its use in cosmetics was only provisionally permitted in the EU, until June 30, 1998. On September 3, 1998, following further scientific tests, the provisional status was removed and this ingredient was permitted for use in cosmetics. It is limited to a maximum of 0.1 percent of the finished product if it is used as a preservative, but may be added in larger quantities if it is used for other stated purposes. The label must state "Avoid contact with the eyes."

Usage: EU/USA

Lauralkonium chloride

Function: Preservative.

Origin: Synthetic compound.

Restrictions and Adverse Effects: The safety of this substance was uncertain and its use in cosmetics was only provisionally permitted in the EU, until June 30, 1998. On September 3, 1998, following further scientific tests, the provisional status was removed and this ingredient was permitted for use in cosmetics. It is limited to a maximum of 0.1 percent of the finished product if it is used as a preservative, but may be added in larger quantities if it is used for other stated purposes. The label must state "Avoid contact with the eyes."

Usage: EU/USA

Lauramide / Myristamide DEA

Function: Surfactant / Foaming agent.

Origin: Semisynthetic or synthetic compound.

Restrictions and Adverse Effects: DEA residues are cancer suspects currently under investigation. See *A–Z of Cosmetic Terms – DEA.*

Usage: EU/USA

Lauramide DEA

Function: Antistatic agent / Viscosity adjuster / Foaming agent /Surfactant.

Origin: Semisynthetic or synthetic compound.

Restrictions and Adverse Effects: DEA residues are cancer suspects currently under investigation. See *A–Z of Cosmetic Terms – DEA.*

Usage: EU/USA

Lauramidopropyl dimethylamine

Function: Antistatic agent.

Origin: Semisynthetic or synthetic compound.

Restrictions and Adverse Effects: May cause contact allergies in some individuals.

Usage: EU/USA

Laureth – Family

Examples include Laureth-2, Laureth-2 benzoate and Laureth-10 carboxylic acid.

Function: Mainly emulsifiers, emollients, moisturizers and surfactants.

Origin: A range of synthetic ingredients manufactured from ethylene oxide. These ethoxylated compounds may be combined with a variety of other molecules to produce a wide range of cosmetic materials. Higher numbers mean higher ethoxylation (bigger molecules), usually resulting in a greater solubility in water.

Restrictions and Adverse Effects: Ethoxylated ingredients are made using ethylene oxide (oxirane), which can form 1,4-dioxane, a carcinogen, as a by-product of manufacture. See *A–Z of Cosmetic Terms – Dioxane.*

Usage: EU/USA

Laurtrimonium bromide

Function: Antistatic agent / Preservative.

Origin: Synthetic compound.

Restrictions and Adverse Effects: This ingredient is limited to 0.1 percent of the finished product if used as a preservative, but it may be added in larger quantities for other stated purposes.

Usage: EU/USA

Laurtrimonium chloride

Function: Preservative.

Origin: Synthetic compound.

Restrictions and Adverse Effects: This ingredient is limited to 0.1 percent of the finished product if used as a preservative, but it may be added in larger quantities for other stated purposes.

Usage: EU/USA

Laurus nobilis

Function: Botanical additive.

Origin: Natural plant extract from members of the laurel family, including bay, which is used as a herb in cooking.

Restrictions and Adverse Effects: Can cause severe allergies.

Usage: EU/USA

Lauryl alcohol

Function: Emollient / Moisturizer / Emulsion stabilizer / Viscosity adjuster.

Origin: Semisynthetic or synthetic compound.

Restrictions and Adverse Effects: Comedogenic (acne promoting, see *A–Z of Cosmetic Terms – Comedogen*).

Usage: EU/USA

Lauryl myristate

Function: Antistatic agent / Emollient / Moisturizer.

Origin: Semisynthetic or synthetic compound.

Restrictions and Adverse Effects: Some myristates are comedogenic (acne promoting, see *A–Z of Cosmetic Terms – Comedogen*).

Usage: EU/USA

Lauryl palmitate

Function: Antistatic agent / Emollient / Moisturizer.

Origin: Semisynthetic or synthetic compound.

Restrictions and Adverse Effects: Some palmitates have been linked to contact dermatitis.

Usage: EU/USA

Lavandula angustifolia

Function: Botanical additive / Aromatherapy oil.

Origin: Plant extract of the lavender family – a fragrant oil.

Restrictions and Adverse Effects: Can cause contact allergies and photosensitivity in some individuals.

Usage: EU/USA

Lavandula hybrida

Function: Emollient / Moisturizer / Aromatherapy oil.

Origin: Plant extract of the lavender family – a fragrant oil.

Restrictions and Adverse Effects: Can cause contact allergies and photosensitivity in some individuals.

Usage: EU/USA

Lead acetate

Function: Progressive hair dye used to gradually change the color of hair.

Origin: Synthetic compound.

Restrictions and Adverse Effects: Irritant. Lead salts are toxic. It is limited to 0.6 percent of lead in the finished product. The label must clearly show the name of this ingredient, and carry the following warnings: "Keep out of the reach of children. Not for use on eyelashes, eyebrows or moustaches. Avoid eye contact. Wash hands after use. Discontinue use if irritation occurs."
Usage: EU/USA

Lecithinamide DEA

Function: Antistatic agent / Viscosity adjuster.
Origin: Semisynthetic or synthetic compound derived from lecithin, a phospholipid (fatty phosphate) obtained from several natural sources, especially soya beans.
Restrictions and Adverse Effects: Some soya beans grown in the USA are genetically modified (GM); these are mixed with natural soya beans resulting in nearly all soya products containing some GM ingredients. There is no scientific reason for these to have any different effects to natural soya ingredients, but many consumers prefer to avoid GM products for a variety of reasons. DEA residues are cancer suspects currently under investigation. See *A–Z of Cosmetic Terms – DEA*.
Usage: EU/USA

Linalool

(Linalol, Linaloöl)
Function: Deodorant / Fragrance.
Origin: A natural fragrant liquid extracted from a variety of essential oils from lavender, bergamot and coriander.
Restrictions and Adverse Effects: Can cause facial psoriasis in some individuals.
Usage: EU/USA

Linoleamide DEA

Function: Antistatic agent / Viscosity adjuster / Foaming agent.
Origin: Semisynthetic or synthetic compound.
Restrictions and Adverse Effects: DEA residues are cancer suspects currently under investigation. See *A–Z of Cosmetic Terms – DEA*.
Usage: EU/USA

Linum usitatissimum

(Linseed oil)
Function: Emollient / Moisturizer.
Origin: Plant extract.
Restrictions and Adverse Effects: Comedogenic (acne promoting, see *A–Z of Cosmetic Terms – Comedogen*).
Usage: EU/USA

Lithium sulfide

Function: Depilatory agent.
Origin: Synthetic compound.
Restrictions and Adverse Effects: Sulfides are toxic. Irritant. May be alkaline (irritant and corrosive). Maximum allowed content is 2 percent of the finished product. The label must carry warnings to avoid contact with the eyes and to keep the product out of the reach of children.
Usage: EU/USA

m-Phenylenediamine

Function: Hair dye.
Origin: Synthetic compound.
Restrictions and Adverse Effects: Irritant. Found to be mutagenic (causes mutation in cells). Limited to 6 percent of the finished product. The label must clearly show the name of this chemical separately from the list of ingredients and it must carry the following warnings: "Can cause an allergic reaction. Do not use to dye eyelashes or eyebrows." Products supplied for professional use should carry the additional warning, "Wear suitable gloves."
Usage: EU/USA

m-Phenylenediamine sulfate

Function: Hair dye.
Origin: Synthetic compound.
Restrictions and Adverse Effects: Irritant. Found to be mutagenic (causes mutation in cells). Limited to 6 percent of the finished product. The label must clearly show the name of this chemical separately from the list of ingredients and it must carry the following warnings: "Can cause an allergic reaction. Do not use to dye eyelashes or eyebrows." Products supplied for professional use should carry the additional warning, "Wear suitable gloves."
Usage: EU/USA

Magnesium benzoate

Function: Preservative.

Origin: Synthetic compound of the benzoate family.

Restrictions and Adverse Effects: Benzoic acid and benzoates have been implicated in a large number of health issues. (See *A–Z of Cosmetic Terms – Benzoates*.) It is limited to 0.5 percent of the finished product if used as a preservative, but it may be added in larger quantities for other stated purposes.

Usage: EU/USA

Magnesium fluoride

Function: Oral care agent.

Origin: Synthetic compound.

Restrictions and Adverse Effects: Fluorides are toxic. They can discolor teeth (fluorosis). Children should only use a small quantity of toothpaste and be discouraged from swallowing it. The total amount of fluoride allowed by EU regulations is 0.15 percent of the finished product. The label must clearly show the name of this ingredient separately from the list of ingredients.

Usage: EU/USA

Magnesium fluorosilicate

Function: Oral care agent.

Origin: Synthetic compound.

Restrictions and Adverse Effects: Fluorides are toxic. They can discolor teeth (fluorosis). Children should only use a small quantity of toothpaste and be discouraged from swallowing it. The total amount of fluoride allowed by EU regulations is 0.15 percent of the finished product.

Usage: EU/USA

Magnesium myristate

Function: Opacifier / Viscosity adjuster.

Origin: Semisynthetic or synthetic compound.

Restrictions and Adverse Effects: Some myristates are comedogenic (acne promoting, see *A–Z of Cosmetic Terms – Comedogen*).

Usage: EU/USA

Magnesium palmitate

Function: Opacifier / Viscosity adjuster.

Origin: Semisynthetic or synthetic compound.

Restrictions and Adverse Effects: Some palmitates have been linked to contact dermatitis.

Usage: EU/USA

Magnesium propionate

Function: Preservative.

Origin: Synthetic compound.

Restrictions and Adverse Effects: Propanoic acid and its salts are limited to 2 percent of the finished product if used as a preservative, but may be added in larger quantities for other stated purposes.

Usage: EU/USA

Magnesium salicylate

Function: Preservative.

Origin: Synthetic compound.

Restrictions and Adverse Effects: This ingredient is limited to 0.5 percent of the finished product if used as a preservative, but may be added in larger quantities for other stated purposes. With the exception of shampoo, it must not be used in preparations intended for children under the age of 3 and must clearly state this restriction on the label.

Usage: EU/USA

Magnesium stearate

Function: White colorant / Opacifier.

Origin: Semisynthetic or synthetic compound.

Restrictions and Adverse Effects: Allowed in all products.

Usage: EU/USA

Magnesium sulfide

Function: Depilatory agent.

Origin: Synthetic compound.

Restrictions and Adverse Effects: Sulfides are toxic. Irritant. May be alkaline (irritant and corrosive). Maximum allowed content is 6 percent of the finished product. The label must carry warnings to avoid contact with the eyes and to keep the product out of the reach of children.

Usage: EU/USA

Malic acid

Function: pH control / Exfoliating agent.

Origin: Natural fruit extract.

Restrictions and Adverse Effects: Malic acid is an alpha-hydroxy acid (AHA), which is used to exfoliate skin. They are also known as skin peelers because they dissolve and remove the outer layer of skin. They can cause increased sensitivity to the sun due to loss of the protective outer layer of skin cells. Do not expose skin to the sun immediately following treatment with AHAs. Test a small area before use and discontinue use if skin irritation, redness, bleeding, or pain is experienced. Not recommended for use on children. May cause exfoliative dermatitis.
Usage: EU/USA

MDM hydantoin
Function: Antimicrobial.
Origin: Synthetic compound.
Restrictions and Adverse Effects: Hydantoins have been linked to contact dermatitis.
Usage: EU/USA

MEA o-phenylphenate
Function: Preservative.
Origin: Synthetic compound.
Restrictions and Adverse Effects: This ingredient is limited to 0.2 percent of the finished product if used as a preservative, but may be added in larger quantities for other stated purposes.
Usage: EU/USA

MEA sulfite
(Monoethanolamine sulfite, Ethanolamine sulfite)
Function: Preservative.
Origin: Synthetic compound.
Restrictions and Adverse Effects: Can cause contact dermatitis and contact allergies.
Usage: USA/Not currently on the EU inventory of cosmetic ingredients.

MEA-benzoate
Function: Preservative.
Origin: Synthetic compound of the benzoate family.
Restrictions and Adverse Effects: Benzoic acid and benzoates have been implicated in a large number of health issues. (See *A–Z of Cosmetic Terms – Benzoates*.) It is limited to 0.5 percent of the finished product if used as a preservative, but may be added

in larger quantities for other stated purposes.
Usage: EU/USA

MEA-borate
Function: Viscosity adjuster.
Origin: Synthetic compound.
Restrictions and Adverse Effects: Borates are toxic and have been linked to fetal malformations.
Usage: EU/USA

MEA-salicylate
Function: Preservative.
Origin: Synthetic compound.
Restrictions and Adverse Effects: This ingredient is limited to 0.5 percent of the finished product if used as a preservative, but may be added in larger quantities for other stated purposes. With the exception of shampoo, it must not be used in preparations intended for children under the age of 3 and must clearly state this restriction on the label.
Usage: EU/USA

MEA-undecylenate
Function: Preservative.
Origin: Synthetic compound.
Restrictions and Adverse Effects: This ingredient is limited to 0.2 percent of the finished product if used as a preservative, but may be added in larger quantities for other stated purposes.
Usage: EU/USA

Mentha piperita
(Peppermint oil)
Function: Botanical additive.
Origin: Plant extract (peppermint).
Restrictions and Adverse Effects: Irritant for some individuals. May cause allergic contact dermatitis.
Usage: EU/USA

Methenamine
Function: Preservative.
Origin: Synthetic compound.
Restrictions and Adverse Effects: Skin irritant. Limited to 0.2 percent of the finished product.
Usage: EU/USA

Methyl alcohol

(Methanol)

Function: Denaturant / Solvent.

Origin: Synthetic compound.

Restrictions and Adverse Effects: Toxic. Can cause contact eczema. Maximum amount allowed is 5 percent of the total alcohol content in the product.

Usage: EU/USA

Methyl benzoate

Function: Preservative.

Origin: Synthetic compound of the benzoate family.

Restrictions and Adverse Effects: Benzoic acid and benzoates have been implicated in a large number of health issues. (See *A–Z of Cosmetic Terms – Benzoates*.) It is limited to 0.5 percent of the finished product if used as a preservative, but may be added in larger quantities for other stated purposes.

Usage: EU/USA

Methyl glucose sesquistearate

Function: Emollient / Moisturizer / Emulsifier.

Origin: Semisynthetic compound.

Restrictions and Adverse Effects: May cause dermatitis in some individuals.

Usage: EU/USA

Methyl glucoside

(Methyl-alpha-d-glycopyranoside)

Function: Additive.

Origin: Semisynthetic compound.

Restrictions and Adverse Effects: May cause contact dermatitis in some individuals.

Usage: USA/Not currently on the EU inventory of cosmetic ingredients.

Methyl methacrylate

Function: Solvent.

Origin: Synthetic compound.

Restrictions and Adverse Effects: Highly flammable. Danger of explosion when mixed with air. Explosive limit – 2.1 to 12.5 percent.

Usage: USA/This ingredient is banned in the EU.

Methyl myristate

Function: Emollient / Moisturizer.

Origin: Semisynthetic or synthetic compound.

Restrictions and Adverse Effects: Some myristates are comedogenic (acne promoting, see *A–Z of Cosmetic Terms – Comedogen*).

Usage: EU/USA

Methyl oleate

Function: Emollient / Moisturizer.

Origin: Semisynthetic or synthetic compound.

Restrictions and Adverse Effects: Comedogenic (acne promoting, see *A–Z of Cosmetic Terms – Comedogen*).

Usage: EU/USA

Methyl palmitate

Function: Emollient / Moisturizer.

Origin: Semisynthetic or synthetic compound.

Restrictions and Adverse Effects: Some palmitates have been linked to contact dermatitis.

Usage: EU/USA

Methyl thioglycolate

Function: Depilatory agent / Reducing agent.

Origin: Synthetic compound.

Restrictions and Adverse Effects: EU regulations require the following mandatory warnings: "May cause sensitization in the event of skin contact. Avoid contact with eyes. In the event of contact with eyes, rinse with plenty of water and seek medical advice. Wear suitable gloves. Follow the instructions. Keep out of reach of children." The label must also state "Contains Thioglycolate." It is limited to 8 percent for general use or 11 percent for professional use, and the pH must be between 6 and 9.5.

Usage: EU/USA

Methylchloroisothiazolinone

Function: Preservative.

Origin: Synthetic compound.

Restrictions and Adverse Effects: Can cause contact dermatitis and contact allergies. Methylchloroisothiazolinone is used in combination with Methylisothiazolinone in the ratio 3:1, with

magnesium chloride and magnesium nitrate added to enhance the effectiveness of this preservative. The mixture is limited to 0.0015 percent of the finished product.
Usage: EU/USA

Methyldibromo glutaronitrile

(Tektamer 38)
Function: Preservative.
Origin: Synthetic compound.
Restrictions and Adverse Effects: Can cause allergic contact dermatitis and contact eczema. It is limited to 0.1 percent of the finished product, or 0.025 percent in suntan and sunscreen preparations, as this compound is activated by sunlight and can cause damage to skin cells and can destroy the UV-absorbing compounds in the suntan lotions, rendering them ineffective as sunscreens.
Usage: EU/USA

Methylethanolamine

Function: pH control.
Origin: Synthetic compound.
Restrictions and Adverse Effects: Harmful. Danger of nitrosamine contamination (see *A–Z of Cosmetic Terms – Nitrosamines*). This product must have a minimum purity of 99 percent, with a maximum secondary alkolamine contamination of 0.5 percent. The maximum allowed content is 0.5 percent of the finished product.
Usage: EU/USA

Methylisothiazolinone

Function: Preservative.
Origin: Synthetic compound.
Restrictions and Adverse Effects: Can cause allergic reactions. Methylisothiazolinone is used in combination with Methylchloroisothiazolinone in the ratio 1:3, with magnesium chloride and magnesium nitrate added to enhance the effectiveness of this preservative. The mixture is limited to 0.0015 percent of the finished product.
Usage: EU/USA

Methylparaben

Function: Preservative.
Origin: Synthetic compound of the benzoate family.
Restrictions and Adverse Effects: Benzoic acid, benzoates and parabens have been implicated in a large number of health issues. (See *A–Z of Cosmetic Terms – Benzoates*.) It is limited to 0.4 percent of the finished product if used on its own as a preservative, or 0.8 percent in total if used in combination with other parabens. Parabens may be added in larger quantities for other stated purposes.
Usage: EU/USA

Methylsilanol elastinate

Function: Antistatic agent.
Origin: A semisynthetic compound derived from elastin, a flexible protein extracted from the layers of skin and artery walls of mammals.
Restrictions and Adverse Effects: No currently known adverse effects. For BSE precautions, see *Chapter 17 – Animal Products and Animal Testing*.
Usage: EU/USA

Mink oil

Function: Emollient / Moisturizer.
Origin: An oil extracted from the subcutaneous fatty tissue of mink.
Restrictions and Adverse Effects: No currently known adverse effects.
Usage: EU/USA

Mink oil PEG-13 esters

Function: Emollient / Moisturizer.
Origin: A semisynthetic compound derived from mink oil obtained from the fatty, subcutaneous tissue of mink.
Restrictions and Adverse Effects: No currently known adverse effects. This ethoxylated ingredient is made using ethylene oxide (oxirane), which can form 1,4-dioxane, a carcinogen, as a by-product of manufacture. See *A–Z of Cosmetic Terms – Dioxane*.
Usage: EU/USA

Minkamide DEA

Function: Surfactant / Foaming agent.

Origin: A semisynthetic compound derived from mink oil obtained from the fatty, subcutaneous tissue of mink.

Restrictions and Adverse Effects: DEA residues are cancer suspects currently under investigation. See *A–Z of Cosmetic Terms – DEA*.

Usage: EU/USA

Minkamidopropalkonium chloride

Function: Antistatic agent.

Origin: A semisynthetic compound derived from mink oil obtained from the fatty, subcutaneous tissue of mink.

Restrictions and Adverse Effects: No currently known adverse effects.

Usage: EU/USA

Minkamidopropyl betaine

Function: Surfactant.

Origin: A semisynthetic compound derived from mink oil obtained from the fatty, subcutaneous tissue of mink.

Restrictions and Adverse Effects: No currently known adverse effects.

Usage: EU/USA

Minkamidopropyl dimethylamine

Function: Antistatic agent / Emulsifier / Surfactant.

Origin: A semisynthetic compound derived from mink oil obtained from the fatty, subcutaneous tissue of mink.

Restrictions and Adverse Effects: No currently known adverse effects.

Usage: EU/USA

Minkamidopropyl ethyldimonium ethosulfate

Function: Antistatic agent.

Origin: A semisynthetic compound derived from mink oil obtained from the fatty, subcutaneous tissue of mink.

Restrictions and Adverse Effects: No currently known adverse effects.

Usage: EU/USA

Minkamidopropylamine oxide

Function: Surfactant.

Origin: A semisynthetic compound derived from mink oil obtained from the fatty, subcutaneous tissue of mink.

Restrictions and Adverse Effects: No currently known adverse effects.

Usage: EU/USA

MIPA-borate

Function: Viscosity adjuster.

Origin: Synthetic compound.

Restrictions and Adverse Effects: Borates are toxic and have been linked to fetal malformations.

Usage: EU/USA

Mixed fruit acids

(Tri-alpha Hydroxy Fruit Acids, Triple Fruit Acids)

Function: Exfoliating agent.

Origin: Mostly natural fruit extracts.

Restrictions and Adverse Effects: These ingredients contain alpha-hydroxy acids (AHAs), which are used to exfoliate skin. They are also known as skin peelers because they dissolve and remove the outer layer of skin. They can cause increased sensitivity to the sun due to loss of the protective outer layer of skin cells. Do not expose skin to the sun immediately following treatment with AHAs. Test a small area before use and discontinue use if skin irritation, redness, bleeding, or pain is experienced. Not recommended for use on children. May cause exfoliative dermatitis.

Usage: USA/Not currently on the EU inventory of cosmetic ingredients.

Mixed isopropanolamines

Function: pH control.

Origin: Synthetic mixture of compounds.

Restrictions and Adverse Effects: Harmful. Danger of nitrosamine contamination (see *A–Z of Cosmetic Terms – Nitrosamines*). This product must have a minimum purity of 99 percent, with a maximum secondary alkolamine contamination of 0.5 percent. The maximum allowed content is 0.5 percent of the finished product.

Usage: EU/USA

Mixed isopropanolamines myristate

Function: Emulsifier / Surfactant.

Origin: Synthetic mixture of compounds.

Restrictions and Adverse Effects: Some myristates are comedogenic (acne promoting, see *A–Z of Cosmetic Terms – Comedogen*).

Usage: EU/USA

Modulan

Function: Additive.

Origin: Synthetic compound.

Restrictions and Adverse Effects: Skin irritant. This ingredient has caused changes in the skin cells of laboratory animals.

Usage: USA/Not currently on the EU inventory of cosmetic ingredients.

Moskene

(Musk moskene)

Function: Fragrance. (Synthetic nitro musk.)

Origin: Synthetic compound made by the nitration of petroleum derivatives.

Restrictions and Adverse Effects: Can cause pigmented contact dermatitis and hyperpigmentation (excessive coloration of the skin). This ingredient was banned from cosmetics sold in the EU with effect from September 3, 1998.

Usage: USA/Banned from cosmetics in the EU.

Musk ambrette

Function: Fragrance. (Synthetic nitro musk.)

Origin: Synthetic compound made by the nitration of petroleum derivatives.

Restrictions and Adverse Effects: Can cause pigmented photoallergic contact dermatitis and has neurotoxic effects. The International Fragrance Association has recommended that musk ambrette should not be used in cosmetics that come into contact with the skin, especially those products that are used on parts of the body that are exposed to sunlight.

Usage: USA/Banned from cosmetics in the EU.

Myreth – Family

Examples include Myreth-10. Myreth-3 caprate and Myreth-5 carboxylic acid.

Function: Mainly emulsifiers, emollients, moisturizers and surfactants.

Origin: A range of synthetic ingredients manufactured from ethylene oxide. These ethoxylated compounds may be combined with a variety of other molecules to produce a wide range of cosmetic materials. Higher numbers mean higher ethoxylation (bigger molecules), usually resulting in a greater solubility in water.

Restrictions and Adverse Effects: Ethoxylated ingredients are made using ethylene oxide (oxirane), which can form 1,4-dioxane, a carcinogen, as a by-product of manufacture. See *A–Z of Cosmetic Terms – Dioxane*.

Usage: EU/USA

Myreth-2 myristate

Function: Emollient / Moisturizer / Surfactant.

Origin: Semisynthetic or synthetic compound.

Restrictions and Adverse Effects: Some myristates are comedogenic (acne promoting). This ethoxylated ingredient is made using ethylene oxide (oxirane), which can form 1,4-dioxane, a carcinogen, as a by-product of manufacture. See *A–Z of Cosmetic Terms – Comedogen; Dioxane*.

Usage: EU/USA

Myreth-3 myristate

Function: Emollient / Moisturizer / Surfactant.

Origin: Semisynthetic or synthetic compound.

Restrictions and Adverse Effects: Some myristates are comedogenic (acne promoting). This ethoxylated ingredient is made using ethylene oxide (oxirane), which can form 1,4-dioxane, a carcinogen, as a by-product of manufacture. See *A–Z of Cosmetic Terms – Comedogen; Dioxane*.

Usage: EU/USA

Myreth-3 palmitate

Function: Emollient / Moisturizer.

Origin: Semisynthetic or synthetic compound.

Restrictions and Adverse Effects: Some palmitates have been linked to contact dermatitis. This ethoxylated ingredient is made using ethylene oxide (oxirane), which can form 1,4-dioxane, a carcinogen, as a by-product of manufacture. See *A–Z of Cosmetic Terms – Dioxane.*
Usage: EU/USA

Myristalkonium chloride

Function: Preservative.
Origin: Semisynthetic or synthetic compound.
Restrictions and Adverse Effects: The safety of this substance was uncertain and its use in cosmetics was only provisionally permitted in the EU, until June 30, 1998. On September 3, 1998, following further scientific tests, the provisional status was removed and this ingredient was permitted for use in cosmetics. It is limited to a maximum of 0.1 percent of the finished product if it is used as a preservative, but may be added in larger quantities if it is used for other stated purposes. The label must state "Avoid contact with the eyes."
Usage: EU/USA

Myristalkonium saccharinate

Function: Preservative.
Origin: Semisynthetic or synthetic compound.
Restrictions and Adverse Effects: The safety of this substance was uncertain and its use in cosmetics was only provisionally permitted in the EU, until June 30, 1998. On September 3, 1998, following further scientific tests, the provisional status was removed and this ingredient was permitted for use in cosmetics. It is limited to a maximum of 0.1 percent of the finished product if it is used as a preservative, but may be added in larger quantities if it is used for other stated purposes. The label must state "Avoid contact with the eyes."
Usage: EU/USA

Myristamide DEA

Function: Antistatic agent / Viscosity adjuster / Foaming agent.
Origin: Semisynthetic or synthetic compound.

Restrictions and Adverse Effects: DEA residues are cancer suspects currently under investigation. See *A–Z of Cosmetic Terms – DEA.*
Usage: EU/USA

Myristamidopropyl dimethylamine

Function: Antistatic agent.
Origin: Semisynthetic or synthetic compound.
Restrictions and Adverse Effects: May cause contact allergies in some individuals.
Usage: EU/USA

Myristyl alcohol

Function: Emollient / Moisturizer / Emulsion stabilizer / Viscosity adjuster.
Origin: Semisynthetic or synthetic compound.
Restrictions and Adverse Effects: May cause contact allergies in some individuals.
Usage: EU/USA

Myristyl myristate

Function: Emollient / Moisturizer / Opacifier.
Origin: Semisynthetic or synthetic compound.
Restrictions and Adverse Effects: Comedogenic (acne promoting, see *A–Z of Cosmetic Terms – Comedogen*).
Usage: EU/USA

Myristyl propionate

Function: Emollient / Moisturizer.
Origin: Semisynthetic or synthetic compound.
Restrictions and Adverse Effects: Comedogenic (acne promoting, see *A–Z of Cosmetic Terms – Comedogen*).
Usage: EU/USA

Myrtrimonium bromide

Function: Preservative.
Origin: Semisynthetic or synthetic compound.
Restrictions and Adverse Effects: This ingredient is limited to 0.1 percent of the finished product if it is used as a preservative, but may be added in larger quantities for other stated purposes.
Usage: EU/USA

N-Butyl alcohol

(Butanol, Butan-1-ol, Butyl alcohol)

Function: Denaturant / Solvent.

Origin: Synthetic compound.

Restrictions and Adverse Effects: Skin irritant. Eye irritant. May cause inflammation.

Usage: EU/USA

N-Phenyl-p-phenylenediamine HCl

Function: Hair dye.

Origin: Synthetic compound.

Restrictions and Adverse Effects: Irritant. This ingredient is limited to 6 percent of the finished product. The label must clearly show the name of this chemical separately from the list of ingredients and it must carry the following warnings: "Can cause an allergic reaction. Do not use to dye eyelashes or eyebrows." Products supplied for professional use should carry the additional warning, "Wear suitable gloves."

Usage: EU/USA

Naphthalene

(Tar camphor)

Function: Insecticide.

Origin: Polyaromatic hydrocarbon extracted from petroleum or coal tar.

Restrictions and Adverse Effects: Cancer suspect. Toxic by inhalation.

Usage: USA/Not currently on the EU inventory of cosmetic ingredients.

Naphthoquinone

(Naphtoquinone)

Function: Oxidizing agent.

Origin: Synthetic compound.

Restrictions and Adverse Effects: Irritant.

Usage: USA/Not currently on the EU inventory of cosmetic ingredients.

Neomycin

Function: Antibiotic.

Available only on prescription in the UK.

Origin: Semisynthetic compound.

Restrictions and Adverse Effects: Can cause contact dermatitis in some individuals.

Usage: USA/Antibiotics are banned from cosmetics in the EU.

Neopentyl glycol dicaprylate / Dicaprate

Function: Emollient / Moisturizer.

Origin: Semisynthetic or synthetic compound.

Restrictions and Adverse Effects: No currently known adverse effects.

Usage: EU/USA

Nickel sulfate

Function: Additive.

Origin: Synthetic compound.

Restrictions and Adverse Effects: Causes contact dermatitis.

Usage: USA/Not currently on the EU inventory of cosmetic ingredients.

Nicomethanol hydrofluoride

Function: Oral care agent.

Origin: Synthetic compound.

Restrictions and Adverse Effects: Fluorides are toxic. They can discolor teeth (fluorosis). Children should only use a small quantity of toothpaste and be discouraged from swallowing it. The total amount of fluoride allowed by EU regulations is 0.15 percent of the finished product. The label must clearly show the name of this additive separately from the list of ingredients.

Usage: EU/USA

Nitrilotriacetic acid

Function: Chelating agent.

Origin: Synthetic compound.

Restrictions and Adverse Effects: Cancer suspect.

Usage: USA/Not currently on the EU inventory of cosmetic ingredients.

Nitromethane

Function: Anticorrosive.

Origin: Synthetic compound.

Restrictions and Adverse Effects: Harmful. Irritant. This ingredient is limited to 3 percent of the finished product.

Usage: EU/USA

Nizoral™

(Ketoconazole)

Function: Antidandruff agent.

Origin: Synthetic compound.

Restrictions and Adverse Effects: No currently known adverse effects.

Usage: USA/Not currently on the EU inventory of cosmetic ingredients.

Nonylphenol

Function: Surfactant / Emulsifier.

Widely used in cleaning products, cosmetics, toiletries, plastics, spermicides, and pesticides.

Origin: Synthetic compound.

Restrictions and Adverse Effects: Skin irritant. Can cause contact dermatitis in some individuals. A known endocrine disrupter chemical (EDC), which mimics estrogen (the female sex hormone) causing feminization of males of all species and resulting in low sperm counts and malformed genitalia. It is persistent in the environment and can accumulate in body tissues. (See *A–Z of Cosmetic Terms – Gender Bender; Biodegradable.*)

Usage: USA/Not currently on the EU inventory of cosmetic ingredients.

Novocain

(Procaine Hydrochloride, Procaine HCl)

Function: Local anesthetic / Pain control.

Origin: Synthetic compound.

Restrictions and Adverse Effects: Can cause contact dermatitis in some individuals.

Usage: USA/Not currently on the EU inventory of cosmetic ingredients.

o-Cymen-5-ol

Function: Preservative.

Origin: Synthetic compound.

Restrictions and Adverse Effects: This ingredient is limited to 0.1 percent of the finished product.

Usage: EU/USA

o-Nitro-p-aminophenol

Function: Hair dye.

Origin: Synthetic compound.

Restrictions and Adverse Effects: Cancer suspect.

Usage: USA/Banned from cosmetics in the EU.

o-Phenylphenol

Function: Preservative.

Origin: Synthetic compound.

Restrictions and Adverse Effects: This ingredient is limited to 0.2 percent of the finished product if used as a preservative, but it may be added in larger quantities for other stated purposes.

Usage: EU/USA

Oak moss

Function: Botanical additive.

Origin: Plant extract.

Restrictions and Adverse Effects: Skin irritant. May cause contact allergies in some individuals.

Usage: USA/Not currently on the EU inventory of cosmetic ingredients.

Octadecenyl-ammonium fluoride

Function: Oral care agent.

Origin: Semisynthetic or synthetic compound.

Restrictions and Adverse Effects: Fluorides are toxic. They can discolor teeth (fluorosis). Children should only use a small quantity of toothpaste and be discouraged from swallowing it. The total amount of fluoride allowed by EU regulations is 0.15 percent of the finished product.

Usage: EU/USA

Octoxyglyceryl palmitate

Function: Emulsifier.

Origin: Semisynthetic or synthetic compound.

Restrictions and Adverse Effects: Some palmitates have been linked to contact dermatitis.

Usage: EU/USA

Octyl dimethyl PABA

(Padimate O)

Function: UV absorber.

Origin: Synthetic compound.

Restrictions and Adverse Effects: The safety of this substance was uncertain and its use in cosmetics was only provisionally permitted in the EU, until June

30, 1998. After this date its safety was still unproven and its provisional status was extended. It is limited to a maximum amount of 8 percent of the finished product. It may be used to protect the ingredients of other cosmetics and toiletries from the detrimental effects of sunlight.

Usage: EU/USA

Octyl isopalmitate

Function: Emollient / Moisturizer.

Origin: Semisynthetic or synthetic compound.

Restrictions and Adverse Effects: Some palmitates have been linked to contact dermatitis.

Usage: EU/USA

Octyl methoxycinnamate

Function: UV absorber.

Origin: Synthetic compound.

Restrictions and Adverse Effects: Cinnamates have been reported to cause a stinging sensation in some people. The safety of this substance was uncertain and its use in cosmetics was only provisionally permitted in the EU, until June 30, 1998. On September 3, 1998, following further scientific tests, the provisional status was removed and this ingredient was permitted for use in cosmetics. It is limited to a maximum amount of 10 percent of the finished product. It may be used to protect the ingredients of other cosmetics and toiletries from the detrimental effects of sunlight.

Usage: EU/USA

Octyl myristate

Function: Emollient / Moisturizer.

Origin: Semisynthetic or synthetic compound.

Restrictions and Adverse Effects: Some myristates are comedogenic (acne promoting, see *A–Z of Cosmetic Terms – Comedogen*).

Usage: EU/USA

Octyl palmitate

Function: Emollient / Moisturizer.

Origin: Semisynthetic or synthetic compound.

Restrictions and Adverse Effects: Comedogenic (acne promoting). Some palmitates have been linked to contact dermatitis. See *A–Z of Cosmetic Terms – Comedogen*.

Usage: EU/USA

Octyl salicylate

Function: UV absorber.

Origin: Semisynthetic or synthetic compound.

Restrictions and Adverse Effects: The safety of this substance was uncertain and its use in cosmetics was only provisionally permitted in the EU, until June 30, 1998. On September 3, 1998, following further scientific tests, the provisional status was removed and this ingredient was permitted for use in cosmetics. It is limited to a maximum amount of 5 percent of the finished product. It may be used to protect the ingredients of other cosmetics and toiletries from the detrimental effects of sunlight.

Usage: EU/USA

Octyl stearate

Function: Emollient / Moisturizer.

Origin: Semisynthetic or synthetic compound.

Restrictions and Adverse Effects: Comedogenic (acne promoting, see *A–Z of Cosmetic Terms – Comedogen*).

Usage: EU/USA

Octyl triazone

Function: UV absorber.

Origin: Synthetic compound.

Restrictions and Adverse Effects: The safety of this substance was uncertain and its use in cosmetics was only provisionally permitted in the EU, until June 30, 1998. On September 3, 1998, following further scientific tests, the provisional status was removed and this ingredient was permitted for use in cosmetics. It is limited to a maximum amount of 5 percent of the finished product. It may be used to protect the ingredients of other cosmetics and toiletries from the detrimental effects of sunlight.

Usage: EU/USA

Octyldodecyl myristate

Function: Emollient / Moisturizer.

Origin: Semisynthetic or synthetic compound.

Restrictions and Adverse Effects: Some myristates are comedogenic (acne promoting, see *A–Z of Cosmetic Terms – Comedogen*).
Usage: EU/USA

Oil of purcellin
(Purcellin, oil of)
Function: Emollient / Moisturizer.
Origin: Natural extract.
Restrictions and Adverse Effects: Skin irritant. Can cause dermatitis in some individuals.
Usage: USA/Not currently on the EU inventory of cosmetic ingredients.

Olea europaea
(Olive oil)
Function: Emollient / Moisturizer / Solvent.
Origin: Plant extract.
Restrictions and Adverse Effects: Comedogenic (acne promoting, see *A–Z of Cosmetic Terms – Comedogen*).
Usage: EU/USA

Olealkonium chloride
Function: Preservative.
Origin: Synthetic compound.
Restrictions and Adverse Effects: The safety of this substance was uncertain and its use in cosmetics was only provisionally permitted in the EU, until June 30, 1998. On September 3, 1998, following further scientific tests, the provisional status was removed and this ingredient was permitted for use in cosmetics. It is limited to a maximum of 0.1 percent of the finished product if it is used as a preservative, but it may be added in larger quantities if it is used for other stated purposes. The label must state "Avoid contact with the eyes."
Usage: EU/USA

Oleamide DEA
Function: Antistatic agent / Viscosity adjuster / Foaming agent.
Origin: Semisynthetic or synthetic compound.
Restrictions and Adverse Effects: DEA residues are cancer suspects currently under investigation. See *A–Z of Cosmetic Terms – DEA*.
Usage: EU/USA

Oleamidopropyl dimethylamine
Function: Antistatic agent.
Origin: Synthetic compound.
Restrictions and Adverse Effects: May cause contact allergies and contact dermatitis in some individuals.
Usage: EU/USA

Oleic acid
Function: Emollient / Moisturizer / Emulsifier.
Origin: Semisynthetic or synthetic compound.
Restrictions and Adverse Effects: Comedogenic (acne promoting, see *A–Z of Cosmetic Terms – Comedogen*).
Usage: EU/USA

Oleyl myristate
Function: Emollient / Moisturizer.
Origin: Semisynthetic or synthetic compound.
Restrictions and Adverse Effects: Some myristates are comedogenic (acne promoting, see *A–Z of Cosmetic Terms – Comedogen*).
Usage: EU/USA

Olivamide DEA
Function: Surfactant / Foaming agent.
Origin: Semisynthetic or synthetic compound derived from olive oil.
Restrictions and Adverse Effects: DEA residues are cancer suspects currently under investigation. See *A–Z of Cosmetic Terms – DEA*.
Usage: EU/USA

Oxalic acid
Function: Chelating agent.
Origin: Synthetic compound.
Restrictions and Adverse Effects: Oxalates are toxic. Maximum allowed content is 5 percent and it is restricted to professional use only.
Usage: EU/USA

Oxybenzone
(Benzophenone-3)
Function: UV absorber.
Origin: Synthetic compound.

Restrictions and Adverse Effects: Irritant. May cause contact dermatitis and photosensitivity in some people. This ingredient is restricted to a maximum of 10 percent of the finished sunscreen product. If used as a sunscreen, the label must state: "Contains Oxybenzone."
Usage: EU/USA

Oxyquinoline
Function: Stabilizer for Hydrogen peroxide.
Origin: Synthetic compound.
Restrictions and Adverse Effects: Irritant. Harmful. This ingredient is limited in amount to 0.3 percent in rinse-off hair care preparations and 0.03 percent in non-rinse off preparations.
Usage: EU/USA

Oxyquinoline sulfate
Function: Antimicrobial / Stabilizer for Hydrogen peroxide.
Origin: Synthetic compound.
Restrictions and Adverse Effects: Irritant. Harmful. This ingredient is limited in amount to 0.3 percent in rinse-off hair care preparations and 0.03 percent in non-rinse off preparations.
Usage: EU/USA

p-Chloro-m-cresol
(Chlorocresol)
Function: Preservative.
Origin: Synthetic compound.
Restrictions and Adverse Effects: Toxic. Harmful by skin absorption. Corrosive to skin. It is limited to 0.2 percent of the finished product if used as a preservative, but it may be added in larger quantities for other stated purposes. It is prohibited from oral hygiene products and any preparations that may come into contact with the mucous membranes (mouth, nose, genitals, and eyelids).
Usage: EU/USA

p-Methylaminophenol
(Aminomethylphenol, Aminomethyl phenol)
Function: Hair dye.
Origin: Synthetic compound.

Restrictions and Adverse Effects: No currently known adverse effects.
Usage: EU/USA

p-Phenylenediamine
(Paraphenylenediamine)
Function: Hair dye.
Origin: Synthetic compound.
Restrictions and Adverse Effects: Strong skin irritant. Toxic by inhalation and ingestion. Demonstrated to be a mutagen. Can cause contact dermatitis. It is limited to 6 percent of the finished product. The label must clearly show the name of this compound separately from the list of ingredients and must carry the following warnings: "Can cause an allergic reaction. Do not use to dye eyelashes or eyebrows." Products supplied for professional use should carry the additional warning, "Wear suitable gloves."
Usage: EU/USA

p-Phenylenediamine HCl
(Paraphenylenediamine hydrochloride)
Function: Hair dye.
Origin: Synthetic compound.
Restrictions and Adverse Effects: Strong skin irritant. Toxic by inhalation and ingestion. The alkaline form has been demonstrated to be a mutagen. Can cause contact dermatitis. It is limited to 6 percent of the finished product. The label must clearly show the name of this compound separately from the list of ingredients and must carry the following warnings: "Can cause an allergic reaction. Do not use to dye eyelashes or eyebrows." Products supplied for professional use should carry the additional warning, "Wear suitable gloves."
Usage: EU/USA

p-Phenylenediamine sulfate
Function: Hair dye.
Origin: Synthetic compound.
Restrictions and Adverse Effects: Strong skin irritant. Toxic by inhalation and ingestion. The alkaline form has been demonstrated to be a mutagen. Can cause contact dermatitis. It is limited to 6 percent of

the finished product. The label must clearly show the name of this compound separately from the list of ingredients and must carry the following warnings: "Can cause an allergic reaction. Do not use to dye eyelashes or eyebrows." Products supplied for professional use should carry the additional warning, "Wear suitable gloves."
Usage: EU/USA

PABA
(p-Aminobenzoic acid, 4-Aminobenzoic acid)
Function: UV absorber.
Origin: Synthetic compound of the benzoate family.
Restrictions and Adverse Effects: Benzoic acid and benzoates have been implicated in a large number of health issues. (See *A–Z of Cosmetic Terms – Benzoates*.) Irritant for some individuals. Can cause contact dermatitis and photosensitivity. This ingredient is restricted to a maximum of 5 percent of the finished product.
Usage: EU/USA

Palm kernelamide DEA
Function: Emulsifier / Emulsion stabilizer / Surfactant / Viscosity adjuster / Foaming agent.
Origin: Semisynthetic compound made from oils derived from the kernels of palm trees.
Restrictions and Adverse Effects: DEA residues are cancer suspects currently under investigation. See *A–Z of Cosmetic Terms – DEA*.
Usage: EU/USA

Palmamide DEA
Function: Emulsifier / Emulsion stabilizer / Surfactant / Viscosity adjuster / Foaming agent.
Origin: Semisynthetic compound.
Restrictions and Adverse Effects: DEA residues are cancer suspects currently under investigation. See *A–Z of Cosmetic Terms – DEA*.
Usage: EU/USA

Palmitamide DEA
Function: Antistatic agent / Viscosity adjuster.
Origin: Semisynthetic compound.

Restrictions and Adverse Effects: DEA residues are cancer suspects currently under investigation. See *A–Z of Cosmetic Terms – DEA*.
Usage: EU/USA

Palmitic acid
(Cetylic acid)
Function: Emollient / Moisturizer / Emulsifier.
Origin: Semisynthetic or synthetic compound.
Restrictions and Adverse Effects: May cause contact dermatitis in some individuals.
Usage: EU/USA

Palmityl trihydroxyethyl propylenediamine dihydrofluoride
Function: Oral care agent.
Origin: Semisynthetic or synthetic compound.
Restrictions and Adverse Effects: Fluorides are toxic. They can discolor teeth (fluorosis). Children should only use a small quantity of toothpaste and be discouraged from swallowing it. The total amount of fluoride allowed by EU regulations is 0.15 percent of the finished product.
Usage: EU/USA

Panthenol
(Pro-vitamin B$_5$, Dexpanthenol)
Function: Antistatic agent / Humectant.
A biologically active substance that is metabolized to vitamin B$_5$ in the skin. It is said to have revitalizing and conditioning effects on the hair and skin. It has humectant-like properties that promote moisture absorption.
Origin: Natural product.
Restrictions and Adverse Effects: No currently known adverse effects.
Usage: EU/USA

Paraffinum liquidum
(Mineral oil, Liquid Paraffin)
Function: Antistatic agent / Emollient / Moisturizer / Solvent.
Origin: Liquid hydrocarbons from petroleum.
Restrictions and Adverse Effects: May cause discoloration of the skin. Carcinogenic and mutagenic

polycyclic aromatic hydrocarbons may be present as impurities.

Usage: EU/USA

Parfum

(Fragrance)

Function: Fragrance.

Origin: A mixture of many synthetic and natural fragrance chemicals, often dissolved in a carrier solvent, e.g., ethanol.

Restrictions and Adverse Effects: May cause contact dermatitis and contact allergies.

Usage: EU/USA

PEG – Family

(Polyethylene glycol, Polyoxyethylene glycol, Poly(ethan-1,2-diol))

Function: This is a large family with a wide range of functions, e.g., PEG-75 Lanolin has protective and emollient properties, while PEG-20 Stearate is an emulsifier. Other uses include surfactants, emulsion stabilizers and viscosity adjusters (often thickeners).

Origin: A range of synthetic polymers made from ethylene oxide. These polymers are combined with a variety of other molecules to produce a wide range of cosmetic materials. Higher numbers mean higher ethoxylation (bigger molecules), usually resulting in a greater solubility in water.

Restrictions and Adverse Effects: The PEG family of ingredients is made using ethylene oxide (oxirane), which can form 1,4-dioxane, a carcinogen, as a by-product of manufacture. See *A–Z of Cosmetic Terms – Dioxane*.

Usage: EU/USA

PEG-3 dipalmitate

Function: Emulsifier.

Origin: Synthetic compound.

Restrictions and Adverse Effects: Some palmitates have been linked to contact dermatitis. This ethoxylated ingredient is made using ethylene oxide (oxirane), which can form 1,4-dioxane, a carcinogen, as a by-product of manufacture. See *A–Z of Cosmetic Terms – Dioxane*.

Usage: EU/USA

PEG-5 DEDM hydantoin

Function: Antimicrobial.

Origin: Synthetic compound.

Restrictions and Adverse Effects: Hydantoins have been linked to contact dermatitis. This ethoxylated ingredient is made using ethylene oxide (oxirane), which can form 1,4-dioxane, a carcinogen, as a by-product of manufacture. See *A–Z of Cosmetic Terms – Dioxane*.

Usage: EU/USA

PEG-5 DEDM hydantoin oleate

Function: Antimicrobial.

Origin: Synthetic compound.

Restrictions and Adverse Effects: Hydantoins have been linked to contact dermatitis. This ethoxylated ingredient is made using ethylene oxide (oxirane), which can form 1,4-dioxane, a carcinogen, as a by-product of manufacture. See *A–Z of Cosmetic Terms – Dioxane*.

Usage: EU/USA

PEG-5 trimethylolpropane trimyristate

Function: Emulsifier.

Origin: Synthetic compound.

Restrictions and Adverse Effects: Some myristates are comedogenic (acne promoting). This ethoxylated ingredient is made using ethylene oxide (oxirane), which can form 1,4-dioxane, a carcinogen, as a by-product of manufacture. See *A–Z of Cosmetic Terms – Comedogen; Dioxane*.

Usage: EU/USA

PEG-6 isopalmitate

Function: Emulsifier.

Origin: Synthetic compound.

Restrictions and Adverse Effects: Some palmitates have been linked to contact dermatitis. This ethoxylated ingredient is made using ethylene oxide (oxirane), which can form 1,4-dioxane, a carcinogen, as a by-product of manufacture. See *A–Z of Cosmetic Terms – Dioxane*.

Usage: EU/USA

PEG-6 palmitate

Function: Emulsifier / Surfactant.

Origin: Synthetic compound.

Restrictions and Adverse Effects: Some palmitates have been linked to contact dermatitis. This ethoxylated ingredient is made using ethylene oxide (oxirane), which can form 1,4-dioxane, a carcinogen, as a by-product of manufacture. See *A–Z of Cosmetic Terms – Dioxane*.

Usage: EU/USA

PEG-8 myristate

Function: Emulsifier.

Origin: Synthetic compound.

Restrictions and Adverse Effects: Some myristates are comedogenic (acne promoting). This ethoxylated ingredient is made using ethylene oxide (oxirane), which can form 1,4-dioxane, a carcinogen, as a by-product of manufacture. See *A–Z of Cosmetic Terms – Comedogen; Dioxane*.

Usage: EU/USA

PEG-13 mink glycerides

Function: Emulsifier.

Origin: A semisynthetic compound derived from mink oil obtained from the fatty, subcutaneous tissue of mink.

Restrictions and Adverse Effects: No currently known adverse effects. This ethoxylated ingredient is made using ethylene oxide (oxirane), which can form 1,4-dioxane, a carcinogen, as a by-product of manufacture. See *A–Z of Cosmetic Terms – Dioxane*.

Usage: EU/USA

PEG-15 DEDM hydantoin

Function: Antimicrobial.

Origin: Synthetic compound.

Restrictions and Adverse Effects: Hydantoins have been linked to contact dermatitis. This ethoxylated ingredient is made using ethylene oxide (oxirane), which can form 1,4-dioxane, a carcinogen, as a by-product of manufacture. See *A–Z of Cosmetic Terms – Dioxane*.

Usage: EU/USA

PEG-15 DEDM hydantoin stearate

Function: Antimicrobial.

Origin: Synthetic compound.

Restrictions and Adverse Effects: Hydantoins have been linked to contact dermatitis. This ethoxylated ingredient is made using ethylene oxide (oxirane), which can form 1,4-dioxane, a carcinogen, as a by-product of manufacture. See *A–Z of Cosmetic Terms – Dioxane*.

Usage: EU/USA

PEG-18 palmitate

Function: Emulsifier.

Origin: Synthetic compound.

Restrictions and Adverse Effects: Some palmitates have been linked to contact dermatitis. This ethoxylated ingredient is made using ethylene oxide (oxirane), which can form 1,4-dioxane, a carcinogen, as a by-product of manufacture. See *A–Z of Cosmetic Terms – Dioxane*.

Usage: EU/USA

PEG-20 myristate

Function: Emulsifier / Surfactant.

Origin: Synthetic compound.

Restrictions and Adverse Effects: Some myristates are comedogenic (acne promoting). This ethoxylated ingredient is made using ethylene oxide (oxirane), which can form 1,4-dioxane, a carcinogen, as a by-product of manufacture. See *A–Z of Cosmetic Terms – Comedogen; Dioxane*.

Usage: EU/USA

PEG-20 palmitate

Function: Emulsifier / Surfactant.

Origin: Synthetic compound.

Restrictions and Adverse Effects: Some palmitates have been linked to contact dermatitis. This ethoxylated ingredient is made using ethylene oxide (oxirane), which can form 1,4-dioxane, a carcinogen, as a by-product of manufacture. See *A–Z of Cosmetic Terms – Dioxane*.

Usage: EU/USA

PEG-25 PABA

Function: UV absorber.

Origin: Synthetic compound.

Restrictions and Adverse Effects: The safety of this substance was uncertain and its use in cosmetics was only provisionally permitted in the EU, until June 30, 1998. On September 3, 1998, following further scientific tests, the provisional status was removed and this ingredient was permitted for use in cosmetics. It is limited to a maximum of 10 percent of the finished product. It may be used to protect the ingredients of other cosmetics and toiletries from the detrimental effects of sunlight. This ethoxylated ingredient is made using ethylene oxide (oxirane), which can form 1,4-dioxane, a carcinogen, as a by-product of manufacture. See *A–Z of Cosmetic Terms – Dioxane*.

Usage: EU/USA

PEG-80 sorbitan palmitate

Function: Emulsifier / Surfactant.

Origin: Synthetic compound.

Restrictions and Adverse Effects: Some palmitates have been linked to contact dermatitis. This ethoxylated ingredient is made using ethylene oxide (oxirane), which can form 1,4-dioxane, a carcinogen, as a by-product of manufacture. See *A–Z of Cosmetic Terms – Dioxane*.

Usage: EU/USA

Pentaerythrityl tetramyristate

Function: Emollient / Moisturizer.

Origin: Semisynthetic or synthetic compound.

Restrictions and Adverse Effects: Some myristates are comedogenic (acne promoting, see *A–Z of Cosmetic Terms – Comedogen*).

Usage: EU/USA

Petrolatum

Function: Antistatic agent / Emollient / Moisturizer.

Origin: Heavy oil extracted from petroleum.

Restrictions and Adverse Effects: May cause discoloration of the skin.

Usage: EU/USA

Phenacetin

(Acetophenetidin, p-Acetylphenetidin, Acetophenetidide, p-Ethoxyacetanilide)

Function: Additive.

Origin: Synthetic compound.

Restrictions and Adverse Effects: Cancer and mutagen suspect. Toxic by ingestion.

Usage: EU/USA

Phenol

Function: Antimicrobial / Denaturant / Deodorant.

Origin: Synthetic compound. May be extracted from coal tar.

Restrictions and Adverse Effects: Phenol is harmful. It corrodes skin. It is a severe irritant. It is limited to 1 percent maximum in the finished product and the label must clearly state the name of this additive separately from the list of ingredients.

Usage: EU/USA

Phenoxyethanol

(2- Phenoxyethanol)

Function: Preservative.

Origin: Synthetic compound.

Restrictions and Adverse Effects: Can cause contact allergies and contact dermatitis. It is limited to 1 percent of the finished product if used as a preservative, but may be added in larger quantities for other stated purposes.

Usage: EU/USA

Phenoxyisopropanol

Function: Preservative / Solvent.

Origin: Synthetic compound.

Restrictions and Adverse Effects: Harmful. Irritant. Maximum allowed amount is 2 percent of the finished product. Prohibited in oral care products. Restricted to rinse-off products only.

Usage: EU/USA

Phenyl benzoate

Function: Preservative.

Origin: Synthetic compound of the benzoate family.

Restrictions and Adverse Effects: Benzoic acid and benzoates have been implicated in a large number of

health issues. (See *A–Z of Cosmetic Terms – Benzoates*.) It is limited to 0.5 percent of the finished product if used as a preservative. It may be added in larger quantities for other stated purposes.
Usage: EU/USA

Phenyl mercuric acetate
Function: Preservative.
Origin: Synthetic compound.
Restrictions and Adverse Effects: Mercury compounds are toxic by skin absorption, cause dermatitis, and accumulate in the body. They are limited to a total mercury content of 0.007 percent in the EU or 0.0065 percent in the USA. The label must carry suitable warnings and mercury salts are restricted to use in eye make-up and make-up removers only in both the EU and USA.
Usage: EU/USA

Phenyl mercuric benzoate
Function: Preservative.
Origin: Synthetic compound.
Restrictions and Adverse Effects: Mercury compounds are toxic by skin absorption, cause dermatitis, and accumulate in the body. They are limited to a total mercury content of 0.007 percent in the EU or 0.0065 percent in the USA. The label must carry suitable warnings and mercury salts are restricted to use in eye make-up and make-up removers only in both the EU and USA. Benzoic acid and benzoates have been implicated in a large number of health issues (see *A–Z of Cosmetic Terms – Benzoates*).
Usage: EU/USA

Phenyl mercuric borate
Function: Preservative.
Origin: Synthetic compound.
Restrictions and Adverse Effects: Mercury compounds are toxic by skin absorption, cause dermatitis, and accumulate in the body. They are limited to a total mercury content of 0.007 percent in the EU or 0.0065 percent in the USA. The label must carry suitable warnings and mercury salts are restricted to use in eye make-up and make-up

removers only in both the EU and USA. Borates are toxic and have been linked to fetal malformations.
Usage: EU/USA

Phenyl mercuric bromide
Function: Preservative.
Origin: Synthetic compound.
Restrictions and Adverse Effects: Mercury compounds are toxic by skin absorption, cause dermatitis, and accumulate in the body. They are limited to a total mercury content of 0.007 percent in the EU or 0.0065 percent in the USA. The label must carry suitable warnings and mercury salts are restricted to use in eye make-up and make-up removers only in both the EU and USA.
Usage: EU/USA

Phenyl mercuric chloride
Function: Preservative.
Origin: Synthetic compound.
Restrictions and Adverse Effects: Mercury compounds are toxic by skin absorption, cause dermatitis, and accumulate in the body. They are limited to a total mercury content of 0.007 percent in the EU or 0.0065 percent in the USA. The label must carry suitable warnings and mercury salts are restricted to use in eye make-up and make-up removers only in both the EU and USA.
Usage: EU/USA

Phenylbenzimidazole sulfonic acid
Function: UV absorber.
Origin: Synthetic compound.
Restrictions and Adverse Effects: Irritant. This ingredient is restricted to a maximum of 8 percent of the finished product.
Usage: EU/USA

Phenylparaben
Function: Preservative.
Origin: Synthetic compound of the benzoate family.
Restrictions and Adverse Effects: Benzoic acid, benzoates and parabens have been implicated in a large number of health issues. (See *A–Z of Cosmetic Terms – Benzoates*.) It is limited to 0.4 percent of the

finished product if used on its own as a preservative, or 0.8 percent in total if used in combination with other parabens. Parabens may be added in larger quantities for other stated purposes.
Usage: EU/USA

Phenylthioglycolic acid

Function: Antioxidant.

Origin: Synthetic compound.

Restrictions and Adverse Effects: Skin contact can cause sensitization. Causes eye damage which may require medical attention.

Usage: EU/USA

Phthalic anhydride / Adipic acid / Castor oil / Neopentyl glycol / PEG-3 / Trimethylolpropane copolymer

Function: Film former.

Origin: Synthetic compound.

Restrictions and Adverse Effects: May contain residues of phthalic acid and phthalates, which have been linked with testicular cancer and cell mutation. This ethoxylated ingredient is made using ethylene oxide (oxirane), which can form 1,4-dioxane, a carcinogen, as a by-product of manufacture. See *A–Z of Cosmetic Terms – Dioxane*.

Usage: EU/USA

Phthalic anhydride / Benzoic acid / Trimethylolpropane copolymer

Function: Film former.

Origin: Synthetic compound.

Restrictions and Adverse Effects: May contain residues of phthalic acid and phthalates, which have been linked with testicular cancer and cell mutation.

Usage: EU/USA

Phthalic anhydride / Butyl benzoic acid / Propylene glycol copolymer

Function: Film former.

Origin: Synthetic compound.

Restrictions and Adverse Effects: May contain residues of phthalic acid and phthalates, which have been linked with testicular cancer and cell mutation.

Usage: EU/USA

Phthalic anhydride / Glycerin / Glycidyl decanoate copolymer

Function: Antistatic agent / Film former / Viscosity adjuster.

Origin: Synthetic compound.

Restrictions and Adverse Effects: May contain residues of phthalic acid and phthalates, which have been linked with testicular cancer and cell mutation.

Usage: EU/USA

Phthalic anhydride / Trimellitic anhydride / Glycols copolymer

Function: Film former.

Origin: Synthetic compound.

Restrictions and Adverse Effects: May contain residues of phthalic acid and phthalates, which have been linked with testicular cancer and cell mutation.

Usage: EU/USA

Piroctone olamine

Function: Preservative.

Origin: Synthetic compound.

Restrictions and Adverse Effects: This ingredient is limited to 1 percent of finished rinse-off products or 0.5 percent for non-rinse off products, but it may be added in larger quantities for other stated purposes.

Usage: EU/USA

Polyacrylamidomethyl benzylidene camphor

Function: UV absorber.

Origin: Synthetic compound.

Restrictions and Adverse Effects: The safety of this substance was originally uncertain and its use in cosmetics was only provisionally permitted in the EU. Following further scientific tests, the provisional status was removed during the 1990s and this ingredient was permitted for use in cosmetics. It is limited to a maximum of 6 percent of the finished product. It may be used to protect the ingredients of other cosmetics and toiletries from the detrimental effects of sunlight.

Usage: EU/USA

Polyaminopropyl biguanide

Function: Preservative.

Origin: Synthetic compound.

Restrictions and Adverse Effects: This ingredient is limited to 0.3 percent of the finished product if used as a preservative, but may be added in larger quantities for other stated purposes.

Usage: EU/USA

Polybutylene terephthalate

Function: Antistatic agent / Film former / Viscosity adjuster.

Origin: Synthetic compound.

Restrictions and Adverse Effects: Phthalic acid and phthalates have been linked with testicular cancer and cell mutation.

Usage: EU/USA

Polyethylene terephthalate

Function: Film former.

Origin: Synthetic compound.

Restrictions and Adverse Effects: Phthalic acid and phthalates have been linked with testicular cancer and cell mutation.

Usage: EU/USA

Polyglyceryl-10 myristate

Function: Emulsifier.

Origin: Synthetic compound.

Restrictions and Adverse Effects: Some myristates are comedogenic (acne promoting, see *A–Z of Cosmetic Terms – Comedogen*).

Usage: EU/USA

Polyglyceryl-2 isopalmitate

Function: Emulsifier.

Origin: Synthetic compound.

Restrictions and Adverse Effects: Some palmitates have been linked to contact dermatitis.

Usage: EU/USA

Polyglyceryl-3 myristate

Function: Emulsifier.

Origin: Synthetic compound.

Restrictions and Adverse Effects: Some myristates are comedogenic (acne promoting, see *A–Z of Cosmetic Terms – Comedogen*).

Usage: EU/USA

Polysorbate – Family

(Examples include Polysorbate 20, Polysorbate 60, Polysorbate 80 acetate, etc.)

Function: Polysorbates are used as emulsifiers and/or surfactants.

Origin: Semisynthetic or synthetic compounds.

Restrictions and Adverse Effects: Some polysorbates have been linked to irritation and sensitization.

Usage: EU/USA

Potassium benzoate

Function: Preservative.

Origin: Synthetic compound of the benzoate family.

Restrictions and Adverse Effects: Benzoic acid and benzoates have been implicated in a large number of health issues. (See *A–Z of Cosmetic Terms – Benzoates.*) It is limited to 0.5 percent of the finished product if used as a preservative, but may be added in larger quantities for other stated purposes.

Usage: EU/USA

Potassium biphthalate

(Potassium Hydrogen Phthalate)

Function: pH control.

Origin: Synthetic compound.

Restrictions and Adverse Effects: Phthalic acid and phthalates have been linked with testicular cancer and cell mutation.

Usage: EU/USA

Potassium borate

Function: pH control.

Origin: Synthetic compound.

Restrictions and Adverse Effects: Borates are toxic and have been linked to fetal malformations.

Usage: EU/USA

Potassium butylparaben

Function: Preservative.

Origin: Synthetic compound of the benzoate family.

Restrictions and Adverse Effects: Benzoic acid, benzoates, and parabens have been implicated in a large number of health issues. (See *A–Z of Cosmetic Terms – Benzoates*.) It is limited to 0.4 percent of the finished product if used on its own as a preservative, or 0.8 percent in total if used in combination with other parabens. Parabens may be added in larger quantities for other stated purposes.

Usage: EU/USA

Potassium chlorate

Function: Oxidizing agent / Bleaching agent.

Origin: Synthetic compound.

Restrictions and Adverse Effects: Maximum allowed content is 5 percent of the finished product in toothpaste and 3 percent in other products.

Usage: EU/USA

Potassium ethylparaben

Function: Preservative.

Origin: Synthetic compound of the benzoate family.

Restrictions and Adverse Effects: Benzoic acid, benzoates, and parabens have been implicated in a large number of health issues. (See *A–Z of Cosmetic Terms – Benzoates*.) It is limited to 0.4 percent of the finished product if used on its own as a preservative, or 0.8 percent in total if used in combination with other parabens. Parabens may be added in larger quantities for other stated purposes.

Usage: EU/USA

Potassium fluoride

Function: Oral care agent.

Origin: Synthetic compound.

Restrictions and Adverse Effects: Fluorides are toxic. They can discolor teeth (fluorosis). Children should only use a small quantity of toothpaste and be discouraged from swallowing it. The total amount of fluoride allowed by EU regulations is 0.15 percent of the finished product.

Usage: EU/USA

Potassium fluorosilicate

Function: Oral care agent.

Origin: Synthetic compound.

Restrictions and Adverse Effects: Fluorides are toxic. They can discolor teeth (fluorosis). Children should only use a small quantity of toothpaste and be discouraged from swallowing it. The total amount of fluoride allowed by EU regulations is 0.15 percent of the finished product.

Usage: EU/USA

Potassium hydroxide

Function: pH control / Cuticle solvent.

Origin: Synthetic compound.

Restrictions and Adverse Effects: Harmful. Irritant. Corrosive to skin in dilute solutions. Maximum total alkali, including other alkalis, is 5 percent in nail cuticle solvents and 2 percent in hair care products (4.5 percent in professional products). In depilatories the pH must not exceed 12.7, and in other products pH must be below 11. Labels must state that the product contains alkali which can cause blindness, therefore, avoid eye contact. The label must also carry the warning "Keep out of the reach of children."

Usage: EU/USA

Potassium metabisulfite

Function: Preservative.

Origin: Synthetic compound.

Restrictions and Adverse Effects: Irritant. It is limited to 0.2 percent of the finished product if used as a preservative, but may be added in larger quantities for other stated purposes.

Usage: EU/USA

Potassium methoxycinnamate

Function: UV absorber.

Origin: Synthetic compound.

Restrictions and Adverse Effects: Cinnamates have been reported to cause a stinging sensation in some people.

Usage: EU/USA

Potassium methylparaben

Function: Preservative.

Origin: Synthetic compound of the benzoate family.

Restrictions and Adverse Effects: Benzoic acid, benzoates, and parabens have been implicated in a large number of health issues. (See *A–Z of Cosmetic Terms – Benzoates*.) It is limited to 0.4 percent of the finished product if used on its own as a preservative, or 0.8 percent in total if used in combination with other parabens. Parabens may be added in larger quantities for other stated purposes.

Usage: EU/USA

Potassium monofluorophosphate

Function: Oral care agent.

Origin: Synthetic compound.

Restrictions and Adverse Effects: Fluorides are toxic. They can discolor teeth (fluorosis). Children should only use a small quantity of toothpaste and be discouraged from swallowing it. The total amount of fluoride allowed by EU regulations is 0.15 percent of the finished product.

Usage: EU/USA

Potassium myristate

Function: Emulsifier / Surfactant.

Origin: Semisynthetic or synthetic compound.

Restrictions and Adverse Effects: Some myristates are comedogenic (acne promoting, see *A–Z of Cosmetic Terms – Comedogen*).

Usage: EU/USA

Potassium o-phenylphenate

Function: Preservative.

Origin: Synthetic compound.

Restrictions and Adverse Effects: It is limited to 0.2 percent of the finished product if used as a preservative, but may be added in larger quantities for other stated purposes.

Usage: EU/USA

Potassium palm kernelate

Function: Surfactant.

A common ingredient in soaps, including baby soap and shaving soap.

Origin: Semisynthetic compound made from coconut oil and palm oil extracted from the kernels of palm trees.

Restrictions and Adverse Effects: No currently known adverse effects.

Usage: EU/USA

Potassium palmitate

Function: Emulsifier / Surfactant.

Origin: Semisynthetic or synthetic compound.

Restrictions and Adverse Effects: Some palmitates have been linked to contact dermatitis.

Usage: EU/USA

Potassium paraben

Function: Preservative.

Origin: Synthetic compound of the benzoate family.

Restrictions and Adverse Effects: Benzoic acid, benzoates, and parabens have been implicated in a large number of health issues. (See *A–Z of Cosmetic Terms – Benzoates*.) It is limited to 0.4 percent of the finished product if used on its own as a preservative, or 0.8 percent in total if used in combination with other parabens. Parabens may be added in larger quantities for other stated purposes.

Usage: EU/USA

Potassium persulfate

(Potassium peroxodisulfate)

Function: Oxidizing agent.

Origin: Synthetic compound.

Restrictions and Adverse Effects: This ingredient has been linked to asthma in hairdressers.

Usage: EU/USA

Potassium phenoxide

Function: Antimicrobial.

Origin: Synthetic compound.

Restrictions and Adverse Effects: Phenols are harmful. They corrode skin. They are severe irritants. This ingredient is limited to 1 percent maximum of the finished product and the label must clearly state its name separately from the list of ingredients.

Usage: EU/USA

Potassium phenylbenzimidazole sulfonate

Function: UV absorber.

Origin: Synthetic compound.

Restrictions and Adverse Effects: Irritant for some individuals. This ingredient is restricted to a maximum of 8 percent of the finished product.

Usage: EU/USA

Potassium propionate

Function: Preservative.

Origin: Synthetic compound.

Restrictions and Adverse Effects: Propanoic acid and its salts are limited to 2 percent of the finished product if used as a preservative, but may be added in larger quantities for other stated purposes.

Usage: EU/USA

Potassium propylparaben

Function: Preservative.

Origin: Synthetic compound of the benzoate family.

Restrictions and Adverse Effects: Benzoic acid, benzoates, and parabens have been implicated in a large number of health issues. (See *A–Z of Cosmetic Terms – Benzoates*.) It is limited to 0.4 percent of the finished product if used on its own as a preservative, or 0.8 percent in total if used in combination with other parabens. Parabens may be added in larger quantities for other stated purposes.

Usage: EU/USA

Potassium salicylate

Function: Preservative.

Origin: Synthetic compound.

Restrictions and Adverse Effects: This ingredient is limited to 0.5 percent of the finished product if used as a preservative, but may be added in larger quantities for other stated purposes. With the exception of shampoo, it must not be used in preparations intended for children under the age of 3 and must clearly state this restriction on the label.

Usage: EU/USA

Potassium sorbate

Function: Preservative.

Origin: Synthetic compound.

Restrictions and Adverse Effects: This ingredient is limited to 0.6 percent of the finished product if used as a preservative but it may be added in larger quantities for other stated purposes.

Usage: EU/USA

Potassium stearate

Function: Emulsifier / Surfactant / Viscosity adjuster. A common ingredient in soaps, including baby soap, shaving soap, and dermatological soap.

Origin: Semisynthetic compound made from animal or vegetable oils.

Restrictions and Adverse Effects: No currently known adverse effects.

Usage: EU/USA

Potassium sulfide

Function: Depilatory agent.

Origin: Synthetic compound.

Restrictions and Adverse Effects: Sulfides are toxic. Irritant. May be alkaline (irritant and corrosive). Maximum allowed content is 2 percent of the finished product. The label must carry warnings to avoid contact with the eyes and to keep the product out of the reach of children.

Usage: EU/USA

Potassium sulfite

Function: Preservative.

Origin: Synthetic compound.

Restrictions and Adverse Effects: Irritant. It is limited to 0.2 percent of the finished product if used as a preservative, but may be added in larger quantities for other stated purposes.

Usage: EU/USA

Potassium tallowate

Function: Emulsifier / Surfactant.

Origin: Semisynthetic compound made by the action of potassium hydroxide on animal fats.

Restrictions and Adverse Effects: Reported to be comedogenic (acne promoting, see *A–Z of Cosmetic*

Terms – Comedogen). May cause contact eczema. For BSE precautions see *Chapter 17 – Animal Products and Animal Testing*.
Usage: EU/USA

Potassium thioglycolate
Function: Depilatory agent / Reducing agent.
Origin: Synthetic compound.
Restrictions and Adverse Effects: Harmful. May be alkaline (irritant and corrosive). In the EU its content is limited to 8 percent in hair perming preparations (11 percent for professional use), 5 percent in depilatories and 2 percent in rinse-off hair care products. The pH must be between 7 and 9.5 in hair care products and between 7 and 12.7 in depilatories. The label must clearly state "Contains Thioglycolate," and it must show the following mandatory warnings: "Follow the instructions. Keep out of reach of children. Avoid contact with eyes. In the event of contact with eyes, rinse with plenty of water and seek medical advice." Additionally, hair care products must state, "Wear suitable gloves."
Usage: EU/USA

Propane
Function: Propellant for aerosol sprays. (Often used in combination with Butane and Isobutane.)
Origin: Petroleum product.
Restrictions and Adverse Effects: A flammable hydrocarbon gas that is used as an alternative to CFCs, which are known to damage the ozone layer. It is a powerful greenhouse gas (contributes to the greenhouse effect causing global warming), and is inhaled by solvent abusers. It is harmless if inhaled in small concentrations. There is a danger of fire or explosion if used near a source of ignition.
Usage: EU/USA

Propantheline bromide
Function: Additive.
Origin: Synthetic compound.
Restrictions and Adverse Effects: Can cause widening of the pupils (unilateral mydriasis).
Usage: USA/Not currently on the EU inventory of cosmetic ingredients.

Propionic acid
Function: Preservative.
Origin: Synthetic compound.
Restrictions and Adverse Effects: Propanoic acid and its salts are limited to 2 percent of the finished product if used as a preservative, but may be added in larger quantities for other stated purposes.
Usage: EU/USA

Propyl benzoate
Function: Preservative.
Origin: Synthetic compound of the benzoate family.
Restrictions and Adverse Effects: Benzoic acid and benzoates have been implicated in a large number of health issues. (See *A–Z of Cosmetic Terms – Benzoates*.) It is limited to 0.5 percent of the finished product if used as a preservative, but it may be added in larger quantities for other stated purposes.
Usage: EU/USA

Propyl gallate
Function: Antioxidant.
Origin: Synthetic compound.
Restrictions and Adverse Effects: May cause contact allergies in some individuals.
Usage: EU/USA

Propylene glycol
(PG, Propan-1,2-diol, Propylenglycolum)
Function: Humectant / Solvent.
Propylene glycol can penetrate the outermost layer of skin cells and carry other ingredients into deeper layers of the epidermis. It is, therefore, an extremely common cosmetic ingredient occurring in a wide range of products. It is used as a humectant in skin products and a solvent for preservatives, essential oils, flavors, and fragrances. It is also used in the preparation of herbal extracts.
Origin: Synthetic compound derived from petroleum.
Restrictions and Adverse Effects: Skin irritant for some people. May cause dermatitis and delayed contact allergies in some individuals.
Usage: EU/USA

Propylene glycol dicaprylate / Dicaprate

Function: Emollient / Moisturizer.

Origin: Semisynthetic or synthetic compound.

Restrictions and Adverse Effects: No currently known adverse effects.

Usage: EU/USA

Propylene glycol myristate

Function: Emollient / Moisturizer / Emulsifier.

Origin: Semisynthetic or synthetic compound.

Restrictions and Adverse Effects: Some myristates are comedogenic (acne promoting, see *A–Z of Cosmetic Terms – Comedogen*).

Usage: EU/USA

Propyleneglycol-2-myristyl propionate

Function: Emollient / Moisturizer / Emulsifier.

Origin: Semisynthetic or synthetic compound.

Restrictions and Adverse Effects: Comedogenic (acne promoting, see *A–Z of Cosmetic Terms – Comedogen*).

Usage: USA/Not currently on the EU inventory of cosmetic ingredients.

Propylparaben

(Propyl-4-hydroxybenzoate)

Function: Preservative.

Common cosmetic preservative that is anti-fungal and antimicrobial. Less water soluble than methylparaben, it preserves the oily components in preparations.

Origin: Synthetic compound of the benzoate family.

Restrictions and Adverse Effects: Benzoic acid, benzoates, and parabens have been implicated in a large number of health issues. (See *A–Z of Cosmetic Terms – Benzoates*.) It is limited to 0.4 percent of the finished product if used on its own as a preservative, or 0.8 percent in total if used in combination with other parabens. Parabens may be added in larger quantities for other stated purposes.

Usage: EU/USA

Prunus dulcis

Function: Emollient.

Origin: An oil extracted from the seeds of sweet almonds.

Restrictions and Adverse Effects: No currently known adverse effects. People with an almond allergy are advised to do a patch test before using products containing almond extracts.

Usage: EU/USA

PVP

(Polyvinylpyrrolidone)

Function: Antistatic agent / Binding agent / Emulsion stabilizer / Film former.

Origin: Synthetic polymer.

Restrictions and Adverse Effects: Cancer suspect. PVP residues may be present in a number of PVP copolymers used widely in decorative cosmetics.

Usage: EU/USA

Pyridoxine dipalmitate

Function: Antistatic agent.

Origin: Semisynthetic or synthetic compound.

Restrictions and Adverse Effects: Some palmitates have been linked to contact dermatitis.

Usage: EU/USA

Pyridoxine tripalmitate

Function: Antistatic agent.

Origin: Semisynthetic or synthetic compound.

Restrictions and Adverse Effects: Some palmitates have been linked to contact dermatitis.

Usage: EU/USA

Quaternium – Family

A large family of cationic compounds used widely in cosmetics, especially hair conditioners and shampoos. Examples include Quaternium-1, Quaternium-15, Quaternium-85, Quaternium-18 / Benzalkonium bentonite, Quaternium-18 methosulfate, Quaternium-79 hydrolyzed collagen, etc.

Function: Quaternium compounds have a variety of uses, such as antistatic agents, antimicrobials, preservatives, surfactants, and viscosity adjusters.

Origin: Synthetic compounds.
Restrictions and Adverse Effects: Rarely, quaternium-n compounds have been linked to serious hypersensitivity and anaphylactic shock. Can cause contact dermatitis.
Usage: EU/USA

Quaternium-15

(Methanine, Methenamine)
Function: Preservative.
Origin: Synthetic compound.
Restrictions and Adverse Effects: Can cause contact dermatitis. It is limited to 0.2 percent of the finished product if used as a preservative, but may be added in larger quantities for other stated purposes. Rarely, quaternium-n compounds have been linked to serious hypersensitivity and anaphylactic shock.
Usage: EU/USA

Quinaldine

(Chinaldine, Alpha-Methylquinoline)
Function: Colorant.
Origin: Synthetic compound.
Restrictions and Adverse Effects: Causes severe irritation of the mucous membranes (mouth, nose, respiratory tract, genitals, and eyelids).
Usage: USA/Not currently on the EU inventory of cosmetic ingredients.

Quinine

Function: Additive / Denaturant.
Origin: Plant extract with an unpleasant, bitter taste in minute concentrations. It was the original treatment for malaria and is used as its sulfate salt to flavor tonic water. It is used in nail paint to deter children from biting their fingernails.
Restrictions and Adverse Effects: Harmful. Maximum allowed content is 0.5 percent of the finished product for rinse-off-shampoos and 0.2 percent for non-rinse-off hair lotions.
Usage: EU/USA

Quinolin-8-ol

Function: Stabilizer for Hydrogen peroxide.
Origin: Synthetic compound.

Restrictions and Adverse Effects: Irritant. Harmful. This ingredient is limited to 0.3 percent in rinse-off hair care preparations and 0.03 percent in non-rinse-off preparations.
Usage: EU/USA

Red petrolatum

Function: Emollient / Moisturizer / UV absorber.
Origin: Petroleum derivative.
Restrictions and Adverse Effects: May cause discoloration of the skin.
Usage: EU/USA

Resorcinol

Function: Hair dye.
Origin: Synthetic compound.
Restrictions and Adverse Effects: Harmful by skin contact. Maximum allowed content is 5 percent of the finished product when used as an oxidizing hair colorant, and 0.5 percent in other hair care products. The label must clearly state the name of this chemical separately from the list of ingredients. If the product contains more than 0.5 percent of this ingredient, the label must also carry the following warnings: "Rinse hair well after use. Not to be used on eyelashes or eyebrows. Avoid eye contact. In the event of eye contact rinse with cold water."
Usage: EU/USA

Retinol

(Vitamin A)
Function: Additive.
A natural vitamin added to cosmetics for marketing reasons.
Origin: Natural extract.
Restrictions and Adverse Effects: No currently known adverse effects.
Usage: EU/USA

Retinyl palmitate

Function: Additive.
Origin: Semisynthetic or synthetic compound.
Restrictions and Adverse Effects: Some palmitates have been linked to contact dermatitis.
Usage: EU/USA

Rhodamine B

Function: Colorant.

Origin: Synthetic compound.

Restrictions and Adverse Effects: Can inhibit skin cell metabolism. Can impair the correct growth of lip tissue, causing decreased collagen content in the fibroblast cell layers of the lips.

Usage: USA/Not currently on the EU inventory of cosmetic ingredients.

Riboflavin

(E101a)

Function: Yellow colorant.

Origin: Natural plant extract.

Restrictions and Adverse Effects: Allowed in all products. No known adverse effects.

Usage: EU/USA

Ricinoleamide DEA

Function: Antistatic agent / Viscosity adjuster.

Origin: Semisynthetic or synthetic compound.

Restrictions and Adverse Effects: DEA residues are cancer suspects currently under investigation. See *A–Z of Cosmetic Terms – DEA*.

Usage: EU/USA

Ricinoleamidopropyl dimethylamine

Function: Antistatic agent.

Origin: Semisynthetic or synthetic compound.

Restrictions and Adverse Effects: May cause contact allergies in some individuals.

Usage: EU/USA

Ricinoleic acid

Function: Emollient / Moisturizer / Emulsifier.

Origin: Semisynthetic or synthetic compound.

Restrictions and Adverse Effects: May cause dermatitis.

Usage: EU/USA

Ricinus communis

(Castor oil, Ricinus oil)

Function: Emollient / Moisturizer.

Origin: Plant extract.

Restrictions and Adverse Effects: Can cause inflammation, cracking, and dryness of the lips (allergic cheilitis).

Usage: EU/USA

Rosin

(Colophonium, Colophony)

Function: Viscosity adjuster.

Origin: A natural extract of terpentine oleoresin.

Restrictions and Adverse Effects: May cause eyelid dermatitis and contact allergies in some individuals.

Usage: USA/Not currently on the EU inventory of cosmetic ingredients.

Rosmarinus officinalis

(Rosemary extract)

Function: Botanical additive. Rosemary oil is used in aromatherapy.

Origin: Plant extract.

Restrictions and Adverse Effects: Irritant. Can cause allergic dermatitis and photosensitivity in some individuals.

Usage: EU/USA

Salicylic acid

Function: Preservative / Antidandruff agent / Exfoliating agent.

Origin: Synthetic compound originally obtained from willow trees.

Restrictions and Adverse Effects: Salicylic acid is a beta-hydroxy acid (BHA), which is used to exfoliate skin. BHAs are also known as skin peelers because they dissolve and remove the outer layer of skin. They can cause increased sensitivity to the sun due to loss of the protective outer layer of skin cells. Do not expose skin to the sun immediately following treatment with BHAs. Test a small area before use and discontinue use if skin irritation, redness, bleeding, or pain is experienced. May cause exfoliative dermatitis.

Salicylic acid is limited to 0.5 percent of the finished product if it is used as a preservative, but it may be added in larger quantities if used as an exfoliant or antidandruff agent. With the exception of shampoo, it must not be used in preparations intended for children under the age of 3 and must clearly state this restriction on the label. Fewer restrictions apply in the USA.

Usage: EU/USA

Scoparone

Function: Additive.

Origin: Synthetic compound.

Restrictions and Adverse Effects: Can cause sensitization of the skin.

Usage: USA/Not currently on the EU inventory of cosmetic ingredients.

Selenium sulfide

Function: Antidandruff agent.

Origin: Synthetic compound.

Restrictions and Adverse Effects: Harmful. Maximum allowed content is 1 percent of the finished product. The label must clearly state the name of this compound separately from the list of ingredients and it must carry the following warning: "Avoid contact with the eyes and damaged skin."

Usage: EU/USA

Sesamide DEA

Function: Surfactant.

Origin: Semisynthetic compound.

Restrictions and Adverse Effects: DEA residues are cancer suspects currently under investigation. See *A–Z of Cosmetic Terms – DEA*.

Usage: EU/USA

Sesquiterpene lactone

Function: Additive.

Origin: Semisynthetic compound.

Restrictions and Adverse Effects: Can cause severe allergic reactions.

Usage: USA/Not currently on the EU inventory of cosmetic ingredients.

Silica

Function: Abrasive / Absorbent / Opacifier / Viscosity adjuster.

Origin: A natural mineral (silicon dioxide).

Restrictions and Adverse Effects: Harmful by inhalation.

Usage: EU/USA

Silk amino acids

Function: Humectant.

Origin: Obtained by the hydrolysis of silk, a natural protein fiber.

Restrictions and Adverse Effects: May cause urticaria (nettle rash or hives).

Usage: EU/USA

Silver nitrate

Function: Hair dye.

Origin: Synthetic compound.

Restrictions and Adverse Effects: Silver nitrate can darken the skin temporarily. It can cause skin sensitivity leading to allergies. Maximum allowed content is 4 percent of the finished product and it is restricted to eyelash and eyebrow colorants only. The label must clearly state the name of this ingredient separately from the other ingredients and must carry the following warnings: "Avoid eye contact. In the event of eye contact rinse with cold water."

Usage: EU/USA

Sodium benzoate

Function: Preservative.

Origin: Synthetic compound of the benzoate family.

Restrictions and Adverse Effects: Benzoic acid and benzoates have been implicated in a large number of health issues. (See *A–Z of Cosmetic Terms – Benzoates*.) It is limited to 0.5 percent of the finished product if used as a preservative, but may be added in larger quantities for other stated purposes.

Usage: EU/USA

Sodium bisulfite

Function: Preservative.

Origin: Synthetic compound.

Restrictions and Adverse Effects: Irritant. This ingredient is limited to 0.2 percent of the finished product if used as a preservative, but may be added in larger quantities for other stated purposes.

Usage: EU/USA

Sodium borate

Function: pH control.

Origin: Synthetic compound.

Restrictions and Adverse Effects: Borates are toxic and have been linked to fetal malformations.

Usage: EU/USA

Sodium butylparaben

Function: Preservative.

Origin: Synthetic compound of the benzoate family.

Restrictions and Adverse Effects: Benzoic acid, benzoates, and parabens have been implicated in a large number of health issues. (See *A–Z of Cosmetic Terms – Benzoates*.) It is limited to 0.4 percent of the finished product if used on its own as a preservative, or 0.8 percent in total if used in combination with other parabens. Parabens may be added in larger quantities for other stated purposes.

Usage: EU/USA

Sodium chlorate

Function: Oxidizing agent.

Origin: Synthetic compound.

Restrictions and Adverse Effects: Maximum allowed content is 5 percent of the finished product for toothpaste and 3 percent in other products.

Usage: EU/USA

Sodium chloride

(Common salt, Sea salt, NaCl)

Function: Viscosity adjuster / Astringent / Isotonic control.

A widely used cosmetic ingredient, common salt is believed to have cleansing, toning, refreshing, and astringent properties.

Origin: Extracted from the sea or from underground salt deposits.

Restrictions and Adverse Effects: No currently known adverse effects.

Usage: EU/USA

Sodium dehydroacetate

Function: Preservative.

Origin: Synthetic compound.

Restrictions and Adverse Effects: Harmful by inhalation. Prohibited from use in aerosol dispensers and sprays and limited to 0.6 percent of the finished product.

Usage: EU/USA

Sodium ethylparaben

Function: Preservative.

Origin: Synthetic compound of the benzoate family.

Restrictions and Adverse Effects: Benzoic acid, benzoates, and parabens have been implicated in a large number of health issues. (See *A–Z of Cosmetic Terms – Benzoates*.) It is limited to 0.4 percent of the finished product if used on its own as a preservative, or 0.8 percent in total if used in combination with other parabens. Parabens may be added in larger quantities for other stated purposes.

Usage: EU/USA

Sodium fluoride

Function: Oral care agent.

Origin: Synthetic compound.

Restrictions and Adverse Effects: Fluorides are toxic. They can discolor teeth (fluorosis). Children should only use a small quantity of toothpaste and be discouraged from swallowing it. The total amount of fluoride allowed by EU regulations is 0.15 percent of the finished product.

Usage: EU/USA

Sodium fluorosilicate

Function: Oral care agent.

Origin: Synthetic compound.

Restrictions and Adverse Effects: Fluorides are toxic. They can discolor teeth (fluorosis). Children should only use a small quantity of toothpaste and be discouraged from swallowing it. The total amount of fluoride allowed by EU regulations is 0.15 percent of the finished product.

Usage: EU/USA

Sodium formate

Function: Preservative / pH control.

Origin: Synthetic compound.

Restrictions and Adverse Effects: This ingredient is limited to 0.5 percent of the finished product if used as a preservative, but may be added in larger quantities for other stated purposes.

Usage: EU/USA

Sodium hydroxide

Function: pH control / Denaturant / Cuticle solvent.

Origin: Synthetic compound.

Restrictions and Adverse Effects: Harmful. Irritant. Corrosive to skin in dilute solutions. Maximum total alkali amount, including other alkalis, is 5 percent in nail cuticle solvents and 2 percent in hair care products (4.5 percent in professional products). In depilatories the pH must not exceed 12.7 and in other products pH must be below 11. Labels must state that the product contains alkali which can cause blindness, therefore, avoid eye contact. The label must also carry the warning "Keep out of the reach of children."

Usage: EU/USA

Sodium hydroxymethylglycinate

Function: Preservative.

Origin: Synthetic compound.

Restrictions and Adverse Effects: The safety of this substance was uncertain and its use in cosmetics was only provisionally permitted in the EU, until June 30, 1998. On September 3, 1998, following further scientific tests, the provisional status was removed and this ingredient was permitted for use in cosmetics. It is limited to a maximum of 0.5 percent of the finished product.

Usage: EU/USA

Sodium hypochlorite

(Sodium Chlorate (I))

Function: Bleaching agent / Antimicrobial.

Origin: Manufactured by the electrolysis of salt solution.

Restrictions and Adverse Effects: Corrosive to skin and eyes. Severe irritant. Sodium hypochlorite will bleach many colors if the cosmetic or toiletry comes into contact with fabrics.

Usage: EU/USA

Sodium iodate

Function: Preservative.

Origin: Synthetic compound.

Restrictions and Adverse Effects: This ingredient is limited to 0.1 percent of the finished, rinse-off product only.

Usage: EU/USA

Sodium laureth sulfate

Function: Surfactant.

A fairly high foaming surfactant, this compound is considered to be less irritating than sodium lauryl sulfate (SLS).

Origin: Synthetic detergent derived from coconut oils.

Restrictions and Adverse Effects: Eye irritant. May cause skin irritation and dermatitis. This ethoxylated ingredient is made using ethylene oxide (oxirane), which can form 1,4-dioxane, a carcinogen, as a by-product of manufacture. See *A–Z of Cosmetic Terms – Dioxane.*

Usage: EU/USA

Sodium laureth-5 sulfate

Function: Surfactant.

Origin: Synthetic detergent derived from coconut oils.

Restrictions and Adverse Effects: Eye irritant. May cause skin irritation and dermatitis. This ethoxylated ingredient is made using ethylene oxide (oxirane), which can form 1,4-dioxane, a carcinogen, as a by-product of manufacture. See *A–Z of Cosmetic Terms – Dioxane.*

Usage: EU/USA

Sodium laureth-7 sulfate

Function: Surfactant.

Origin: Synthetic detergent derived from coconut oils.

Restrictions and Adverse Effects: Eye irritant. May cause skin irritation and dermatitis. This ethoxylated ingredient is made using ethylene oxide (oxirane), which can form 1,4-dioxane, a carcinogen, as a by-product of manufacture. See *A–Z of Cosmetic Terms – Dioxane.*

Usage: EU/USA

Sodium laureth-12 sulfate

Function: Surfactant.

Origin: Synthetic detergent derived from coconut oils.

Restrictions and Adverse Effects: Eye irritant. May cause skin irritation and dermatitis. This ethoxylated ingredient is made using ethylene oxide (oxirane),

which can form 1,4-dioxane, a carcinogen, as a by-product of manufacture. See *A–Z of Cosmetic Terms – Dioxane*.
Usage: EU/USA

Sodium lauryl sulfate

(Sodium dodecyl sulfate, SLS)
Function: Denaturant / Emulsifier / Surfactant.
SLS is one of the most widely used surfactants and occurs in a large variety of shampoos, cleansing lotions, foaming bath oils, toothpastes, and liquid soaps.
Origin: Synthetic detergent derived from coconut oils.
Restrictions and Adverse Effects: Can cause contact eczema in some individuals. Eye irritant. Prolonged contact with this ingredient can cause skin irritation. When used in foaming bath oils, the prolonged contact can cause irritation of the mucous membranes of the genitals, resulting in urinary tract and vaginal inflammation and infection. In 1983, the *Journal of the American College of Toxicology* reported that animals exposed to SLS experienced eye damage, along with depression, labored breathing, diarrhea, severe skin irritation and corrosion, and death. Studies suggest SLS prevents children's eyes from developing properly, possibly by denaturing proteins in the eye and inhibiting correct structural formation. This damage is permanent, and there is also significant evidence that SLS retards the healing process of eye damage, especially in infants and children. The protein denaturing properties of SLS have been linked to immune system impairment within the skin.
Usage: EU/USA

Sodium metabisulfite

Function: Preservative.
Origin: Synthetic compound.
Restrictions and Adverse Effects: Irritant. This ingredient is limited to 0.2 percent of the finished product if used as a preservative, but it may be added in larger quantities for other stated purposes.
Usage: EU/USA

Sodium methylparaben

Function: Preservative.
Origin: Synthetic compound of the benzoate family.
Restrictions and Adverse Effects: Benzoic acid, benzoates, and parabens have been implicated in a large number of health issues. (See *A–Z of Cosmetic Terms – Benzoates*.) It is limited to 0.4 percent of the finished product if used on its own as a preservative, or 0.8 percent in total if used in combination with other parabens. Parabens may be added in larger quantities for other stated purposes.
Usage: EU/USA

Sodium monofluorophosphate

Function: Oral care agent.
Origin: Synthetic compound.
Restrictions and Adverse Effects: Fluorides are toxic. They can discolor teeth (fluorosis). Children should only use a small quantity of toothpaste and be discouraged from swallowing it. The total amount of fluoride allowed by EU regulations is 0.15 percent of the finished product.
Usage: EU/USA

Sodium myristate

Function: Emulsifier / Surfactant.
Origin: Semisynthetic or synthetic compound.
Restrictions and Adverse Effects: Some myristates are comedogenic (acne promoting, see *A–Z of Cosmetic Terms – Comedogen*).
Usage: EU/USA

Sodium nitrite

Function: Anticorrosive.
Origin: Synthetic compound.
Restrictions and Adverse Effects: Maximum allowed amount is 0.2 percent of the finished product. If it comes into contact with secondary or tertiary amine ingredients, carcinogenic nitrosamines may be formed. See *A–Z of Cosmetic Terms – Nitrosamines*.
Usage: EU/USA

Sodium o-phenylphenate

Function: Preservative.

Origin: Synthetic compound.

Restrictions and Adverse Effects: It is limited to 0.2 percent of the finished product if used as a preservative, but may be added in larger quantities for other stated purposes.

Usage: EU/USA

Sodium oxalate

Function: Chelating agent.

Origin: Synthetic compound.

Restrictions and Adverse Effects: Oxalates are toxic. Maximum allowed content is 5 percent and it is restricted to professional use only.

Usage: EU/USA

Sodium palm kernelate

Function: Surfactant.

A common ingredient in soaps, including baby soap and shaving soap.

Origin: Semisynthetic compound made from coconut oil and palm oil extracted from the kernels of palm trees.

Restrictions and Adverse Effects: No currently known adverse effects.

Usage: EU/USA

Sodium palmitate

Function: Emulsifier / Surfactant / Viscosity adjuster.

Origin: Semisynthetic or synthetic compound.

Restrictions and Adverse Effects: Some palmitates have been linked to contact dermatitis.

Usage: EU/USA

Sodium paraben

Function: Preservative.

Origin: Synthetic compound of the benzoate family.

Restrictions and Adverse Effects: Benzoic acid, benzoates, and parabens have been implicated in a large number of health issues. (See *A–Z of Cosmetic Terms – Benzoates*.) It is limited to 0.4 percent of the finished product if used on its own as a preservative, or 0.8 percent in total if used in combination with other parabens. Parabens may be added in larger quantities for other stated purposes.

Usage: EU/USA

Sodium persulfate

(Sodium peroxodisulfate)

Function: Oxidizing agent.

Origin: Synthetic compound.

Restrictions and Adverse Effects: This ingredient has been linked to asthma in hairdressers.

Usage: EU/USA

Sodium phenoxide

Function: Antimicrobial.

Origin: Synthetic compound.

Restrictions and Adverse Effects: Phenols are harmful. They corrode skin. They are severe irritants. This ingredient is limited to 1 percent maximum in the finished product and the label must clearly state its name separately from the list of ingredients.

Usage: EU/USA

Sodium phenylbenzimidazole sulfonate

Function: UV absorber.

Origin: Synthetic compound.

Restrictions and Adverse Effects: Irritant. This ingredient is restricted to a maximum of 8 percent of the finished product.

Usage: EU/USA

Sodium phthalate stearyl amide

Function: Emulsifier.

Origin: Semisynthetic or synthetic compound.

Restrictions and Adverse Effects: Phthalic acid and phthalates have been linked with testicular cancer and cell mutation.

Usage: EU/USA

Sodium propionate

Function: Preservative.

Origin: Synthetic compound.

Restrictions and Adverse Effects: Propanoic acid and its salts are limited to 2 percent of the finished

product if used as a preservative, but it may be added in larger quantities for other stated purposes.
Usage: EU/USA

Sodium propylparaben

Function: Preservative.

Origin: Synthetic compound of the benzoate family.

Restrictions and Adverse Effects: Benzoic acid, benzoates, and parabens have been implicated in a large number of health issues. (See *A–Z of Cosmetic Terms – Benzoates*.) It is limited to 0.4 percent of the finished product if used on its own as a preservative, or 0.8 percent in total if used in combination with other parabens. Parabens may be added in larger quantities for other stated purposes.

Usage: EU/USA

Sodium salicylate

Function: Preservative.

Origin: Synthetic compound.

Restrictions and Adverse Effects: This ingredient is limited to 0.5 percent of the finished product if used as a preservative, but may be added in larger quantities for other stated purposes. With the exception of shampoo, it must not be used in preparations intended for children under the age of 3 and must clearly state this restriction on the label.

Usage: EU/USA

Sodium sorbate

Function: Preservative.

Origin: Semisynthetic or synthetic compound.

Restrictions and Adverse Effects: This ingredient is limited to 0.6 percent of the finished product if used as a preservative, but may be added in larger quantities for other stated purposes.

Usage: EU/USA

Sodium stearate

Function: Emulsifier / Surfactant / Viscosity adjuster. A common ingredient in deodorant sticks and soaps, including baby soap, shaving soap, and dermatological soap.

Origin: Semisynthetic compound made by the action of caustic soda (sodium hydroxide) on animal or vegetable oils.

Restrictions and Adverse Effects: No currently known adverse effects. For BSE precautions see *Chapter 17 – Animal Products and Animal Testing*.

Usage: EU/USA

Sodium sulfide

Function: Depilatory agent.

Origin: Synthetic compound.

Restrictions and Adverse Effects: Sulfides are toxic. Irritant. May be alkaline (irritant and corrosive). Maximum allowed content is 2 percent of the finished product. The label must carry warnings to avoid contact with the eyes and to keep the product out of the reach of children.

Usage: EU/USA

Sodium sulfite

Function: Preservative.

Origin: Synthetic compound.

Restrictions and Adverse Effects: Irritant. This ingredient is limited to 0.2 percent of the finished product if used as a preservative, but may be added in larger quantities for other stated purposes.

Usage: EU/USA

Sodium tallowate

Function: Emulsifier / Surfactant.

Origin: Semisynthetic compound.

Restrictions and Adverse Effects: Reported to be comedogenic (acne promoting). May cause contact eczema. See *A–Z of Cosmetic Terms – Comedogen*. For BSE precautions see *Chapter 17 – Animal Products and Animal Testing*.

Usage: EU/USA

Sodium thioglycolate

Function: Depilatory agent / Reducing agent.

Origin: Synthetic compound.

Restrictions and Adverse Effects: Harmful. May be alkaline (irritant and corrosive). In the EU its content is limited to 8 percent in hair perming preparations (11 percent for professional use), 5 percent in depilatories and 2 percent in rinse-off hair care products. The pH must be between 7 and 9.5 in hair care products and between 7 and 12.7 in depilatories. The label must clearly state "Contains

Thioglycolate," and it must show the following mandatory warnings: "Follow the instructions. Keep out of reach of children. Avoid contact with eyes. In the event of contact with eyes, rinse with plenty of water and seek medical advice." Additionally, hair care products must state, "Wear suitable gloves."
Usage: EU/USA

Sodium undecylenate

Function: Preservative.
Origin: Semisynthetic or synthetic compound.
Restrictions and Adverse Effects: This ingredient is limited to 0.2 percent of the finished product if used as a preservative, but may be added in larger quantities for other stated purposes.
Usage: EU/USA

Sorbic acid

(2,4-Hexanedioic acid)
Function: Preservative.
Origin: Semisynthetic or synthetic compound.
Restrictions and Adverse Effects: Can cause urticaria (nettle rash or hives). It is limited to 0.6 percent of the finished product if used as a preservative, but may be added in larger quantities for other stated purposes.
Usage: EU/USA

Sorbitan laurate

Function: Emulsifier.
Origin: Semisynthetic or synthetic compound.
Restrictions and Adverse Effects: May cause contact urticaria (nettle rash or hives) in some individuals.
Usage: EU/USA

Sorbitan oleate

Function: Emulsifier.
Origin: Semisynthetic or synthetic compound.
Restrictions and Adverse Effects: May cause contact urticaria (nettle rash or hives) in some individuals.
Usage: EU/USA

Sorbitan palmitate

Function: Emulsifier.
Origin: Semisynthetic or synthetic compound.
Restrictions and Adverse Effects: May cause contact dermatitis in some individuals.
Usage: EU/USA

Sorbitan sesquioleate

Function: Emulsifier.
Origin: Semisynthetic or synthetic compound.
Restrictions and Adverse Effects: May cause contact dermatitis in some individuals.
Usage: EU/USA

Sorbitan stearate

Function: Emulsifier.
Origin: Semisynthetic or synthetic compound.
Restrictions and Adverse Effects: May cause contact urticaria (nettle rash or hives) in some individuals.
Usage: EU/USA

Sorbitol

(Glucitol, Hexan-1,2,3,4,5,6-hexol)
Function: A humectant believed to leave skin with a velvety feel. Sorbitol is similar to, but less expensive than naturally occurring glycerin and is rapidly taking its place as the most common cosmetic humectant.
Origin: Derived from fruits, seaweed, and algae or by the chemical reduction of glucose.
Restrictions and Adverse Effects: No currently known adverse effects.
Usage: EU/USA

Soyamide DEA

Function: Emulsifier / Emulsion stabilizer / Surfactant / Viscosity adjuster.
Origin: Semisynthetic compound derived from soya oil.
Restrictions and Adverse Effects: Some soya beans grown in the USA are genetically modified (GM) and these are mixed with natural soya beans, resulting in nearly all soya products containing some GM ingredients. There is no scientific reason for these to have any different effects to natural soya ingredients

but many consumers prefer to avoid GM products for a variety of reasons. DEA residues are cancer suspects currently under investigation. See *A–Z of Cosmetic Terms – DEA*.

Usage: EU/USA

Stannous fluoride

Function: Oral care agent.
Origin: Synthetic compound.
Restrictions and Adverse Effects: Fluorides are toxic. They can discolor teeth (fluorosis). Children should only use a small quantity of toothpaste and be discouraged from swallowing it. The total amount of fluoride allowed by EU regulations is 0.15 percent of the finished product.
Usage: EU/USA

Stearalkonium chloride

Function: Preservative.
Origin: Synthetic compound.
Restrictions and Adverse Effects: The safety of this substance was uncertain and its use in cosmetics was only provisionally permitted in the EU, until June 30, 1998. On September 3, 1998, following further scientific tests, the provisional status was removed and this ingredient was permitted for use in cosmetics. It is limited to a maximum of 0.1 percent of the finished product if it is used as a preservative, but may be added in larger quantities if it is used for other stated purposes. The label must state "Avoid contact with the eyes."
Usage: EU/USA

Stearamide DEA

Function: Antistatic agent / Viscosity adjuster.
Origin: Semisynthetic or synthetic compound.
Restrictions and Adverse Effects: DEA residues are cancer suspects currently under investigation. See *A–Z of Cosmetic Terms – DEA*.
Usage: EU/USA

Stearamide DEA-distearate

Function: Opacifier / Viscosity adjuster.
Origin: Semisynthetic or synthetic compound.

Restrictions and Adverse Effects: DEA residues are cancer suspects currently under investigation. See *A–Z of Cosmetic Terms – DEA*.
Usage: EU/USA

Stearamidoethyl diethanolamine

Function: Antistatic agent.
Origin: Synthetic compound.
Restrictions and Adverse Effects: DEA residues are cancer suspects currently under investigation. See *A–Z of Cosmetic Terms – DEA*.
Usage: EU/USA

Stearamidoethyl diethylamine phosphate

Function: Antistatic agent.
Origin: Synthetic compound.
Restrictions and Adverse Effects: May cause allergic contact dermatitis in some individuals.
Usage: EU/USA

Stearamidopropyl dimethylamine

Function: Antistatic agent / Emulsifier / Surfactant.
Origin: Synthetic compound.
Restrictions and Adverse Effects: Cancer suspect. May cause allergic dermatitis in some individuals.
Usage: EU/USA

Steareth – Family

Examples include Steareth-14 and Steareth-2 phosphate.
Function: Mainly emulsifiers and surfactants.
Origin: A range of synthetic ingredients manufactured from ethylene oxide. These ethoxylated compounds may be combined with a variety of other molecules to produce a wide range of cosmetic materials. Higher numbers mean higher ethoxylation (bigger molecules), usually resulting in a greater solubility in water.
Restrictions and Adverse Effects: Ethoxylated ingredients are made using ethylene oxide (oxirane), which can form 1,4-dioxane, a carcinogen, as a by-product of manufacture. See *A–Z of Cosmetic Terms – Dioxane*.
Usage: EU/USA

Stearic acid

(n-Octadecanoic acid, Octadecanoic acid)

Function: Emulsifier / Emulsion stabilizer.
Origin: Semisynthetic or synthetic compound.
Restrictions and Adverse Effects: Linked to skin allergies.
Usage: EU/USA

Steartrimonium chloride

Function: Preservative.
Origin: Synthetic compound.
Restrictions and Adverse Effects: This ingredient is limited to 0.1 percent of the finished product if used as a preservative, but may be added in larger quantities for other stated purposes.
Usage: EU/USA

Stearyl alcohol

Function: Emollient / Moisturizer / Emulsion stabilizer / Opacifier / Viscosity adjuster.
Origin: Semisynthetic or synthetic compound.
Restrictions and Adverse Effects: May cause contact dermatitis and contact allergies in some individuals.
Usage: EU/USA

Stearyl benzoate

Function: Emollient / Moisturizer.
Origin: Synthetic compound of the benzoate family.
Restrictions and Adverse Effects: Benzoic acid and benzoates have been implicated in a large number of health issues. (See *A–Z of Cosmetic Terms – Benzoates*.)
Usage: EU/USA

Stearyl trihydroxyethyl propylenediamine dihydrofluoride

Function: Oral care agent.
Origin: Synthetic compound.
Restrictions and Adverse Effects: Fluorides are toxic. They can discolor teeth (fluorosis). Children should only use a small quantity of toothpaste and be discouraged from swallowing it. The total amount of fluoride allowed by EU regulations is 0.15 percent of the finished product.
Usage: EU/USA

Strontium acetate

Function: Oral care agent.
Origin: Synthetic compound.
Restrictions and Adverse Effects: Strontium compounds are toxic. Maximum allowed content is 3.5 percent total strontium in the finished oral care product or 2.1 percent in shampoo or face care products. The label must clearly state the name of this ingredient separately from the list of other ingredients. The label must also state that frequent use by children is not advised.
Usage: EU/USA

Strontium chloride

Function: Oral care agent.
Origin: Synthetic compound.
Restrictions and Adverse Effects: Strontium compounds are toxic. Maximum allowed content is 3.5 percent total strontium in the finished oral care product or 2.1 percent in shampoo or face care products. The label must clearly state the name of this ingredient separately from the list of other ingredients. The label must also state that frequent use by children is not advised.
Usage: EU/USA

Strontium dioxide

Function: Bleaching agent.
Origin: Synthetic compound.
Restrictions and Adverse Effects: Strontium compounds are toxic. This ingredient is harmful by skin contact and damaging to eyes. It is limited to 4.5 percent total strontium in rinse-off hair preparations, and is restricted to professional use only.
Usage: EU/USA

Strontium hydroxide

Function: pH control / Depilatory agent.
Origin: Synthetic compound.
Restrictions and Adverse Effects: Strontium compounds are toxic. Maximum allowed content is 3.5 percent of the finished product, with a maximum pH of 12.7. The label must carry the following warnings: "Avoid eye contact. Keep out of the reach of children."
Usage: EU/USA

Strontium peroxide

Function: Antimicrobial / Bleaching agent.

Origin: Synthetic compound.

Restrictions and Adverse Effects: Strontium compounds are toxic. This ingredient is harmful by skin contact and damaging to eyes. It is limited to 4.5 percent total strontium in rinse-off hair preparations, and is restricted to professional use only.

Usage: EU/USA

Strontium sulfide

Function: Depilatory agent.

Origin: Synthetic compound.

Restrictions and Adverse Effects: Sulfides are toxic. Irritant. May be alkaline (irritant and corrosive). Maximum allowed content is 6 percent of the finished product. The label must carry warnings to avoid contact with the eyes and to keep the product out of the reach of children.

Usage: EU/USA

Strontium thioglycolate

Function: Depilatory agent / Reducing agent.

Origin: Synthetic compound.

Restrictions and Adverse Effects: Harmful. May be alkaline (irritant and corrosive). In the EU its content is limited to 8 percent in hair perming preparations (11 percent for professional use), 5 percent in depilatories and 2 percent in rinse-off hair care products. The pH must be between 7 and 9.5 in hair care products and between 7 and 12.7 in depilatories. The label must clearly state "Contains Thioglycolate," and it must show the following mandatory warnings: "Follow the instructions. Keep out of reach of children. Avoid contact with eyes. In the event of contact with eyes, rinse with plenty of water and seek medical advice." Additionally, hair care products must state, "Wear suitable gloves."

Usage: EU/USA

Styrene / Acrylates / Acrylonitrile copolymer

Function: Film former / Viscosity adjuster.

Origin: Synthetic compound.

Restrictions and Adverse Effects: Some nitriles have been linked to allergic reactions and contact eczema.

Usage: EU/USA

Sucrose benzoate / Sucrose acetate isobutyrate / Butyl benzyl phthalate / Methyl methacrylate copolymer

Function: Film former / Viscosity adjuster.

Origin: Synthetic compound.

Restrictions and Adverse Effects: Phthalic acid and phthalates have been linked with testicular cancer and cell mutation.

Usage: EU/USA

Sucrose benzoate / Sucrose acetate isobutyrate / Butyl benzyl phthalate copolymer

Function: Film former / Viscosity adjuster.

Origin: Synthetic compound.

Restrictions and Adverse Effects: Phthalic acid and phthalates have been linked with testicular cancer and cell mutation.

Usage: EU/USA

Sucrose myristate

Function: Emulsifier.

Origin: Semisynthetic compound.

Restrictions and Adverse Effects: Some myristates are comedogenic (acne promoting, see *A–Z of Cosmetic Terms – Comedogen*).

Usage: EU/USA

Sucrose palmitate

Function: Emulsifier / Surfactant.

Origin: Semisynthetic compound derived from sugar.

Restrictions and Adverse Effects: Some palmitates have been linked to contact dermatitis.

Usage: EU/USA

Sugar cane extract

Function: Exfoliating agent.

Origin: Natural extract of sugar cane.

Restrictions and Adverse Effects: Sugar cane extract contains alpha-hydroxy acids (AHAs), which are used to exfoliate skin. They are also known as skin peelers because they dissolve and remove the outer layer of skin. They can cause increased sensitivity to the sun due to loss of the protective outer layer of skin cells. Do not expose skin to the sun immediately following treatment with AHAs. Test a small area before use and discontinue use if skin irritation, redness, bleeding, or pain is experienced. Not recommended for use on children. May cause exfoliative dermatitis.

Usage: USA/Not currently on the EU inventory of cosmetic ingredients.

t-Butyl hydroquinone

Function: Antioxidant.

Origin: Synthetic compound.

Restrictions and Adverse Effects: Can cause allergic contact dermatitis when used in lip make-up.

Usage: EU/USA

Talc

Function: Absorbent.

Origin: Natural mineral (Hydrated magnesium silicate).

Restrictions and Adverse Effects: Inhalation of talc dust can cause lung disease. Baby powders must carry a warning to keep the powder away from the infant's nose and mouth. Concerns that natural mineral powders may contain tetanus, a microbe that is found in soil, are largely unwarranted. Some samples of talc have been found to contain asbestos fibers. Talc has been linked to ovarian cancer (see *Chapter 7 – Deodorants and Antiperspirants* for details). It has been demonstrated to cause human and animal soft tissues to form scar tissue.

Usage: EU/USA

Tallamide DEA

Function: Antistatic agent / Viscosity adjuster.

Origin: Semisynthetic compound.

Restrictions and Adverse Effects: DEA residues are cancer suspects currently under investigation. See *A–Z of Cosmetic Terms – DEA*.

Usage: EU/USA

Tallowamide DEA

Function: Antistatic agent / Emulsifier / Emulsion stabilizer / Viscosity adjuster.

Origin: Semisynthetic compound derived from tallow (animal fat).

Restrictions and Adverse Effects: DEA residues are cancer suspects currently under investigation. See *A–Z of Cosmetic Terms – DEA*. For BSE precautions see *Chapter 17 – Animal Products and Animal Testing*.

Usage: EU/USA

Tallowamidopropyl dimethylamine

Function: Surfactant.

Origin: Semisynthetic compound derived from tallow (animal fat).

Restrictions and Adverse Effects: May cause contact allergies in some individuals. For BSE precautions see *Chapter 17 – Animal Products and Animal Testing*.

Usage: EU/USA

TEA-carbomer

Function: Viscosity adjuster.

Origin: Synthetic compound.

Restrictions and Adverse Effects: Can cause severe facial dermatitis.

Usage: EU/USA

TEA-cocoyl glutamate

Function: Surfactant.

Origin: Synthetic compound.

Restrictions and Adverse Effects: Can cause severe facial dermatitis.

Usage: EU/USA

TEA-cocoyl hydrolyzed collagen

Function: Antistatic agent / Surfactant.

Origin: Semisynthetic compound derived from collagen, an animal protein.

Restrictions and Adverse Effects: Can cause severe facial dermatitis. For BSE precautions see *Chapter 17 – Animal Products and Animal Testing*.

Usage: EU/USA

TEA-cocoyl hydrolyzed soy protein

Function: Antistatic agent

Origin: Semisynthetic compound derived from soybeans.

Restrictions and Adverse Effects: Some soybeans grown in the USA are genetically modified (GM) and these are mixed with natural soybeans, resulting in nearly all soybean products containing some GM ingredients. There is no scientific reason for these to have any different effects to natural soybean ingredients but many consumers prefer to avoid GM products for a variety of reasons. Can cause severe facial dermatitis.

Usage: EU/USA

TEA-myristate

Function: Emulsifier / Surfactant.

Origin: Semisynthetic or synthetic compound.

Restrictions and Adverse Effects: Some myristates are comedogenic (acne promoting, see *A–Z of Cosmetic Terms – Comedogen*).

Usage: EU/USA

TEA-palmitate

Function: Emulsifier / Surfactant.

Origin: Semisynthetic or synthetic compound.

Restrictions and Adverse Effects: Some palmitates have been linked to contact dermatitis.

Usage: EU/USA

TEA-phenylbenzimidazole sulfonate

Function: UV absorber.

Origin: Synthetic compound.

Restrictions and Adverse Effects: Irritant for some individuals. This ingredient is restricted to a maximum of 8 percent of the finished product.

Usage: EU/USA

TEA-stearate

Function: Emulsifier / Surfactant.

Origin: Semisynthetic or synthetic compound.

Restrictions and Adverse Effects: Can cause severe facial dermatitis.

Usage: EU/USA

Terephthalylidene dicamphor sulfonic acid

Function: UV absorber.

Origin: Synthetic compound.

Restrictions and Adverse Effects: Irritant. This ingredient is restricted to a maximum of 10 percent of the finished product.

Usage: EU/USA

Tetrahydronaphthalene

Function: Additive.

Origin: Synthetic compound.

Restrictions and Adverse Effects: Skin and eye irritant.

Usage: USA/Not currently on the EU inventory of cosmetic ingredients.

Tetrapotassium etidronate

Function: Chelating agent / Preservative.

Origin: Synthetic compound.

Restrictions and Adverse Effects: Harmful. A skin and mucous membrane irritant for some individuals. It is limited to 1.5 percent in hair care preparations and 0.2 percent in soap.

Usage: EU/USA

Tetrasodium EDTA

(Tetrasodium edetate)

Function: Chelating agent / Preservative.
Softens water and bonds with minerals essential to microbial growth, thus acting as a preservative.

Origin: Synthetic compound.

Restrictions and Adverse Effects: No currently known adverse effects.

Usage: EU/USA

Tetrasodium etidronate

Function: Chelating agent / Emulsion stabilizer / Viscosity adjuster / Preservative.
This is by far the most commonly used preservative in bars of soap.

Origin: Synthetic compound.

Restrictions and Adverse Effects: Harmful. Skin and mucous membrane irritant for some individuals. It is limited to 1.5 percent in hair care preparations and 0.2 percent in soap.

Usage: EU/USA

Theobroma cacao

(Cocoa butter)

Function: Botanical additive.

Origin: Natural plant extract.

Restrictions and Adverse Effects: Comedogenic (acne promoting, see *A–Z of Cosmetic Terms – Comedogen*).

Usage: EU/USA

Thimerosal

Function: Preservative.

Originally used as an antiseptic, this is a highly poisonous, creamy-white compound of mercury, sulfur and salicylic acid.

Origin: Synthetic compound.

Restrictions and Adverse Effects: Mercury compounds are toxic by skin absorption, cause dermatitis, and accumulate in the body. They are limited to a total mercury content of 0.007 percent in the EU and 0.0065 percent in the USA. The label must carry suitable warnings and mercury salts are restricted to use in eye make-up and make-up removers only in both the EU and USA.

Usage: EU/USA

Thioglycolic acid

Function: Depilatory agent / Reducing agent.

Origin: Synthetic compound.

Restrictions and Adverse Effects: Harmful. May be alkaline (irritant and corrosive). In the EU its content is limited to 8 percent in hair perming preparations (11 percent for professional use), 5 percent in depila-tories and 2 percent in rinse-off hair care products. The pH must be between 7 and 9.5 in hair care prod-ucts and between 7 and 12.7 in depilatories. The label must clearly state "Contains Thioglycolate," and it must show the following mandatory warnings: "Follow the instructions. Keep out of reach of children. Avoid contact with eyes. In the event of contact with eyes, rinse with plenty of water and seek medical advice." Additionally, hair care products must state, "Wear suitable gloves."

Usage: EU/USA

Thymus vulgaris

(Thyme extract)

Function: Botanical additive.

Origin: Plant extract.

Restrictions and Adverse Effects: May cause contact allergies in some individuals.

Usage: EU/USA

Titanium dioxide

(TiO_2, Titanium (IV) oxide)

Function: Opacifier / Absorbent / White colorant. A commonly used inorganic oxide occurring in nature, brilliant white in color with many times the covering power of zinc oxide. It is the main pigment in white and light-colored paints.

Origin: Natural mineral.

Restrictions and Adverse Effects: No currently known adverse effects.

Usage: EU/USA

Tocophereth – Family

Examples include Tocophereth-10, Tocophereth-12 and Tocophereth-18.

Function: Mainly surfactants.

Origin: A range of synthetic ingredients manufactured from tocopherol (vitamin E) and ethylene oxide. These ethoxylated compounds may be combined with a variety of other molecules to produce a wide range of cosmetic materials. Higher numbers mean higher ethoxylation (bigger molecules), usually resulting in a greater solubility in water.

Restrictions and Adverse Effects: Ethoxylated ingredients are made using ethylene oxide (oxirane), which can form 1,4-dioxane, a carcinogen, as a by-product of manufacture. See *A–Z of Cosmetic Terms – Dioxane*.

Usage: EU/USA

Tocopherol

(Vitamin E)

Function: Antioxidant.

Origin: May be naturally extracted or prepared synthetically.

Restrictions and Adverse Effects: Cancer suspect. May cause contact dermatitis in some individuals.
Usage: EU/USA

Tocopheryl linoleate

Function: Antioxidant.
A substance that is said to help prevent stiffening and aging of the skin as a result of UV exposure. It is thought to provide the skin with linoleic acid, one of the major essential fatty acids.
Origin: Chemically modified Vitamin E.
Restrictions and Adverse Effects: No currently known adverse effects.
Usage: EU/USA

Toluene-2,5-diamine

(Methylphenylene-2,5-diamine)
Function: Hair dye.
Origin: Synthetic compound.
Restrictions and Adverse Effects: Irritant for some individuals. This dye is limited to 10 percent of the finished product. The label must clearly state "Contains phenylenediamines" and it must carry the following warnings: "Can cause an allergic reaction. Do not use to dye eyelashes or eyebrows." Products supplied for professional use must carry the additional warning, "Wear suitable gloves."
Usage: EU/USA

Toluene-2,5-diamine sulfate

(Methylphenylene-2,5-diamine sulfate)
Function: Hair dye.
Origin: Synthetic compound.
Restrictions and Adverse Effects: Irritant for some individuals. This dye is limited to 10 percent of the finished product. The label must clearly state "Contains phenylenediamines" and it must carry the following warnings: "Can cause an allergic reaction. Do not use to dye eyelashes or eyebrows." Products supplied for professional use must carry the additional warning, "Wear suitable gloves."
Usage: EU/USA

Toluenesulfonamide-formaldehyde resin

Function: Film former / Viscosity adjuster.
Origin: Synthetic compound.
Restrictions and Adverse Effects: May cause contact dermatitis in some individuals. Formaldehyde residues may be present. Formaldehyde is a cancer suspect.
Usage: USA/Not currently on the EU inventory of cosmetic ingredients.

Trethocanic acid

Function: Exfoliating agent.
Origin: Chemically modified natural acid.
Restrictions and Adverse Effects: This ingredient is a beta-hydroxy acid (BHA), which is used to exfoliate skin. BHAs are also known as skin peelers because they dissolve and remove the outer layer of skin. They can cause increased sensitivity to the sun due to loss of the protective outer layer of skin cells. Do not expose skin to the sun immediately following treatment with BHAs. Test a small area before use and discontinue use if skin irritation, redness, bleeding, or pain is experienced. Not recommended for use on children. May cause exfoliative dermatitis.
Usage: USA/Not currently on the EU inventory of cosmetic ingredients.

Trichloroacetic acid

Function: Exfoliating agent.
In general this is a powerfully corrosive acid and is used as an exfoliant only by cosmetic surgeons.
Origin: Synthetic compound.
Restrictions and Adverse Effects: Highly corrosive. Severe skin and eye irritant.
Usage: USA/Not currently on the EU inventory of cosmetic ingredients.

Triclocarban

Function: Preservative.
Origin: Synthetic compound.
Restrictions and Adverse Effects: This ingredient is limited to 0.2 percent of the finished product if used as a preservative, but may be added in larger quantities for other stated purposes. The

manufacturing process produces two extremely harmful by-products which must be reduced in amount to at least 1 ppm before this ingredient may be used.

Usage: EU/USA

Triclosan

Function: Preservative / Deodorant.

A commonly used deodorant found in a vast majority of roll-on deodorants and deodorant sticks and gels. It is occasionally used as a preservative in other cosmetics.

Origin: Synthetic compound.

Restrictions and Adverse Effects: This ingredient is limited to 0.3 percent of the finished product if used as a preservative, but may be added in larger quantities for other stated purposes, such as a deodorant.

Usage: EU/USA

Tridecyl myristate

Function: Emollient / Moisturizer.

Origin: Semisynthetic or synthetic compound.

Restrictions and Adverse Effects: Some myristates are comedogenic (acne promoting, see A–Z of Cosmetic Terms – Comedogen).

Usage: EU/USA

Triethanolamine

(Triolamine, Trolamine, TEA)

Function: pH control.

A commonly used ingredient in skin lotions, eye gels, moisturizing creams, shaving foams, shampoos (including baby shampoos), and dermatological soaps.

Origin: A synthetic compound made from ammonia and ethylene oxide.

Restrictions and Adverse Effects: Harmful. Can cause severe facial dermatitis and contact dermatitis. Danger of nitrosamine contamination (see A–Z of Cosmetic Terms – Nitrosamines). This product must have a minimum purity of 99 percent, with a maximum secondary alkolamine contamination of 0.5 percent. The maximum allowed content is 2.5 percent of the finished non-rinse off product. It is known to contain the carcinogenic impurity

N-nitrosodialkanolamine, which must not exceed 5 ppm in the ingredient.

Usage: EU/USA

Triisopropanolamine

Function: pH control.

Origin: Synthetic compound.

Restrictions and Adverse Effects: Harmful. Danger of nitrosamine contamination (see A–Z of Cosmetic Terms – Nitrosamines). This product must have a minimum purity of 99 percent, with a maximum secondary alkolamine contamination of 0.5 percent. The maximum allowed content is 2.5 percent of the finished non-rinse off product. It is known to contain the carcinogen N-nitrosodialkanolamine, which must not exceed 5 ppm in the ingredient.

Usage: EU/USA

Trimyristin

Function: Emollient / Moisturizer / Solvent / Viscosity adjuster.

Origin: Semisynthetic or synthetic compound.

Restrictions and Adverse Effects: Some myristates are comedogenic (acne promoting, see A–Z of Cosmetic Terms – Comedogen).

Usage: EU/USA

Trioctyldodecyl borate

Function: Additive.

Origin: Synthetic compound.

Restrictions and Adverse Effects: Borates are toxic and have been linked to fetal malformations.

Usage: EU/USA

Tripalmitin

Function: Emollient / Moisturizer / Solvent / Viscosity adjuster.

Origin: Semisynthetic or synthetic glyceryl ester.

Restrictions and Adverse Effects: Both glyceryl esters and palmitates have been linked to contact dermatitis.

Usage: EU/USA

Trisodium NTA

Function: Chelating agent.
Origin: Synthetic compound.
Restrictions and Adverse Effects: The acid form of Trisodium NTA is a cancer suspect.
Usage: EU/USA

Tropic acid

Function: Exfoliating agent.
Origin: Chemically modified natural extract.
Restrictions and Adverse Effects: Tropic acid is a beta-hydroxy acid (BHA), which is used to exfoliate skin. BHAs are also known as skin peelers because they dissolve and remove the outer layer of skin. They can cause increased sensitivity to the sun due to loss of the protective outer layer of skin cells. Do not expose skin to the sun immediately following treatment with BHAs. Test a small area before use and discontinue use if skin irritation, redness, bleeding, or pain is experienced. Not recommended for use on children. May cause exfoliative dermatitis.
Usage: USA/Not currently on the EU inventory of cosmetic ingredients.

Turpentine oils

Function: Fragrance / Solvent.
Origin: Natural extract.
Restrictions and Adverse Effects: Can cause contact dermatitis.
Usage: USA/Not currently on the EU inventory of cosmetic ingredients.

Undecylenamide DEA

Function: Antidandruff agent / Antimicrobial / Antistatic agent / Viscosity adjuster.
Origin: Synthetic compound.
Restrictions and Adverse Effects: DEA residues are cancer suspects currently under investigation. See *A–Z of Cosmetic Terms – DEA*.
Usage: EU/USA

Undecylenic acid

Function: Preservative.
Origin: Synthetic compound.

Restrictions and Adverse Effects: This ingredient is limited to 0.2 percent of the finished product if used as a preservative, but may be added in larger quantities for other stated purposes.
Usage: EU/USA

Urea

Function: Antistatic agent / Humectant.
Origin: A natural substance but usually prepared synthetically.
Restrictions and Adverse Effects: Can cause thinning of the epidermis and may impair skin function.
Usage: EU/USA

Urocanic acid

Function: UV absorber.
Origin: Synthetic compound.
Restrictions and Adverse Effects: Phototoxin. This substance is considered harmful and has been banned from use in cosmetics in the EU.
Usage: USA

Vitamin B

(Inositol, Hexahydroxocyclohexane)
Function: Emollient.
Inositol can exist in eight different forms, which occur in plants as hexaphosphoric esters, and are known as phytins. One of these forms is part of the Vitamin B complex. It appears to have growth-promoting properties in chicks and anti-alopecia (anti-hair loss) effects in mice.
Origin: A natural plant extract.
Restrictions and Adverse Effects: No currently known adverse effects.
Usage: EU/USA

Wheat germamide DEA

Function: Surfactant.
Origin: Semisynthetic compound derived from wheat.
Restrictions and Adverse Effects: DEA residues are cancer suspects currently under investigation. See *A–Z of Cosmetic Terms – DEA*.
Usage: EU/USA

Witch hazel extract

Function: Fragrance / Astringent.
Origin: Natural extract of the witch hazel tree.
Restrictions and Adverse Effects: May cause allergic contact dermatitis in some individuals.
Usage: USA/Not currently on the EU inventory of cosmetic ingredients.

Xanthene

(Dibenzopyran)
Function: Solvent.
Origin: Synthetic compound.
Restrictions and Adverse Effects: Comedogenic (acne promoting, see *A–Z of Cosmetic Terms – Comedogen*). Has been shown to inhibit cell metabolism.
Usage: USA/Not currently on the EU inventory of cosmetic ingredients.

Zea mays (oil)

Function: Antistatic agent / Emollient / Moisturizer / Solvent.
Origin: Corn oil extracted from corn or maize kernels.
Restrictions and Adverse Effects: Comedogenic (acne promoting, see *A–Z of Cosmetic Terms – Comedogen*). May be derived from genetically modified (GM) crops.
Usage: EU/USA

Zea mays (starch)

Function: Absorbent / Viscosity adjuster.
Used as the main ingredient in talc-free absorbent powders, and is often mixed with talc in other absorbent powders. Some baby powders may contain talc mixed with zea mays.
Origin: Corn starch (cornflour) from ground corn grains or maize.
Restrictions and Adverse Effects: No known adverse effects. May be derived from genetically modified (GM) crops.
Usage: EU/USA

Zinc acetate

Function: Antimicrobial.
Origin: Synthetic compound.
Restrictions and Adverse Effects: Soluble zinc salts are toxic and are limited to a maximum zinc content of 1 percent of the finished product.
Usage: EU/USA

Zinc aspartate

Function: Biological additive.
Origin: Semisynthetic or synthetic compound.
Restrictions and Adverse Effects: Soluble zinc salts are toxic and are limited to a maximum zinc content of 1 percent of the finished product.
Usage: EU/USA

Zinc borate

Function: Antimicrobial.
Origin: Synthetic compound.
Restrictions and Adverse Effects: Borates are toxic and have been linked to fetal malformations.
Usage: EU/USA

Zinc chloride

Function: Oral care agent.
Origin: Synthetic compound.
Restrictions and Adverse Effects: Soluble zinc salts are toxic and are limited to a maximum zinc content of 1 percent of the finished product.
Usage: EU/USA

Zinc citrate

Function: Additive / Preservative.
Origin: Synthetic compound.
Restrictions and Adverse Effects: Soluble zinc salts are toxic and are limited to a maximum zinc content of 1 percent of the finished product.
Usage: EU/USA

Zinc gluconate

Function: Deodorant.
Origin: Synthetic compound.
Restrictions and Adverse Effects: Soluble zinc salts are toxic and are limited to a maximum zinc content of 1 percent of the finished product.
Usage: EU/USA

Zinc glutamate

Function: Deodorant.

Origin: Semisynthetic or synthetic compound.

Restrictions and Adverse Effects: Soluble zinc salts are toxic and are limited to a maximum zinc content of 1 percent of the finished product.

Usage: EU/USA

Zinc myristate

Function: Opacifier / Viscosity adjuster.

Origin: Semisynthetic or synthetic compound.

Restrictions and Adverse Effects: Some myristates are comedogenic (acne promoting, see *A–Z of Cosmetic Terms – Comedogen*).

Usage: EU/USA

Zinc palmitate

Function: Deodorant.

Origin: Semisynthetic or synthetic compound.

Restrictions and Adverse Effects: Some palmitates have been linked to contact dermatitis.

Usage: EU/USA

Zinc PCA

Function: Humectant.

Origin: Synthetic compound.

Restrictions and Adverse Effects: Soluble zinc salts are toxic and are limited to a maximum zinc content of 1 percent of the finished product.

Usage: EU/USA

Zinc pentadecene tricarboxylate

Function: Surfactant.

Origin: Synthetic compound.

Restrictions and Adverse Effects: Soluble zinc salts are toxic and are limited to a maximum zinc content of 1 percent of the finished product.

Usage: EU/USA

Zinc phenolsulfonate

Function: Antimicrobial / Deodorant.

Origin: Synthetic compound.

Restrictions and Adverse Effects: Soluble zinc salts are toxic. Harmful to eyes. This ingredient is limited to a maximum zinc content of 6 percent of the finished product. The label must carry a warning to avoid contact with the eyes.

Usage: EU/USA

Zinc pyrithione

(Pyrithione zinc)

Function: Preservative / Antimicrobial / Antidandruff agent.

Origin: Synthetic compound.

Restrictions and Adverse Effects: This ingredient is limited to 0.5 percent of the finished rinse-off products only, but it may be added in larger quantities for other stated purposes. If used in antidandruff shampoos, 1 percent is typically added. It is prohibited in oral hygiene products.

Usage: EU/USA

Zinc stearate

Function: White colorant / Opacifier.

Origin: Semisynthetic or synthetic compound.

Restrictions and Adverse Effects: Allowed in all products.

Usage: EU/USA

Zinc sulfate

Function: Antimicrobial / Oral care agent.

Origin: Synthetic compound.

Restrictions and Adverse Effects: Soluble zinc salts are toxic and are limited to a maximum zinc content of 1 percent of the finished product.

Usage: EU/USA

Zinc sulfide

Function: Depilatory agent.

Origin: Synthetic compound.

Restrictions and Adverse Effects: Soluble zinc salts are toxic and are limited to a maximum zinc content of 1 percent of the finished product.

Usage: EU/USA

Zinc yeast derivative

Function: Biological additive.

Origin: Synthetic compound.

Restrictions and Adverse Effects: Soluble zinc salts are toxic and are limited to a maximum zinc content of 1 percent of the finished product.

Usage: EU/USA

index of alternative names

Alternative Names	INCI / Common Name
1,2-Diaminoethane	Ethylenediamine
2,4-Hexanedioic acid	Sorbic acid
2-Phenoxyethanol	Phenoxyethanol
2-ethoxyethyl-p-methoxy cinnamate	Cinoxate
2-hydroxy-2-phenylacetophenone	Benzoin
2-Hydroxybutanoic acid	Beta-hydroxybutanoic acid
3,7-Dimethyl-7-hydroxyoctenal	Hydroxycitronella
4-Aminobenzoic acid	PABA
4-MMPD	2,4-Diaminoanisole
4-MMPD sulfate	2,4-Diaminoanisole sulfate
4-NOPD	4-Nitro-o-phenylenediamine
4-NOPD hydrochloride	4-Nitro-o-phenylenediamine HCl
5-Chloro-3-methyl-4-isothiazolin-3-one	Methylchloroisotiazolinone
5-Chloro-3-methylisothiazolone	Methylchloroisotiazolinone
Acetophenetidide	Phenacetin
Acetophenetidin	Phenacetin
Alcohol	Alcohol denat.
Aloe extract	Aloe barbadensis
Aloe juice	Aloe barbadensis
Aloe vera gel	Aloe barbadensis
Aloe vera oil	Aloe barbadensis
Alpha-hydroxycaprylic acid	Alpha-hydroxy octanoic acid
Alpha-methylquinoline	Quinaldine

Aluminum monostearate	Aluminum stearate
Amaranth	CI 16185 and CI 16185:1
Aminocyclohexane	Cyclohexylamine
Aminomethyl phenol	p-Methylaminophenol
Aminomethylphenol	p-Methylaminophenol
Ammonium peroxodisulfate	Ammonium persulfate
Allura Red	CI 16035
Avobenzone	Butyl methoxydibenzoylmethane
Barium sulfate	CI 77120
Beetroot red	Beta vulgaris
Benzopyrone	Coumarin
Benzoylphenyl carbinol	Benzoin
Bergamot oil	Citrus bergamia
Beta carotene	CI 40800
Beta carotene	CI 75130
Bronopol	2-Bromo-2-nitropropane-1,3-diol
Butan-1-ol	N-Butyl alcohol
Butanol	N-Butyl alcohol
Butyl alcohol	N-Butyl alcohol
Butyl-4-hydroxybenzoate	Butpylparaben
Butylated hydroxyanisole	BHA
Butylated hydroxytoluene	BHT
Butylparahydroxybenzoate	Butylparaben
C12-15 alcohols benzoate	C12-15 alkyl benzoate
Calcium carbonate	CI 77220
Calcium sulfate	CI 77231
Calendula extract	Calendula officinalis
Calgon S	Calgon
Carbon black	CI 77266
Carboxymethyl cellulose sodium	Cellulose gum
Carmellose	Cellulose gum
Carnauba wax	Carnauba
Castor oil	Ricinus communis
Centaurea cyanus	Cornflower extract

Cera carnauba	Carnauba
Cera flava	Cera alba
Cetylic acid	Palmitic acid
Chamomile extract	Chamomilla recutita
Chinaldine	Quinaldine
Chlorocresol	p-Chloro-m-cresol
Chloromethylisotiazolinone	Methylchloroisotiazolinone
CI 10020	Acid Green 1
CI 10316	Acid Yellow 1
CI 11154	Basic Blue 41
CI 12245	Basic Red 76
CI 12250	Basic Brown 16
CI 12251	Basic Brown 17
CI 12719	Basic Yellow 57
CI 14270	Acid Orange 6
CI 14720	Acid Red 14
CI 15510	Acid Orange 7
CI 15711	Acid Black 52
CI 16185	Acid Red 27
CI 16255	Acid Red 18
CI 17200	Acid Red 33
CI 18065	Acid Red 35
CI 19140	Acid Yellow 23
CI 20170	Acid Orange 24
CI 21010	Basic Brown 4
CI 27290	Acid Red 73
CI 42045	Acid Blue 1
CI 42051	Acid Blue 3
CI 42090	Acid Blue 9
CI 42510	Basic Violet 14
CI 44045	Basic Blue 26
CI 44090	Acid Green 50
CI 45100	Acid Red 52
CI 45350	Acid Yellow 73 sodium salt
CI 45380	Acid Red 95
CI 45380	Acid Red 87

CI 45410	Acid Red 92
CI 45430	Acid Red 51
CI 60730	Acid Violet 43
CI 61570	Acid Green 25
CI 62045	Acid Blue 62
CI 73015	Acid Blue 74
Cinnamaldehyde	Cinnamal
Citronellal hydrate	Hydroxycitronella
Cocoa butter	Theobroma cacao
Coconut oil	Cocos nucifera
Colophonium	Rosin
Colophony	Rosin
Common salt	Sodium chloride
Cornflower distillate	Cornflower extract
Cumarin	Coumarin
D&C Blue #9	CI 69825
D&C Green #5	CI 61570
D&C Green #6	CI 61565
D&C Green #8	CI 59040
D&C Orange #4	CI 15510
D&C Red #6	CI 15850
D&C Red #7	CI 15850
D&C Red #17	CI 26100
D&C Red #27	CI 45410
D&C Red #28	CI 45410
D&C Red #30	CI 73360
D&C Red #31	CI 15800
D&C Red #34	CI 15880
D&C Red #36	CI 12085
D&C Yellow #7	CI 45350:1
D&C Yellow #8	CI 45350
DEA	Diethanolamine
DEET	Diethyl toluamide
Denatured alcohol	Alcohol denat.
Dexpanthenol	Panthenol

DHA	Dihydroxyacetone
Diammonium peroxodisulfate	Ammonium persulfate
Dibenzopyran	Xanthene
Dichlorophen	Dichlorophene
Dichromium trioxide	CI 77288
Diethanolamine	DEA
Dimethicon	Dimethicone
Dimethyl polysiloxane	Dimethicone
Dioxybenzone	Benzophenone-8
Disodium edetate	Disodium EDTA
E100	CI 75300
E101	Lactoflavin
E101a	Riboflavin
E102	CI 19140
E105	CI 13015
E105	CI 47005
E110	CI 15985
E111	CI 15980
E120	CI 75470
E122	CI 14720
E123	CI 16185 and CI 16185:1
E124	CI 16255
E125	CI 14815
E126	CI 16290
E127	CI 45430
E130	CI 69800
E131	CI 42051
E132	CI 73015
E133	CI 42090
E140	CI 75810
E140	CI 75810
E142	CI 44090
E150	Caramel
E152	CI 27755
E153	CI 77268:1

E160a	CI 75130
E160b	CI 75120
E160c	Capsanthin / Capsorubin
E160d	CI 75125
E160e	CI 40820
E160f	CI 40825
E160g	CI 40850
E161d	CI 75135
E162	Beta vulgaris
E163	Anthocyanins
E170	CI 77220
E171	CI 77891
E172	CI 77489, CI 77491, CI 77492, CI 77499
E175	CI 77480
E320	BHA
E321	BHT
E900	Dimethicone
Eosin (Y)	Acid Red 87
Erythrosine	CI 45430
Erythrosine	Acid Red 51
Ethan-1,2-diol	Glycol
Ethanol	Alcohol
Ethanolamine sulfite	MEA sulfite
Ethyl-4-hydroxybenzoate	Ethylparaben
Ethyl-p-aminobenzoate	Benzocain
Ethylene glycol	Glycol
Ethylparahydroxybenzoate	Ethylparaben
Ext. D & C Violet #2	CI 60730
Ext. D & C Yellow #7	CI 10316
Fast Green FCF	CI 42053
FD&C Blue #1	CI 42090
FD&C Blue #2	CI 73015
FD&C Green #3	CI 42053
FD&C Red #3	CI 45430
FD&C Red #4	CI 14700

FD&C Red #40	CI 16035
FD&C Yellow #5	CI 19140
FD&C Yellow #6	CI 15985
Fluorescein sodium	CI 45350
Fluorescein sodium	Acid Yellow 73 sodium salt
Fuchsin	CI 42510
Geranium extract	Geranium
Glucitol	Sorbitol
Glycerine	Glycerin
Glycerol	Glycerin
Glyceryl monolaurate	Glyceryl laurate
Glyceryl monostearate	Glyceryl stearate
Gypsum	CI 77231
Hedera helix	Ivy
Hetaflur	Cetylamine hydrofluoride
Hexadecanol	Cetyl alcohol
Hexahydroxocyclohexane	Vitamin B
Hexan-1,2,3,4,5,6-hexol	Sorbitol
Homomenthyl salicylate	Homosalate
Hydrazine	Diamine
Hydroxycaprylic acid	Alpha-hydroxy octanoic acid
Hydroxyoctanoic acid	Alpha-hydroxy octanoic acid
Indigo carmine	CI 73015
Indigotine	CI 73015
Inositol	Vitamin B
Ketoconazole	Nizoral™
Lemon oil	Citrus limonum
Linalol	Linalool
Linseed oil	Linum usitatissimum
Liquid paraffin	Paraffinum liquidum

m-TD	2,4-Toluenediamine
m-Toluenediamine	2,4-Toluenediamine
MEA	Ethanolamine
Methanine	Quaternium-15
Methanol	Methyl alcohol
Methenamine	Quaternium-15
Methlparahydroxybenzoate	Methylparaben
Methoxsalen	8-Methoxpsoralen
Methoxymethane	Dimethyl ether
Methyl-4-hydroxybenzoate	Methylparaben
Methyl-alpha-d-glycopyranoside	Methyl glucoside
Methylene chloride	Dichloromethane
Methylphenylene-2,5-diamine	Toluene-2,5-diamine
Methylphenylene-2,5-diamine sulfate	Toluene-2,5-diamine sulfate
Mexenone	Benzophenone-10
Mineral oil	Paraffinum liquidum
MIPA	Isopropanolamine
Monoethanolamine sulfite	MEA sulfite
Musk moskene	Moskene
n-Octadecanoic acid	Stearic acid
NaCl	Sodium chloride
Naphthol	1-Naphthol
Naphtoquinone	Naphthoquinone
o-Phenylenediamine	1,2-Phenylenediamine
Octabenzone	Benzophenone-12
Octadecanoic acid	Stearic acid
Olive oil	Olea europaea
Oxybenzone	Benzophenone-3
p-Acetylphenetidin	Phenacetin
p-Aminobenzoic acid	PABA
p-Ethoxyacetanilide	Phenacetin
Padimate O	Octyl dimethyl PABA
Palmityl alcohol	Cetyl alcohol

Paraphenylenediamine	p-Phenylenediamine
Paraphenylenediamine hydrochloride	p-Phenylenediamine HCl
Parsley extract	Carum petroselinum
Parsley seed oil	Carum petroselinum
Peppermint oil	Mentha piperita
PG	Propylene glycol
Phenylbenzoyl carbinol	Benzoin
Pigment Red 4	CI 12085
Pigment Red 57	CI 15850
Pigment Red 57:1	CI 15850
Pigment Red 63:1	CI 15880
Pigment Red 64:1	CI 15800
Polyethan-1,2-diol	PEG – Family
Polyethylene glycol	PEG – Family
Polyoxyethylene glycol	PEG – Family
Polyvinylpyrrolidone	PVP
Potassium hydrogen phthalate	Potassium biphthalate
Potassium peroxodisulfate	Potassium persulfate
Pro-vitamin A	Beta-carotene
Pro-vitamin A, synthetic	Carotene
Pro-vitamin B$_5$	Panthenol
Procaine HCl	Novocain
Procaine hydrochloride	Novocain
Propan-1,2,3-triol	Glycerin
Propan-1,2-diol	Propylene glycol
Propanone	Acetone
Propyl-4-hydroxybenzoate	Propylparaben
Propylenglycolum	Propylene glycol
Propylparahydroxybenzoate	Propylparaben
Purcellin, oil of	Oil of purcellin
Pyrithione zinc	Zinc pyrithione
Ricinus oil	Ricinus communis
Rosemary extract	Rosmarinus officinalis
Saffron	CI 75100

Salt	Sodium chloride
Sea salt	Sodium chloride
Silver	CI 77820
SLS	Sodium lauryl sulfate
Sodium chlorate (I)	Sodium hypochlorite
Sodium dodecyl sulfate	Sodium lauryl sulfate
Sodium peroxodisulfate	Sodium persulfate
Sodium phosphate, dibasic	Disodium phosphate
Solvent Green 3	CI 61565
Solvent Green 7	CI 59040
Solvent Red 23	CI 26100
Solvent Red 28	CI 45410
Solvent Yellow 94	CI 45350:1
Sulisobenzone	Benzophenone-4
Sunset yellow	CI 15985
t-Butyl-4-methoxydibenzoylmethane	Butyl methoxydibenzoylmethane
Tar camphor	Naphthalene
Tartrazine	CI 19140
TCP	Chlorinated phenols
TEA	Triethanolamine
Tektamer 38	Methyldibromo glutaronitrile
Tetrasodium edetate	Tetrasodium EDTA
Thyme extract	Thymus vulgaris
TiO_2	Titanium dioxide
Titanium (IV) oxide	Titanium dioxide
Titanium dioxide	CI 77891
Toluene-2,4-diamine	2,4-Toluenediamine
Tosylchloramide sodium	Chloramine-T
Tri-alpha hydroxy fruit acids	Mixed fruit acids
Triolamine	Triethanolamine
Triple fruit acids	Mixed fruit acids
Trolamine	Triethanolamine
Vat Red 1	CI 73360
Vitamin A	Retinol

Vitamin B complex	Biotin
Vitamin E	Tocopherol
Wool fat	Lanolin
Zinc oxide	CI 77947